Multidisciplinary Approach to Oral Cancer: The Way to Improve Expectancy and Quality of Life

Multidisciplinary Approach to Oral Cancer: The Way to Improve Expectancy and Quality of Life

Editors

Carlo Lajolo
Gaetano Paludetti
Romeo Patini

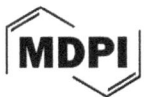

Basel • Beijing • Wuhan • Barcelona • Belgrade • Novi Sad • Cluj • Manchester

Editors
Carlo Lajolo
Head, Neck and Sense Organs
Catholic University of Sacred Heart
Rome, Italy

Gaetano Paludetti
Head, Neck and Sense Organs
Catholic University of Sacred Heart
Rome, Italy

Romeo Patini
Head, Neck and Sense Organs
Catholic University of Sacred Heart
Rome, Italy

Editorial Office
MDPI
St. Alban-Anlage 66
4052 Basel, Switzerland

This is a reprint of articles from the Special Issue published online in the open access journal *Cancers* (ISSN 2072-6694) (available at: https://www.mdpi.com/journal/cancers/special_issues/MAOC).

For citation purposes, cite each article independently as indicated on the article page online and as indicated below:

Lastname, A.A.; Lastname, B.B. Article Title. *Journal Name* **Year**, *Volume Number*, Page Range.

ISBN 978-3-0365-9244-2 (Hbk)
ISBN 978-3-0365-9245-9 (PDF)
doi.org/10.3390/books978-3-0365-9245-9

Cover image courtesy of Carlo Lajolo

© 2023 by the authors. Articles in this book are Open Access and distributed under the Creative Commons Attribution (CC BY) license. The book as a whole is distributed by MDPI under the terms and conditions of the Creative Commons Attribution-NonCommercial-NoDerivs (CC BY-NC-ND) license.

Contents

Preface vii

Jorge Pamias-Romero, Manel Saez-Barba, Alba de-Pablo-García-Cuenca, Pablo Vaquero-Martínez, Joan Masnou-Pratdesaba and Coro Bescós-Atín
Quality of Life after Mandibular Reconstruction Using Free Fibula Flap and Customized Plates: A Case Series and Comparison with the Literature
Reprinted from: *Cancers* 2023, 15, 2582, doi:10.3390/cancers15092582 1

Katharina El-Shabrawi, Katharina Storck, Jochen Weitz, Klaus-Dietrich Wolff and Andreas Knopf
Comparison of T1/2 Tongue Carcinoma with or without Radial Forearm Flap Reconstruction Regarding Post-Therapeutic Function, Survival, and Gender
Reprinted from: *Cancers* 2023, 15, 1885, doi:10.3390/cancers15061885 15

Rex H. Lee, Cara Evans, Joey Laus, Cristina Sanchez, Katherine C. Wai, P. Daniel Knott, et al.
Patterns of Postoperative Trismus Following Mandibulectomy and Fibula Free Flap Reconstruction
Reprinted from: *Cancers* 2023, 15, 536, doi:10.3390/cancers15020536 33

Qingkang Meng, Feng Wu, Guoqi Li, Fei Xu, Lei Liu, Denan Zhang, et al.
Exploring Precise Medication Strategies for OSCC Based on Single-Cell Transcriptome Analysis from a Dynamic Perspective
Reprinted from: *Cancers* 2022, 14, 4801, doi:10.3390/cancers14194801 43

Cosimo Rupe, Gioele Gioco, Giovanni Almadori, Jacopo Galli, Francesco Micciché, Michela Olivieri, et al.
Oral *Candida* spp. Colonisation Is a Risk Factor for Severe Oral Mucositis in Patients Undergoing Radiotherapy for Head & Neck Cancer: Results from a Multidisciplinary Mono-Institutional Prospective Observational Study
Reprinted from: *Cancers* 2022, 14, 4746, doi:10.3390/cancers14194746 63

Xiaokun Li, Siyuan Luan, Yushang Yang, Jianfeng Zhou, Qixin Shang, Pinhao Fang, et al.
Trimodal Therapy in Esophageal Squamous Cell Carcinoma: Role of Adjuvant Therapy Following Neoadjuvant Chemoradiation and Surgery
Reprinted from: *Cancers* 2022, 14, 3721, doi:10.3390/cancers14153721 79

Yu-Hsiang Tsai, Wan-Ming Chen, Ming-Chih Chen, Ben-Chang Shia, Szu-Yuan Wu and Chun-Chi Huang
Effect of Pre-Existing Sarcopenia on Oncological Outcomes for Oral Cavity Squamous Cell Carcinoma Undergoing Curative Surgery: A Propensity Score-Matched, Nationwide, Population-Based Cohort Study
Reprinted from: *Cancers* 2022, 14, 3246, doi:10.3390/cancers14133246 93

Cosimo Rupe, Alessia Basco, Anna Schiavelli, Alessandra Cassano, Francesco Micciche', Jacopo Galli, et al.
Oral Health Status in Patients with Head and Neck Cancer before Radiotherapy: Baseline Description of an Observational Prospective Study
Reprinted from: *Cancers* 2022, 14, 1411, doi:10.3390/cancers14061411 111

Roosa Hujanen, Rabeia Almahmoudi, Tuula Salo and Abdelhakim Salem
Comparative Analysis of Vascular Mimicry in Head and Neck Squamous Cell Carcinoma: In Vitro and In Vivo Approaches
Reprinted from: *Cancers* 2021, 13, 4747, doi:10.3390/cancers13194747 129

Roberta Gasparro, Elena Calabria, Noemi Coppola, Gaetano Marenzi, Gilberto Sammartino, Massimo Aria, et al.
Sleep Disorders and Psychological Profile in Oral Cancer Survivors: A Case-Control Clinical Study
Reprinted from: *Cancers* **2021**, *13*, 1855, doi:10.3390/cancers13081855 . . . . **145**

Romeo Patini, Massimo Cordaro, Denise Marchesini, Francesco Scilla, Gioele Gioco, Cosimo Rupe, et al.
Is Systemic Immunosuppression a Risk Factor for Oral Cancer? A Systematic Review and Meta-Analysis
Reprinted from: *Cancers* **2023**, *15*, 3077, doi:10.3390/cancers15123077 . . . . **161**

Carlo Lajolo, Cosimo Rupe, Gioele Gioco, Giuseppe Troiano, Romeo Patini, Massimo Petruzzi, et al.
Osteoradionecrosis of the Jaws Due to Teeth Extractions during and after Radiotherapy: A Systematic Review
Reprinted from: *Cancers* **2021**, *13*, 5798, doi:10.3390/cancers13225798 . . . . **189**

Diana Russo, Pierluigi Mariani, Vito Carlo Alberto Caponio, Lucio Lo Russo, Luca Fiorillo, Khrystyna Zhurakivska, et al.
Development and Validation of Prognostic Models for Oral Squamous Cell Carcinoma: A Systematic Review and Appraisal of the Literature
Reprinted from: *Cancers* **2021**, *13*, 5755, doi:10.3390/cancers13225755 . . . . **201**

Preface

The progress achieved using new techniques and therapies in HN cancers has influenced chemotherapy, surgery and radiotherapy, facilitating considerable improvement in the life expectancy and in some cases even complete healing. The consequent life elongation of affected patients means that they must face the post-surgical consequences of the interventions for the excision of neoplasms and side effects of radiotherapy for a long time. The surgical treatment of these neoplasms, in fact, unfortunately often exposes patients to disabilities that impair function, aesthetics and psychology.

Among HN cancers, OSCCs still have a poor prognosis, and survivors suffer from heavy aesthetic and functional impairments since oncologic therapies, especially surgery and radiotherapy, can damage important structures in the oral cavity. Recently, scientific research in OSCCs has focused mainly on preventive strategies, early diagnosis and reconstructive techniques of the jaws after demolition surgery [1].

In recent years, however, research has also shifted to the evaluation of the life expectancy and quality of life of patients with OSCC, trying to provide new elements to better evaluate the therapeutic strategies available for the treatment of these cancers.

This Special Issue collects in vitro experiments, clinical papers (either observational or experimental) and systematic reviews to promote the spread of precision and tailored medicine. New evidence strongly supports the idea that the use of molecular diagnostic techniques for early diagnosis could improve the life expectancy and that more tailored therapies could favour better quality of live in affected patients [2].

For the abovementioned reasons, the final objective of this editorial and the associated Special Issue is to spread the most recent knowledge on OSCC patient care, with attention to prevention, early diagnosis, therapy and quality of life. The accepted topics include all the branches of oral oncology, and multidisciplinary research is encouraged.

References

1. Gharat, S.A.; Momin, M.; Bhavsar, C. Oral Squamous Cell Carcinoma: Current Treatment Strategies and Nanotechnology-Based Approaches for Prevention and Therapy. *Crit. Rev. Ther. Drug. Carrier Syst.* **2016**, *33*, 363–400.
2. Sasahira, T.; Kirita, T. Hallmarks of Cancer-Related Newly Prognostic Factors of Oral Squamous Cell Carcinoma. *Int. J. Mol. Sci.* **2018**, *16*, 2413.

Carlo Lajolo, Gaetano Paludetti, and Romeo Patini
Editors

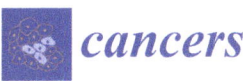

Article

Quality of Life after Mandibular Reconstruction Using Free Fibula Flap and Customized Plates: A Case Series and Comparison with the Literature

Jorge Pamias-Romero [1,2], Manel Saez-Barba [1,2], Alba de-Pablo-García-Cuenca [1,2], Pablo Vaquero-Martínez [1,2], Joan Masnou-Pratdesaba [3] and Coro Bescós-Atín [1,2,4,*]

[1] Service of Oral and Maxillofacial Surgery, Hospital Universitari Vall d'Hebron, Vall d'Hebron Barcelona Hospital Campus, Passeig Vall d'Hebron 119-129, E-08035 Barcelona, Spain; jorge.pamias@vallhebron.cat (J.P.-R.); manuel.saez@vallhebron.cat (M.S.-B.); alba.depablo@vallhebron.cat (A.d.-P.-G.-C.); pablo.vaquero@vallhebron.cat (P.V.-M.)

[2] CIBBM-Nanomedicine, Noves Tecnologies i Microcirurgia Craniofacial, Vall d'Hebron Institut de Reserca (VHIR), Hospital Universitari Vall d'Hebron, Vall d'Hebron Barcelona Hospital Campus, E-08035 Barcelona, Spain

[3] Radiology Department, Hospital Universitari Vall d'Hebron, Vall d'Hebron Barcelona Hospital Campus, Passeig Vall d'Hebron 119-129, E-08035 Barcelona, Spain; joan.masnou@vallhebron.cat

[4] Unitat Docent Vall d'Hebron, Facultat de Medicina UAB, Universitat Autònoma de Barcelona, E-08035 Barcelona, Spain

* Correspondence: mariasocorro.bescos@vallhebron.cat

Simple Summary: The health-related quality of life was evaluated in 23 patients undergoing mandibular reconstruction with free fibula flap and titanium customized plates. A computer-aided design and computer-aided manufacturing technology were used. The University of Washington Quality of Life questionnaire for head and neck cancer patients is a widely used and validated tool, which was self-completed by the patients after 12 months of surgery. In the 12 single question domains, the highest scores were obtained in the domains of taste, shoulder function, anxiety, and pain. The lowest scores corresponded to chewing, appearance, saliva, and mood. The global quality of life was rated as good, very good, or outstanding by 81% of patients. The present results compared favorably with previous studies of mandibular reconstruction using the same questionnaire published in literature.

Abstract: A single-center retrospective study was conducted to assess health-related quality of life (HRQoL) in 23 consecutive patients undergoing mandibular reconstruction using the computer-aided design (CAD) and computer-aided manufacturing (CAM) technology, free fibula flap, and titanium patient-specific implants (PSIs). HRQoL was evaluated after at least 12 months of surgery using the University of Washington Quality of Life (UW-QOL) questionnaire for head and neck cancer patients. In the 12 single question domains, the highest mean scores were found for "taste" (92.9), "shoulder" (90.9), "anxiety" (87.5), and "pain" (86.4), whereas the lowest scores were observed for "chewing" (57.1), "appearance" (67.9), and "saliva" (78.1). In the three global questions of the UW-QOL questionnaire, 80% of patients considered that their HRQoL was as good as or even better than it was compared to their HRQoL before cancer, and only 20% reported that their HRQoL had worsened after the presence of the disease. Overall QoL during the past 7 days was rated as good, very good or outstanding by 81% of patients, respectively. No patient reported poor or very poor QoL. In the present study, restoring mandibular continuity with free fibula flap and patient-specific titanium implants designed with the CAD-CAM technology improved HRQoL.

Keywords: quality of life; mandibular reconstruction; free fibula flap; patient-specific implant; plates; University of Washington Quality of Life Questionnaire

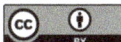

1. Introduction

Refinements in surgical techniques have led to significant improvement in oncological, functional, and aesthetic outcomes in oral cancer. Currently, one of the main goals of mandibular defect reconstruction is to provide patients with the best possible health-related quality of life (HRQoL) [1]. Assessment of results of treatment is a key aspect for the accurate selection of patients and the choice of the most appropriate reconstruction technique [2,3].

The microvascular or free fibula flap, originally described by Hidalgo et al. [4] in 1989, is considered the "gold standard" flap for the reconstruction of mandibular defects. More recently, the use of computer-aided design (CAD) and computer-aided manufacturing (CAM) (CAD-CAM) technology [5] promoted a paradigm shift in the diagnostic and therapeutic approach of defects in the maxillofacial region. Further introduction of 3D-printed titanium using direct metal laser sintering (DMLS) as an additive manufacturing technique allowed the development of custom-made plates or patient-specific implants (PSIs), improving accuracy and efficiency in mandibular reconstruction procedures. PSIs could provide the missing link in the digital flow process for mandibular reconstruction, and in doing so they would avoid potential shortcomings that are inherent to pre-modelled reconstruction plates and improve final precision [6,7]. Thus, computer-generated PSIs would be the next logical step in the digital planning and design flow rather than an independent device, as they represent the metallic cast that accurately reflects the surface of the reconstructed bone compounds and keeps geometry stable [8].

The evidence of PSI printed titanium implants for reconstruction of mandibular continuity defects is scarce. In a systematic review of the literature of 31 clinical studies with 139 patients, benefits identified included finite element analysis of the digital design, dimensional accuracy, shorter duration of surgery, augmenting dental/masticatory function, and capacity for dental implant rehabilitation, although the evidence predominantly was low level and at moderate-to-high risk of bias [9]. The published articles provided valuable evidence of the use of 3D-printed titanium PSIs with reported benefits seemingly outweighing their limitations and of the important role to be played by such implants in mandibular reconstruction for improving patient outcomes. However, in none of the studies included in the review was HRQoL evaluated. Improvements in different domains of HRQoL and patient satisfaction after free fibula flap reconstruction of segmental mandibulectomy have been rarely reported [10–15], but as far as we are aware, no studies have specifically assessed HRQoL outcomes in the setting of mandibular reconstruction using free fibula flaps combined with 3D-customized titanium plates.

Therefore, the aim of this study was to assess the impact of using free fibula flaps associated with CAD-CAM technology and PSI titanium plates on HRQoL in patients with mandibular pathology undergoing reconstruction for continuity defects.

2. Materials and Methods

2.1. Study Design and Participants

This was a retrospective study of all consecutive patients undergoing mandibular reconstruction with free fibula flaps using CAD-CAM technology and titanium PSI for the repair of mandibular defects of malignant or benign etiology operated on at the Service of Oral and Maxillofacial Surgery of Hospital Universitari Vall d'Hebron in Barcelona (Spain) between October 2015 and July 2019. Inclusion criteria were as follows: adult patients scheduled for primary or secondary mandibular reconstruction due to benign or malignant pathology, whether diseases had been treated previously or not; use of CAD-CAM technology including virtual planning, mandibular resection, fibula cutting guides for modelling, and PSI; use of free fibula flap for the reconstruction of the mandibular bone defect; and follow-up for at least 1 year after surgery. Patients were excluded if one or several components of the CAD-CAM technology were lacking (such as virtual planning, mandibular resection guides, fibula cutting guides for modelling), PSI was not used, or the free fibula flap failed.

The study protocol was approved by the Clinical Research Ethics Committee of Hospital Universitari Vall d'Hebron (codes PR(AG)93/2016, approval date 1 March 2016) (Barcelona, Spain). Written informed consent was obtained from all participants.

2.2. Protocol for Mandibular Reconstruction with Free Fibula Flap

Briefly, the presurgical stage included the following steps: (a) virtual planning (image processing, segmentation, resection, cutting, and reconstruction planning); (b) CAD (mandibular resection guides, fibula cutting guides, custom-made reconstruction plates, and custom-made prostheses); and (c) manufacturing stage (polyamide models from StereoLitography (STL) file format for resection and cutting guides for the mandible and fibula, STL model for the mandible, 3D printing and manufacturing titanium plates [PSI], and custom-made polyetheretherketone [PEEK] prosthesis) (Figure 1). Custom-made plates were manufactured using direct metal laser sintering using an EOSINT M270 system (EOS GmbH, Electro Optical Systems Company, Munich, Germany).

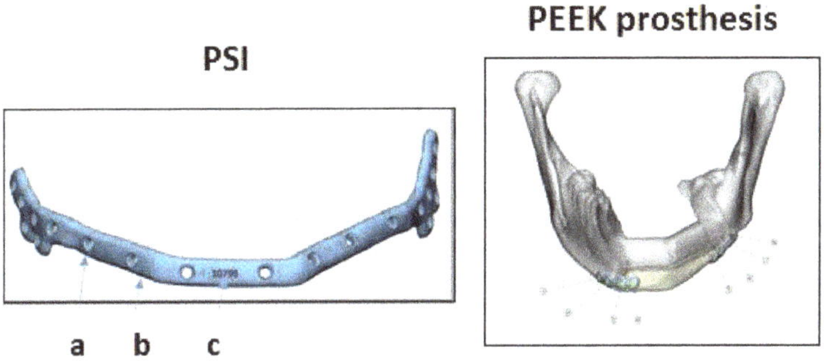

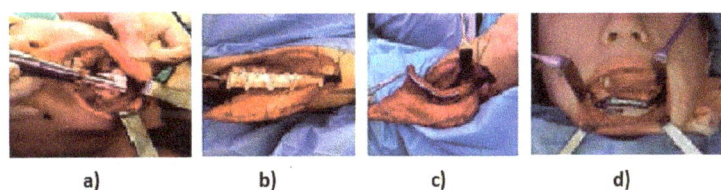

Figure 1. Patient-specific implant (PSI): (**a**) screw hole with thread; it contains information on the screw angle; (**b**) an enveloping design to help place the plate in the optimal position; and (**c**) patient's information code (left). PEEK prosthesis. Positioning of the PSI in the remaining healthy bone (right).

The surgical procedure (Figure 2) included the following steps: (1) mandibular resection using resection guides; (2) modelling of the fibula flap using cutting guides and placement of immediate implants (if required); (3) plate binding in the donor zone before sectioning the vascular pedicle; (4) positioning and binding of the flap in the mandibular defect; (5) microsurgical anastomosis; (6) positioning and binding of the PEEK prosthesis with miniplates and screws (if required); and (7) final repositioning of soft tissues and wound closure. All plates were customized for each patient. In all cases, PSI modelling was performed in the limb while the flap remained vascularized.

Figure 2. Details of the surgical procedure: (**a**) mandibular resection; (**b**) fibula flap modelling; (**c**) plate binding in the donor zone; and (**d**) positioning and binding of the flap in the mandibular defect.

Anatomical models, surgical guides, and custom-made plates were designed using the specific design software "D-matic Medical ® 10.0 by Materialise". Biomodels were manufactured directly using a rapid prototyping machine that used tridimensional solid support technology (Stratasys, Eden Prairie, MN, USA). Plates were manufactured using direct sintering with metal laser using an EOSINT M270 system (Electro-Optical Systems, GmbH, Munich, Germany).

2.3. Evaluation and Follow-up

Patients were visited postoperatively by the same investigator (J.P.-R.) during their stay in the hospital, after 1 week of hospital discharge, and at 1, 3, 6, and 12 months thereafter. Postoperative complications were evaluated using the Clavien–Dindo classification [16]. Complications related to PSI (presence or absence of intraoral or extraoral exposure) and the PEEK prosthesis (stability) were evaluated clinically. Prosthesis failure was determined when the prosthesis was extra-orally exposed and had to be removed. Other variables were evaluated by orthopantomography and computed tomography (CT) scan performed at least 6 months after mandibular reconstruction, including merging of fibula fragments (between different fibula fragments and between the fibula fragments and the remaining mandible), stability of screws, plate adjustment (defined as the presence of close contact between the PSI, the fibula, and the mandible), and presence or absence of PSI fracture.

Esthetical evaluation included photographs of the patients before and after surgery. Additionally, pre- and post-surgical panoramic radiographs and 3D-cone-beam computed tomography (CBCT) scans were acquired, and image superposition was used to assess the correlation between virtual planning and the results obtained.

2.4. Health-Related Quality of Life

At least 12 months after surgery, patients were contacted by phone and were appointed for a face-to-face visit to assess HRQoL. After signing the informed consent, they completed the University of Washington Quality of Life Questionnaire (UW-QOL v4) for head and neck cancer patients [17,18]. A Spanish validation version of the UW-QOL instrument was used [19]. The UW-QOL is a self-administered questionnaire specifically for head and neck cancer patients that measures health and quality of life (QoL) over the past 7 days. The questionnaire includes 12 single question domains (pain, appearance, activity, recreation, swallowing, chewing, speech, shoulder function, taste, saliva, mood, and anxiety) and 3 global questions, one about how patients feel relative to before they developed their cancer, one about their HRQoL, and one about their overall QoL. A free-text box is also included, so that the patient may write down any other comment he or she wishes to make on QoL that had not come forth in the previous questions. Domains are scaled from 0 (worst possible response) to 100 (best possible response). Domain scores include the mean (SD), the percentage of patients selecting the best possible response (100), and the percentage of patients choosing each domain. The domains can also be ranked by order.

2.5. Study Outcomes

The primary outcome was HRQoL assessed by means of the UW-QOL questionnaire at least 12 months after mandibular reconstruction using free fibula flap and titanium PSI based on the CAD-CAM technology. Secondary outcomes were complications related to the PSI and the PEEK prosthesis.

2.6. Statistical Analysis

Categorical variables are expressed as frequencies and percentages, and continuous variables are expressed as mean and standard deviation (SD) or median and interquartile range (IQR) (25th–75th percentile) or range (maximum–minimum). The chi-square test or the Fisher's exact test were used for the comparison of categorical variables, and the Student's t-test or the Mann–Whitney U test were used for the comparison of quantitative variables according to conditions of application. Statistical significance was set at $p < 0.05$.

3. Results

3.1. Clinical and Surgical Characteristics

The study population consisted of 23 patients (56.5% men) with a mean age of 52.8 (14.2) years. Fifteen patients (65.2%) had malignant tumors and locally advanced disease. Four patients had received neoadjuvant radiotherapy or combined radiochemotherapy.

Central defects according to the classification of Boyd et al. [20] were the most common (56.5%). PSIs were inserted in the occlusal zone in 15 patients and in the basal zone in the remaining 8. The skin flap was used as an internal intraoral layer in 20 patients, as an external skin layer in 2, and both as internal and external layers in 1. One patient required bilateral nasolabial flaps because of a defect that involved a large amount of soft tissue. Arterial anastomosis was most frequently performed with the facial artery and venous anastomosis with the thyrolinguofacial trunk. Osseointegrated dental implants were placed immediately in 2 patients and in a second step in 3.

The mean (SD) ischemia time was 122 (4) minutes, and the mean duration of surgery was 10.2 (1.4) hours. Immediate postoperative complications were recorded in 11 patients, which were classified as grade I in 7 and grade IIIb in 4 (2 cases of cervical bleeding and 2 of compartment syndromes in the donor limb). These 4 patients were reoperated under general or local anesthesia. In all cases, complications were solved. The mean length of hospital stay was 23 days (range 10–55 days), without significant differences between patients without and with complications (17 [4.4] vs. 26.3 [12.9] days, $p = 0.062$).

The microvascular fibula flap survived in 100% of the patients. Postoperatively, 12 patients received chemotherapy and/or radiotherapy adjuvant treatment. Table 1 shows the main clinical characteristics of patients and surgery-related data.

Table 1. Clinical and surgical data of the 23 patients included in the study.

Variables	Number (%)
Men/women	13 (56.5)/10 (43.5)
Age, years, mean (SD)	52.8 (14.2)
Type of pathology	
Malignant	15 (65.2)
Benign	8 (34.8)
Histological type	
Oral squamous cell carcinoma	10 (43.5)
Odontogenic tumors (benign and malignant)	7 (30.4)
Sarcoma	2 (8.7)
Secondary deformity	1 (4.3)
Osteoradionecrosis	1 (4.3)
Infiltrating verrucous carcinoma	1 (4.3)
TNM stage of malignant tumors	15 (65.2)
T4N0	9 (39.1)
T4N1	3 (13.0)
T4N2a	3 (13.0)
Neoadjuvant treatment (RT or QT/RT)	4 (17.4)
Mandibular defect	
Type C (LCL, CL, LC, and CH)	13 (56.5)
Type H	4 (17.4)
Type L	6 (26.1)

Table 1. Cont.

Variables	Number (%)
Fibula skin flap positioning	
Intraoral internal	20 (87.0)
Extraoral external	3 (13.0)
Closure of the lower limb defect	
Direct	3 (13.0)
Skin graft	20 (87.0)
Postoperative complications (Clavien–Dindo)	
Grade I	7 (30.4)
Grade IIIb	4 (17.4)
Adjuvant treatment	12 (52.2)

SD: standard deviation; TNM: tumor node metastasis; T: tumor; N: node; RT: radiotherapy; CT: chemotherapy; type C: defect consisting of the entire central segment containing four incisors and two canines; LCL: lateral defect-to-bilateral angle defect; CL, LC: lateral angle-to-bilateral canines; CH: lateral segment defect including the condyle and central defect; type H: lateral defect of any length, including the condyle but not significantly crossing the midline; type L: defect of the same type without the condyle.

Image superposition studies showed a high correlation (greater than 92% in most patients) between preoperative virtual surgical plan and the results obtained.

The mean length of follow-up was 26 months (range 12–50 months). Twenty-two patients (95.6%) were alive at 12 months after surgery. One patient developed a recurrence of their oral cancer and the other patient died due to cancer progression.

3.2. Health-Related Quality of Life

Twenty-one patients (91.3%) completed the UW-QOL questionnaire, after a median of 27 months (IQR 19–41 months) after primary surgery. Two patients did not complete the questionnaire; one patient had an advanced stage of the oral cancer due to recurrence, and the other patient had died.

Table 2 shows the results obtained in the 12 single question domains of the UW-QOL questionnaire. The highest mean scores were found for "taste" (92.9 [13.1]), "shoulder" (90.9 [18.4]), "anxiety" (87.5 [24.5]), and "pain" (86.4 [12.8]). In contrast, the lowest mean scores were observed in the domains of "chewing" (57.1 [39.6]), "appearance" (67.9 [19.6]), and "saliva" (78.1 [27.3]).

Table 2. Results obtained in the 12 single question domains of the UW-QOL questionnaire.

Domain	Patients Number	Mean (SD)	Median (Range)	% Best Score (of 100)	Importance of Domain *	Rank Order
Pain	21	86.9 (12.8)	75 (75–100)	48	10	6
Appearance	21	67.9 (19.6)	75 (25–100)	10	48	2
Activity	21	83.3 (16.5)	75 (50–100)	43	29	4
Recreation	21	84.5 (20.1)	100 (25–100)	52	5	7
Swallowing	21	84.5 (20.1)	100 (30–100)	67	10	6
Chewing	21	57.1 (39.6)	50 (0–100)	38	62	1
Speech	20	83.0 (19.5)	85 (30–100)	50	43	3
Shoulder	21	90.9 (18.4)	100 (30–100)	76	5	7

Table 2. Cont.

Domain	Patients Number	Mean (SD)	Median (Range)	% Best Score (of 100)	Importance of Domain *	Rank Order
Taste	21	92.9 (13.1)	100 (70–100)	76	10	6
Saliva	21	78.1 (27.3)	100 (30–100)	52	24	5
Mood	20	82.6 (21.6)	87.5 (25–100)	50	24	5
Anxiety	20	87.5 (24.5)	100 (25–100)	70	10	6

* This asks about which three domain issues were the most important during the past 7 days, and results expressed as the percentage of patients choosing each domain.

The highest percentages of patients selecting the best possible response (100) were 76% for "shoulder" and "taste", 70% for "anxiety", 67% for "swallowing", and 52% for "recreation" and "saliva". The lowest percentages corresponded to 10% for "appearance", 38% for "chewing", and 43% for "activity".

In relation to importance of domain, "chewing", "appearance", and "speech" were selected by 62%, 48%, and 43% of patients, respectively. "Recreation" and "shoulder" were chosen by only 5% of patients, respectively. The rank order of domains was consistent with the importance already assigned to the different domains.

In the three global questions of the UW-QOL questionnaire (Table 3), 80% of patients considered that their HRQoL was as good as or even better than it was compared with their HRQoL before cancer, and only 20% reported that their HRQoL had worsened after the presence of the disease. Additionally, HRQoL and overall QoL during the past 7 days were rated as good, very good, or outstanding by 81% of patients, respectively. No patient reported poor or very poor QoL.

Table 3. Responses to three global questions of the UW-QOL questionnaire.

Questions	Mean (SD)	% Best Scores *
A. Health-related QoL compared to month before had cancer	60.0 (34.8)	80
B. Health-related QoL during the past 7 days	73.3 (22.2)	81
C. Overall QoL during the past 7 days	71.4 (22.4)	81

Key to ratings: A: (0) much worse, (25) somewhat worse, (50) about the same, (75) somewhat better, (100) much better. B: (0) very poor, (20) poor, (40) fair, (60) good, (80) very good, (100) outstanding. C: (0) very poor, (20) poor, (40) fair, (60) good, (80) very good, (100) outstanding. * Best scores: A = % of scoring 50, 75, or 100; B and C = % scoring 60, 80, or 100.

Thirteen patients (61.9%) provided an answer in the free-text box of the questionnaire. Four patients explicitly stated their satisfaction with the outcomes of surgery, but 9 patients would like to undergo dental rehabilitation for improving chewing and aesthetic functions. Other complaints were the possibility of a secondary reconstruction to improve appearance (3 cases), reduction in the extension of mouth opening (1 case), decreased saliva output and taste alterations (1 case), paresthesia (1 case), and delayed wound healing and/or paresthesia in the graft area of the lower limb.

3.3. PSI-Related Complications

At 6 months after surgery, 22 out of 23 patients (95.6%) underwent clinical and radiological assessment. One patient moved to another city and was lost to follow-up. The fibula fragments were properly consolidated in all 22 patients. In 19 patients (86.4%), PSI-related complications did not occur, whereas complications were recorded in the remaining

3 patients (13.6%). Extraoral and intraoral exposure of the PSI was clinically documented in 2 patients, and in both cases, the plate was removed, but the segments of the microvascularized fibula flap were found to be well consolidated. In the remaining patient, there was a lack of consolidation between the fibula and the remaining mandible, with screw instability and plate mobility. In this patient, removal of both the plate and the remaining segment of the mandibular ramus were performed.

3.4. PEEK Prosthesis-Related Complications

A PEEK prosthesis for the reconstruction of the mandibular inferior border was performed in 14 patients (60.9%) (immediate reconstruction in 13 cases and at a later stage in 1). In 6 patients (42.8%), the prosthesis became exposed and had to be removed. Five of these 6 patients had received radiotherapy (RT) in the neoadjuvant or adjuvant setting. Removal of the PEEK prosthesis was significantly more common in patients treated with RT than in those who had not received RT (83.3% vs. 16.7%, $p = 0.031$).

4. Discussion

This study shows that in patients undergoing extensive mandibular resection leading to wide mandibular continuity defects, the use of a surgical procedure based on CAD-CAM technology with free fibula flap and titanium PSI was associated with high scores in the UW-QOL questionnaire at least 12 months after surgery. In the 12 single question domains, mean scores were higher than 80 (with 100 being the highest possible response) in 9 domains (75%), with only 3 domains scoring below 80%. In the three global questions of the UW-QOL instrument, HRQoL before diagnosis of malignancy and overall QoL in the previous 7 days, high scores were achieved, as 80% and 81% of patients selected the options of much better and good, very good, or outstanding, respectively.

Assessment of QoL is a clinically relevant outcome in monitoring the treatment success and the sequelae of illness in patients with oral cancer. Subjective measures of health status can be evaluated by generic or disease-specific instruments, but due to the complex anatomy of the oral cavity, it is desirable to use specific HRQoL measures. These measures are more sensitive in assessing the impact of oral conditions on daily life activities. The relatively large number of questionnaires that are specific for diseases of the oral cavity (e.g., 14-item Oral Health Impact Profile [OHIP-14], Oral Impacts on Daily Performances [OIDP], Oral Health-Related Quality of Life [OHRQoL], European Organization for Research and Treatment of Cancer Head and Neck cancer questionnaire [EORTC-H&N35]) [21], underscores the fact that there is no gold standard tool. The UW-QOL instrument is one of the most used and validated questionnaires for patients with head and neck cancer and has shown good psychometric properties that have been specifically developed for this pathology [17,18]. Furthermore, the incorporation of importance-rating domains makes UW-QOL unique among head and neck cancer instruments [22,23]. The Spanish version of this questionnaire was validated by Nazar et al. [19] in 2010. In fact, the following characteristics of the UW-QOL questionnaire stand out: (1) it provides a specific "appearance" item related to disfigurement; (2) it allows for the evaluation of appearance problems through "recreation", "anxiety", and "mood" domains; and (3) it is quick and simple for patients to complete (it may take 5 minutes) and is easy to process.

Despite the advantages of the UW-QOL questionnaire, few studies have used this instrument for assessing HRQoL after mandibular reconstruction using free fibula flaps. In 2019, Petrovic et al. [24] conducted a systematic review of the literature and found only 6 studies in which QoL outcomes following mandible reconstruction using free fibula flap had been evaluated using the UW-QOL questionnaire. All these studies were retrospective case series. Apart from these 6 publications, we did not find any subsequent publication of the use of this questionnaire after free fibula flap reconstruction of the mandible. Therefore, the present results are compared with data reported in these 6 studies [14,15,25–28]. As shown in Table 4, mean scores obtained in our study were higher than those reported by others, except for "appearance". Overall, "chewing" was the domain with the lowest mean values in all studies followed by "appearance", "anxiety", "speech", and "swallowing".

Table 4. Mean scores of the 12 single question domains of the UW-QOL questionnaire.

Domain	Present Series (n = 21)	Li et al., 2014 [15] (n = 35)	Yang et al., 2014 [27] (n = 34)	Zhu et al., 2014 [25] (n = 33)	Luo et al., 2014 [28] (n = 32)	Zhang 2013 [14] (n = 31)	Wang 2009 [26] (n = 15)
Pain	86.9 (12.8)	82.2 (5.8)	67.4 (7.5)	76.4 (6.5)	80.6 (7.5)	87.6 (10.2)	86.7 (16.0)
Appearance	67.9 (19.6)	78.1 (11.6)	70.1 (6.6)	74.6 (9.6)	76.3 (8.7)	58.5 (2.1)	66.7 (29.4)
Activity	83.3 (16.5)	69.5 (7.6)	56.5 (9.1)	64.1 (8.3)	66.2 (9.1)	72.4 8.5)	76.7 (22.1)
Recreation	84.5 (20.1)	68.2 (10.6)	60.1 (9.1)	65.6 (8.7)	69.4 (7.1)	75.9 (6.1)	65.0 (33.8)
Swallowing	84.5 (20.1)	77.3 (6.8)	52.8 (9.0)	79.2 (7.2)	78.1 (5.1)	83.7 (1.6)	48.7 (26.9)
Chewing	57.1 (39.6)	28.5 (3.2)	33.1 (16.1)	32.4 (1.8)	30.3 (2.7)	42.2 (2.6)	36.7 (22.8)
Speech	83.0 (19.5)	71.3 (12.6)	55.3 (10.3)	68.8 (9.9)	66.4 (7.8)	47.9 (1.2)	53.3 (34.1)
Shoulder	90.9 (18.4)	80.3 (9.0)	65.9 (7.1)	81.1 (5.5)	82.3 (3.1)	92.4 (3.1)	82.0 (15.2)
Taste	92.9 (13.1)	71.2 (8.8)	55.6 (6.0)	80.5 (5.5)	78.7 (7.5)	90.3 (1.9)	80.7 (24.9)
Saliva	78.1 (27.3)	60.0 (7.6)	47.8 (8.9)	75.0 (9.7)	74.1 (8.0)	70.8 (1.5)	58.7 (28.2)
Mood	82.6 (21.6)	67.1 (1.2)	73.4 (11.5)	67.1 (1.2)	60.1 (3.0)	85.3 (7.9)	71.7 (31.1)
Anxiety	87.5 (24.5)	55.8 (8.2)	50.8 (14.3)	65.2 (8.6)	45.3 (9.6)	69.8 (6.3)	64.7 (66.7)

SD: standard deviation.

In relation to the domains in which the best score (of 100) was obtained, data were reported in four studies, with "pain", "shoulder function", "activity", and "recreation" as those with the most favorable evaluation (Table 5).

Table 5. Best scores obtained in the 12 single question domains of the UW-QOL questionnaire.

Domain	Present Series (n = 21)	Li et al., 2014 [15] (n = 35)	Zhu et al., 2014 [25] (n = 33)	Luo et al., 2014 [28] (n = 32)	Wang 2009 [26] (n = 15)
Pain	48	43	42	44	53
Appearance	10	26	36	31	20
Activity	43	9	6	NR	40
Recreation	52	0	3	6	33
Swallowing	67	29	49	28	7
Chewing	38	0	0	0	0
Speech	50	23	15	3	20
Shoulder	76	40	46	44	40
Taste	76	26	33	40	53
Saliva	52	42	42	22	13
Mood	50	11	9	3	40
Anxiety	70	0	0	6	40

Data as % best score (of 100) for each domain; NR: not reported.

A remarkable finding was that the "chewing" domain had the lowest score both in our study and in the 6 studies analyzed. Additionally, this domain showed a rate of importance of 62% in the present study as compared with 76.8% in the remaining studies. On the other hand, when considering the rank order assigned to the different domains, "chewing" ranked first in all studies but one (Table 6).

Table 6. Importance of domain and rank order assigned to the 12 single question domains of the UW-QOL questionnaire.

Domain	First Author, Year [Reference] (Number of Patients)						
	Present Series (n = 21)	Li et al., 2014 [15] (n = 35)	Yang et al., 2014 [27] (n = 34)	Zhu et al., 2014 [25] (n = 33)	Luo et al., 2014 [28] (n = 32)	Zhang 2013 [14] (n = 31)	Wang 2009 [26] (n = 15)
Pain	10% (6)	0% (11)	5.9% (9)	0% (9)	0% (8)	7% (8)	7% (6)
Appearance	48% (2)	49% (3)	18% (7)	67% (2)	50% (3)	55% (3)	20% (5)
Activity	29% (4)	17% (7)	41% (4)	58% (3)	38% (4)	0% (11)	0% (8)
Recreation	5% (7)	14% (8)	0% (10)	15% (7)	13% (6)	0% (11)	0% (8)
Swallowing	10% (6)	6% (10)	47% (3)	0% (9)	3% (7)	13% (7)	93% (1)
Chewing	62% (1)	77% (1)	71% (1)	76% (1)	94% (1)	90% (1)	53% (2)
Speech	43% (3)	54% (2)	53% (2)	30% (4)	25% (5)	68% (2)	46% (3)
Shoulder	5% (7)	0% (11)	0% (10)	0% (9)	0% (8)	3% (9)	0% (8)
Taste	10% (6)	11% (9)	29% (5)	0% (9)	3% (7)	3% (9)	NR
Saliva	24% (5)	23% (5)	24% (6)	12% (8)	0% (8)	26% (4)	40% (4)
Mood	24% (5)	20% (6)	0% (10)	18% (6)	13% (6)	16% (6)	0% (8)
Anxiety	10% (6)	29% (4)	12% (8)	24% (5)	63% (2)	19% (5)	7% (6)

Data as percentage of patients choosing which three domains were the most important during the past 7 days. Rank order of domains in parenthesis; NR: not reported.

Chewing has been shown to score worse after segmental mandibulectomy and reconstruction using composite free tissue transfer [29]. In these patients, rehabilitation with implant-supported prosthesis appears to improve QoL outcomes [30–32]. In a pilot study of 10 patients of early loaded implant-supported fixed dental prosthesis following mandibular reconstruction, patient satisfaction improved significantly after dental rehabilitation as compared to mandibular reconstruction alone [33]. Dental implants were placed in only 5 patients in our series, but 9 of the 13 patients (69.2%) reported the desire to undergo dental rehabilitation for improving chewing and aesthetic functions in the free-text box. Prosthetic rehabilitation, however, should be indicated on a case-by-case basis [31]. This decision should be based on several considerations including the medical history, prognosis, comorbidities and, particularly, the patient's desires and expectations. In addition, special attention should be paid to the surgical planning of implants, soft tissue management, and prosthodontics in order to avoid complications and achieve stable long-term results. We also believe that tests of swallowing function could help identify patients with a preserved swallowing function, which are in fact those who would benefit most from this kind of rehabilitation.

"Appearance" in the preceding 7 days was another domain selected as one of the most important by 48% of our patients, which is consistent with percentages between 49% and 67% reported in other studies [14,15,25,28]. Although "appearance" was considered an important factor, 71.4% of our patients stated in the questionnaire that their appearance had suffered slight or no changes, 19% a moderate change, and only 9.5% (2 patients) reported feeling disfigured. However, appearance did not seem to be a reason for social isolation, as "recreation" was rated as only 5% in the importance of domain and in the 7th position of the rank order. As for the overall QoL during the past 7 days, 81% reported that it was good, very good, or outstanding, and only 4 patients (20%) considered that QoL was fair. Poor or very poor ratings were not observed.

In relation to secondary outcomes, only 3 patients presented PSI-related complications, with a rate of 13.6%, which is consistent with 12.2% reported in the systematic review of Goodson et al. [9]. Plate removal was required by only 2 patients because of exposure, but no deficiencies in the consolidation process between the fibula fragment and the mandible were found.

A PEEK prosthesis was used in 14 patients for the correction of mandibular asymmetry after free fibula flap reconstruction [34]. In 6 patients (42.8%), the prosthesis was exposed and had to be removed. It should be noted that 5 of these 6 patients had received RT for the treatment of their oncological disease. Patients in whom the PEEK prosthesis was not exposed to RT did not present complications, with satisfactory aesthetic results and stability of the mandibular contour.

Esthetical evaluation was performed using pre- and post-surgical photographs, panoramic radiographs, and 3D-CBCT scans showing a high correlation between virtual surgical plan and the results obtained. Other techniques, such as cephalometric analysis and photogrammetry, were not used as the study was focused on the assessment of QoL as a primary subjective domain.

Limitations of the study include the single-center characteristics, retrospective design, and a small study population. Additionally, patients with malignant and benign conditions were included, which may have different risk factors related to QoL, particularly the use of radiation therapy and chemotherapy. However, the aim of the study was to assess the impact of the reconstructive process of the mandible (CAD-CAM, free fibula flap, and customized titanium plates) on QoL rather than the pathology itself, and in this respect, the population was homogeneous. Patients included in other series reported in the literature with which a comparison was made (Table 6) also included patients with ameloblastoma, osteoradionecrosis, and oral squamous cell carcinoma. Preoperative data of HRQoL using the same UW-QOL questionnaire was not obtained, so a within-group comparison of QoL before and after surgery was not feasible. Although only 4 patients received neoadjuvant or adjuvant RT and/or chemotherapy, the impact of this oncological treatment (e.g., impairment of salivary gland, trismus, mucositis, mouth opening limitation, etc.) was not evaluated. Other risk factors, such as oral health status, smoking, or age were not evaluated either. However, the use of a validated HRQoL instrument, such as the UW-QOL questionnaire, after a period of at least 12 months after surgery is a strength of this study. Moreover, a detailed comparison of the present findings with other studies published in the literature in which the UW-QOL questionnaire was completed by patients undergoing similar mandibular reconstruction procedures with free fibula flap is an interesting and distinctive aspect of the study.

5. Conclusions

Restoring mandibular continuity with free fibula flap and patient-specific titanium implants designed with the CAD-CAM technology improved HRQoL. High scores in most specific domains of the UW-QOL questionnaire were obtained at 12 months after surgery, except for "chewing" which had the lowest score. The global QoL was considered good, very good, or outstanding by 81% of the patients. Further studies with a larger study population are necessary to confirm the present findings.

Author Contributions: Conceptualization, J.P.-R. and C.B.-A.; methodology, J.P.-R.; software, J.P.-R.; validation, J.P.-R. and C.B.-A.; formal analysis, J.P.-R.; investigation, J.P.-R., M.S.-B., A.d.-P.-G.-C., P.V-M., J.M.-P. and C.B.-A.; data curation, J.P.-R. and C.B.-A.; writing—original draft preparation, C.B.-A.; writing—review and editing, J.P.-R., M.S.-B., A.d.-P.-G.-C. and P.V.-M.; supervision, J.P.-R. The authors decline the use of artificial intelligence, language models, machine learning, or similar technologies to create content or assist with writing or editing of the manuscript. All authors have read and agreed to the published version of the manuscript.

Funding: This research received no external funding.

Institutional Review Board Statement: The study was conducted in accordance with the Declaration of Helsinki and approved by the Clinical Research Ethics Committee of Hospital Universitari Vall d'Hebron (codes PR(AG)93/2016, approval date 1 March 2016), Barcelona, Spain.

Informed Consent Statement: Informed consent was obtained from all subjects involved in the study.

Data Availability Statement: Study data are available from the corresponding author upon request.

Acknowledgments: The authors thank Marta Pulido, for editing the manuscript and editorial assistance.

Conflicts of Interest: The authors declare no conflict of interest.

References

1. Chandu, A.; Smith, A.C.; Rogers, S.N. Health-related quality of life in oral cancer: A review. *J. Oral Maxillofac. Surg.* **2006**, *64*, 495–502. [CrossRef]
2. Komisar, A. The functional result of mandibular reconstruction. *Laryngoscope* **1990**, *100*, 364–374. [CrossRef] [PubMed]
3. Gal, T.J.; Futran, N.D. Outcomes research in head and neck reconstruction. *Facial Plast. Surg.* **2002**, *18*, 113–117. [CrossRef] [PubMed]
4. Hidalgo, D.A. Fibula free flap: A new method of mandible reconstruction. *Plast. Reconstr. Surg.* **1989**, *84*, 71–79. [CrossRef] [PubMed]
5. Levine, J.P.; Patel, A.; Saadeh, P.B.; Hirsch, D.L. Computer-aided design and manufacturing in craniomaxillofacial surgery: The new state of the art. *J. Craniofac. Surg.* **2012**, *23*, 288–293. [CrossRef]
6. Ciocca, L.; Mazzoni, S.; Fantini, M.; Persiani, F.; Marchetti, C.; Scotti, R. CAD/CAM guided secondary mandibular reconstruction of a discontinuity defect after ablative cancer surgery. *J. Craniomaxillofac. Surg.* **2012**, *40*, e511–e515. [CrossRef] [PubMed]
7. Tarsitano, A.; Mazzoni, S.; Cipriani, R.; Scotti, R.; Marchetti, C.; Ciocca, L. The CAD-CAM technique for mandibular reconstruction: An 18 patients oncological case-series. *J. Craniomaxillofac. Surg.* **2014**, *42*, 1460–1464. [CrossRef]
8. Wilde, F.; Cornelius, C.P.; Schramm, A. Computer-assisted mandibular reconstruction using a patient-specific reconstruction plate fabricated with computer-aided design and manufacturing techniques. *Craniomaxillofac. Trauma Reconstr.* **2014**, *7*, 158–166. [CrossRef]
9. Goodson, A.M.; Kittur, M.A.; Evans, P.L.; Williams, E.M. Patient-specific, printed titanium implants for reconstruction of mandibular continuity defects: A systematic review of the evidence. *J. Craniomaxillofac. Surg.* **2019**, *47*, 968–976. [CrossRef]
10. Löfstrand, J.; Nyberg, M.; Karlsson, T.; Thórarinsson, A.; Kjeller, G.; Lidén, M.; Fröjd, V. Quality of life after free fibula flap reconstruction of segmental mandibular defects. *J. Reconstr. Microsurg.* **2018**, *34*, 108–120.
11. Zavalishina, L.; Karra, N.; Zaid, W.S.; El-Hakim, M. Quality of life assessment in patients after mandibular resection and free fibula flap reconstruction. *J. Oral Maxillofac. Surg.* **2014**, *72*, 1616–1626. [CrossRef] [PubMed]
12. Maciejewski, A.; Szymczyk, C. Fibula free flap for mandible reconstruction: Analysis of 30 consecutive cases and quality of life evaluation. *J. Reconstr. Microsurg.* **2007**, *23*, 1–10. [CrossRef] [PubMed]
13. Hundepool, A.C.; Dumans, A.G.; Hofer, S.O.; Fokkens, N.J.; Rayat, S.S.; van der Meij, E.H.; Schepman, K.P. Rehabilitation after mandibular reconstruction with fibula free-flap: Clinical outcome and quality of life assessment. *Int. J. Oral Maxillofac. Surg.* **2008**, *37*, 1009–1013. [CrossRef] [PubMed]
14. Zhang, X.; Li, M.J.; Fang, Q.G.; Li, Z.N.; Li, W.L.; Sun, C.F. Free fibula flap: Assessment of quality of life of patients with head and neck cancer who have had defects reconstructed. *J. Craniofac. Surg.* **2013**, *24*, 2010–2013. [CrossRef]
15. Li, X.; Zhu, K.; Liu, F.; Li, H. Assessment of quality of life in giant ameloblastoma adolescent patients who have had mandible defects reconstructed with a free fibula flap. *World J. Surg. Oncol.* **2014**, *12*, 201. [CrossRef]
16. Dindo, D.; Demartines, N.; Clavien, P.A. Classification of surgical complications: A new proposal with evaluation in a cohort of 6336 patients and results of a survey. *Ann. Surg.* **2004**, *240*, 205–213. [CrossRef]
17. Lowe, D.; Rogers, S.N. University of Washington Quality of Life Questionnaire (UW-QOL v4 and v4.1). Guidance for Scoring and Presentation. Available online: http://www.hancsupport.com/sites/default/files/assets/pages/UW-QOL-update_2012.pdf (accessed on 16 March 2023).
18. Hassan, S.J.; Weymuller, E.A., Jr. Assessment of quality of life in head and neck cancer patients. *Head Neck* **1993**, *15*, 485–496. [CrossRef]
19. Nazar, G.; Garmendia, M.L.; Royer, M.; McDowell, J.A.; Weymuller, E.A., Jr.; Yueh, B. Spanish validation of the University of Washington Quality of Life questionnaire for head and neck cancer patients. *Otolaryngol. Head Neck Surg.* **2010**, *143*, 801–807.e1–2. [CrossRef] [PubMed]
20. Boyd, J.B.; Gullane, P.J.; Rotstein, L.E.; Brown, D.H.; Irish, J.C. Classification of mandibular defects. *Plast. Reconstr. Surg.* **1993**, *92*, 1266–1275. [PubMed]
21. Rogers, S.N.; Fisher, S.E.; Woolgar, J.A. A review of quality of life assessment in oral cancer. *Int. J. Oral Maxillofac. Surg.* **1999**, *28*, 99–117. [CrossRef]

22. Rogers, S.N.; Lowe, D.; Brown, J.S.; Vaughan, E.D. A comparison between the University of Washington Head and Neck Disease-Specific measure and the Medical Short Form 36, EORTC QOQ-C33 and EORTC Head and Neck 35. *Oral Oncol.* **1998**, *34*, 361–371. [CrossRef] [PubMed]
23. Rogers, S.N.; Laher, S.H.; Overend, L.; Lowe, D. Importance-rating using the University of Washington quality of life questionnaire in patients treated by primary surgery for oral and oro-pharyngeal cancer. *J. Craniomaxillofac. Surg.* **2002**, *30*, 125–132. [CrossRef]
24. Petrovic, I.; Panchal, H.; De Souza Franca, P.D.; Hernandez, M.; McCarthy, C.C.; Shah, J.P. A systematic review of validated tools assessing functional and aesthetic outcomes following fibula free flap reconstruction of the mandible. *Head Neck* **2019**, *41*, 248–255. [CrossRef]
25. Zhu, J.; Yang, Y.; Li, W. Assessment of quality of life and sociocultural aspects in patients with ameloblastoma after immediate mandibular reconstruction with a fibular free flap. *Br. J. Oral Maxillofac. Surg.* **2014**, *52*, 163–167. [CrossRef]
26. Wang, L.; Su, Y.X.; Liao, G.Q. Quality of life in osteoradionecrosis patients after mandible primary reconstruction with free fibula flap. *Oral Surg. Oral Med. Oral Pathol. Oral Radiol. Endod.* **2009**, *108*, 162–168. [CrossRef]
27. Yang, W.; Zhao, S.; Liu, F.; Sun, M. Health-related quality of life after mandibular resection for oral cancer: Reconstruction with free fibula flap. *Med. Oral Patol. Oral Cir. Bucal* **2014**, *19*, e414–e418. [CrossRef]
28. Luo, R.L.P.; Li, W.; Li, Y.; Qi, J. Measures of health-related quality of life in huge ameloblastoma young patients after mandible reconstruction with free fibula flap. *J. Hand Tissue Biol.* **2014**, *23*, 261–266. [CrossRef]
29. Rogers, S.N.; Devine, J.; Lowe, D.; Shokar, P.; Brown, J.S.; Vaugman, E.D. Longitudinal health-related quality of life after mandibular resection for oral cancer: A comparison between rim and segment. *Head Neck* **2004**, *26*, 54–62. [CrossRef]
30. Kumar, V.V.; Jacob, P.C.; Ebenezer, S.; Kuriakose, M.A.; Kekatpure, V.; Baliarsing, A.S.; Al-Nawas, B.; Wagner, W. Implant supported dental rehabilitation following segmental mandibular reconstruction- quality of life outcomes of a prospective randomized trial. *J. Craniomaxillofac. Surg.* **2016**, *44*, 800–810. [CrossRef] [PubMed]
31. Patel, S.Y.; Kim, D.D.; Ghali, G.-E. Maxillofacial reconstruction using vascularized fibula free flaps and endosseous implants. *Oral Maxillofac. Surg. Clin. North. Am.* **2019**, *31*, 259–284. [CrossRef]
32. Jacobsen, H.C.; Wahnschaff, F.; Trenkle, T.; Sieg, P.; Hakim, S.G. Oral rehabilitation with dental implants and quality of life following mandibular reconstruction with free fibular flap. *Clin. Oral Investig.* **2016**, *20*, 187–192. [CrossRef] [PubMed]
33. Barbier, L.; Pottel, L.; De Ceulaer, J.; Lamoral, P.; Duyck, J.; Jacobs, R.; Abeloos, J. Evaluation of quality of life after mandibular reconstruction using a novel fixed implant-supported dental prosthesis concept: A pilot study. *Int. J. Prosthodont.* **2019**, *32*, 162–173. [CrossRef] [PubMed]
34. Berrone, M.; Aldiano, C.; Pentenero, M.; Berrone, S. Correction of a mandibular asymmetry after fibula reconstruction using a custom-made polyetheretherketone (PEEK) onlay after implant supported occlusal rehabilitation. *Acta Otorhinolaryngol. Ital.* **2015**, *35*, 285–288. [PubMed]

Disclaimer/Publisher's Note: The statements, opinions and data contained in all publications are solely those of the individual author(s) and contributor(s) and not of MDPI and/or the editor(s). MDPI and/or the editor(s) disclaim responsibility for any injury to people or property resulting from any ideas, methods, instructions or products referred to in the content.

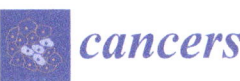

Article

Comparison of T1/2 Tongue Carcinoma with or without Radial Forearm Flap Reconstruction Regarding Post-Therapeutic Function, Survival, and Gender

Katharina El-Shabrawi [1,2,*], Katharina Storck [2], Jochen Weitz [3,4], Klaus-Dietrich Wolff [3] and Andreas Knopf [1,2]

1. Department of Otorhinolaryngology, Head and Neck Surgery, Faculty of Medicine, Medical Centre, University of Freiburg, 79106 Freiburg, Germany
2. Department of Otorhinolaryngology, Head and Neck Surgery, Klinikum rechts der Isar, Technical University, 81675 Munich, Germany
3. Clinic and Policlinic for Oro-Maxillofacial Surgery, Klinikum rechts der Isar, Technical University, 81675 Munich, Germany
4. Department of Oral and Maxillofacial Surgery, Josefinum, Augsburg and Private Practice Oral and Maxillofacial Surgery im Pferseepark, 86157 Augsburg, Germany
* Correspondence: katharina.el-shabrawi@uniklinik-freiburg.de

Simple Summary: Surgical therapy for tongue carcinoma is challenging due to the various important functions of the tongue. In order to compensate for loss of tongue tissue and function, flap reconstruction has been firmly established. Interestingly, a large number of early-stage tongue cancer receive flap reconstruction despite minor tissue loss. This study aims to investigate functional and survival differences as well as epidemiologic characteristics in tongue carcinoma patients with or without flap reconstruction. Our retrospective and prospective analyses show no significant survival or functional differences between the groups with or without flap reconstruction. Still, we were able to demonstrate that the possibility of flap reconstruction leads to a more generous tumor resection, less frequent presence of close margin, and subsequently less frequent use of toxic adjuvant therapy regimens. Moreover, for the first time, a significantly higher female ratio could be depicted in the reconstruction group ($p = 0.02$). These findings suggest that, apart from oncologic and functional factors, proportional aspects should be taken into consideration for future decisions on the optimal reconstruction method.

Abstract: Background: Flap reconstruction is commonly used in advanced tongue carcinoma in order to compensate for the loss of tongue tissue and function. Surprisingly, a large number of reconstructed early-stage tongue cancer can be found. Survival or functional benefits in these cases remain unclear. Methods: A retrospective data analysis of 384 surgically treated tongue carcinoma patients was conducted aiming to find epidemiologic and survival differences between patients with ($n = 158$) or without flap reconstruction ($n = 226$). A prospective functional analysis was performed on 55 early-stage tongue cancer patients, 33 without and 22 with radial-forearm flap reconstruction, focusing on post-therapeutic swallowing function as the primary endpoint, speech as the secondary endpoint, xerostomia, quality of life, and mouth opening. Results: Consistent with the current literature, we demonstrated the significantly more frequent use of flap grafts in advanced tongue carcinomas. For the first time, we depicted a higher female ratio in the reconstructed group ($p = 0.02$). There were no significant differences in survival or functional outcomes between the groups. The none-reconstructed group showed more frequent use of adjuvant C/RT despite presenting fewer N+ stages. Conclusions: The higher female ratio in the reconstruction group is plausible due to the anatomically smaller oral cavity and relatively larger carcinoma in women. A higher presence of close margins in the none-reconstruction group may explain the more frequent use of adjuvant C/RT. Since we found no survival or functional differences between the groups, we propose a critical approach toward flap reconstruction in T1/2 tongue carcinoma. At the same time, proportional aspects and adequate resection margins should be taken into account.

Citation: El-Shabrawi, K.; Storck, K.; Weitz, J.; Wolff, K.-D.; Knopf, A. Comparison of T1/2 Tongue Carcinoma with or without Radial Forearm Flap Reconstruction Regarding Post-Therapeutic Function, Survival, and Gender. *Cancers* **2023**, *15*, 1885. https://doi.org/10.3390/cancers15061885

Academic Editors: Romeo Patini, Carlo Lajolo and Gaetano Paludetti

Received: 6 February 2023
Revised: 17 March 2023
Accepted: 19 March 2023
Published: 21 March 2023

Copyright: © 2023 by the authors. Licensee MDPI, Basel, Switzerland. This article is an open access article distributed under the terms and conditions of the Creative Commons Attribution (CC BY) license (https://creativecommons.org/licenses/by/4.0/).

Keywords: tongue cancer; primary closure; flap reconstruction; functional outcome; survival outcome; gender distribution

1. Introduction

Tongue cancer represents one of the most common subtypes of oral cancer, with the majority of it being squamous cell cancer [1]. Annually, there are estimated 354,900 new cases and 177,400 deaths associated with oral cancer worldwide [2]. In addition, an increasing incidence of tongue cancer has been reported over the last few years [3]. The two major risk factors for developing tongue cancer are tobacco and alcohol abuse. Despite its growing significance in the development of oropharyngeal cancer, human papilloma virus (HPV) does not show major relevance in the etiology of tongue cancer [4]. Apart from radiation and chemotherapy, primary surgical resection holds the greatest importance in the therapy of tongue cancer. In a randomized, prospective trial, Iyer et al. showed the significant advantage of surgery compared to primary chemo/radiotherapy (C/RT) regarding survival in oral cancer patients [5]. While surgical treatment remains the first-choice therapy for tongue cancer, a higher focus on its functional outcome must be established. The anatomical reduction in tongue tissue evolves into a functional loss and impairs essential abilities such as speaking, swallowing, and eating, as well as the overall quality of life [6,7]. Furthermore, deteriorated tongue functionality can lead to a decline in survival through complications such as aspiration. For this reason, especially for wide tumor resections in advanced tumor stages, flap reconstruction has been firmly established in order to compensate for the loss of tongue volume and function [6]. However, for early-stage tongue cancer (T1/2), there is an inconsistent opinion on the necessity of flap reconstruction [8,9]. In the literature, there is poor data concerning the functional or survival benefits of performing flap reconstruction after smaller resections of tongue tissue. However, a large number of flap-reconstructed early-stage tongue cancers can be observed. Oncologically, the possibility of flap reconstruction during tumor resection might allow an extension of safety margins and thus better survival outcomes. Consequently, the higher rate of tumor-free margins could result in less use of adjuvant therapy in nodal-negative patients. Considering postoperative functionality, flap reconstruction could improve tongue mobility and thus have a positive effect on speech and swallowing function. These aspects prompted us to investigate not only functional but also survival outcomes after partial glossectomy in patients with or without flap reconstruction. We performed a retrospective analysis on a cohort of 384 surgically treated tongue cancer patients regarding therapeutic modalities and survival as well as epidemiological characteristics. Based on this retrospectively analyzed cohort, we recruited patients with surgically treated T1 and T2 tongue carcinomas for further prospective analyses of their functional outcomes. To receive conclusive results, we defined clear inclusion criteria and recruited only patients in tumor stages T1 and T2 with carcinomas of only the mobile tongue to exclude the possible involvement of the floor of the mouth. To form comparable cohorts, only patients who received reconstruction with or without radial-forearm flaps were included. Postoperative functionality was assessed in swallowing as the primary study endpoint, speech as the secondary endpoint, sicca symptoms, mouth-opening, and overall quality of life. The null hypothesis was that flap reconstruction improves functional outcomes.

2. Materials and Methods

2.1. Retrospective Analysis

To get a rough breakdown of patients' epidemiology, therapeutic regimes, and particularly the type of tongue reconstruction, a total of 384 patients with surgically treated tongue carcinoma were analyzed retrospectively. Patients from both the department of otorhinolaryngology and the clinic for oro-maxillofacial surgery were included. Epidemiological data, e.g., age, gender, therapy, reconstruction method, as well as survival data (death/loss to follow-up), were analyzed according to the UICC manual, 7th edition. Patients with a known history of head and neck cancer were excluded from the study. Retrospective data collection and analysis were confirmed by the local ethical committee.

2.2. Patient Selection

A homogeneous sub-cohort of T1/2 cancer patients was chosen for further functional assessment. To avoid surgical bias, only patients with T1/2 cancer of the mobile tongue and without the involvement of the floor of the mouth were included. Patients were divided into two groups: patients with and without radial forearm flap reconstruction (RFF).

From the 384 retrospectively identified patients, there were 204 T1/2 patients without flap reconstruction and 111 T1/2 patients who received any flap reconstruction. To receive reliable results regarding swallowing function, we excluded all patients with secondary tumors in the head and neck area. To build comparable groups, we additionally excluded all patients who received other flaps than RFF. Finally, 143 T1/2 patients without flap reconstruction or radial forearm flap reconstruction remained. RFF was selected because it is considered the first choice for small defects of the tongue [10]. A total number of 55 patients who had undergone partial glossectomy agreed to participate in the study, the other 88 patients could not be recruited due to residential distance, missing contact information, personal reasons, their medical condition, or were already deceased (Figure 1). Informed consent was obtained from all 55 patients.

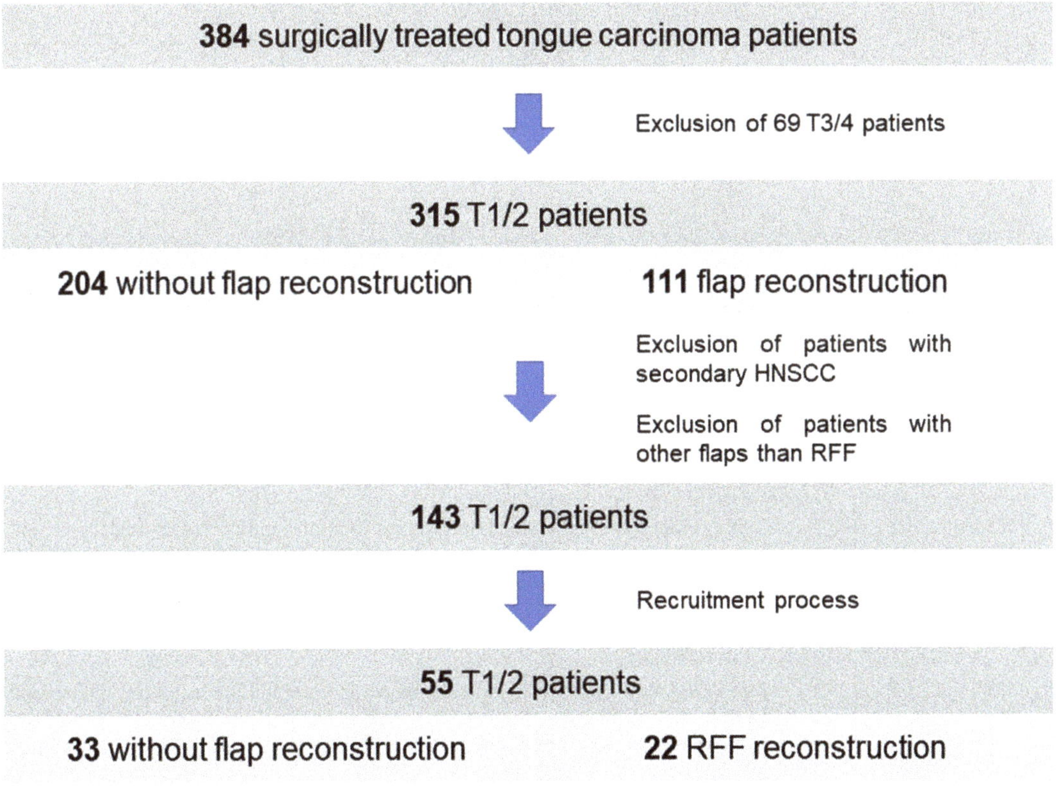

384 surgically treated tongue carcinoma patients

Exclusion of 69 T3/4 patients

315 T1/2 patients

204 without flap reconstruction   **111** flap reconstruction

Exclusion of patients with secondary HNSCC

Exclusion of patients with other flaps than RFF

143 T1/2 patients

Recruitment process

55 T1/2 patients

33 without flap reconstruction   **22** RFF reconstruction

Figure 1. Patient selection.

Reconstruction with an RFF was performed on 22 patients. Thirty-three patients underwent surgery with primary closure or healing by secondary intention. The date of surgical intervention and the date of functional analysis were defined and calculated as delta therapy analysis in months. Additionally, clinical parameters on age, sex, height, and weight, TNM-staging (referring to the UICC 7th edition), grading, and treatment modalities, as well as personal risk factors such as nicotine consumption in pack years and alcohol consumption in quantity and quality, were collected. Furthermore, histopathological data on maximum tumor diameter, maximum depth of penetration, minimal tumor-free margin, as well as tumor-free margins at first pass or by follow-up resection were gathered retrospectively. At least two experienced pathologists histologically reviewed all tumor samples.

The local ethical committee approved the study (289/16S).

2.3. Swallowing Assessment

To assess the extent of dysphagia, patients completed the 100 mL water swallowing test (WST) [11], which portrays the primary endpoint of the study. The WST previously proved to be a valuable tool to assess post-treatment swallowing performance in head and neck cancer patients [12,13]. In addition, swallowing dysfunction was determined by the M.D. Anderson Dysphagia Inventory (MDADI) [14], which contained 20 dysphagia-related questions and was self-completed by the patients. A score between 0 and 100 could be achieved, with lower scores indicating higher levels of dysphagia. Moreover, a score for changes in eating habits was developed based on the Toxicity Criteria of the Radiation Therapy Oncology Group (RTOG) and the European Organization for Research and Treatment of Cancer (EORTC) [15]. Patients were categorized into five different groups by the examiner according to their dietary changes (Table 1).

Table 1. Dietary changes.

Scheme	Dietary Changes
0	No changes
1	Mild dysphagia with slight changes of eating habits (mild diet), slight difficulties in swallowing solid food.
2	Moderate dysphagia with necessary changes of eating habits to pureed or liquid food, solid food can't be swallowed.
3	Severe dysphagia with changes of eating habits to only liquid food.
4	Complete obstruction, nutrition requires N-G feeding tube, i.v. fluids or hyperalimentation

2.4. Speech Assessment

Speech problems were evaluated using the Speech Handicap Index (SHI) [16], which was self-completed by the patients. The questionnaire consisted of 30 items dealing with daily impairments in social interactions. A score between 0 (no problems) and 120 (high grade of speech problems) could be obtained.

2.5. Xerostomia Assessment

Mouth dryness was assessed in patients performing the Saxon Test [17]. To quantify saliva production, patients insalivated a 5×5 cm sterile sponge for 2 min. The sponge was weighed before and after salivation. Additionally, all patients completed the Visual Analogue Scale xerostomia questionnaire (VAS) for salivary dysfunction [18], which contained eight items dealing with problems caused by mouth dryness. For each item, a symptom severity scale between 0 and 100 was calculated; higher levels indicating more symptoms. The test included the following questions:

Q1. Rate your difficulty in talking due to dryness
Q2. Rate your difficulty in chewing due to dryness

Q3. Rate your difficulty in swallowing solid food due to dryness
Q4. Rate the frequency of your sleeping problems due to dryness
Q5. Rate your mouth or throat dryness when eating food
Q6. Rate your mouth or throat dryness while not eating
Q7. Rate the frequency of sipping liquids to aid swallowing food
Q8. Rate the frequency of sipping liquids for oral comfort when not eating

2.6. Mouth-Opening

Due to surgery and radiotherapy in tongue cancer patients, problems with mouth opening are frequently reported [19]. We assessed mouth opening in all patients as the maximal distance from the upper alveolar ridge to the lower alveolar ridge using a measuring compass. Measurements were taken in millimeters. Furthermore, we determined the Mallampati score in all patients.

2.7. Quality of Life Assessment

In order to assess the physical and psychosocial quality of life after cancer surgery, patients completed the Head and Neck module of the EORTC Quality of Life Questionnaire (QLQ-H&N35) [20]. The questionnaire contained 35 items and portrayed frequently reported health and lifestyle changes in patients diagnosed with head and neck cancer face, including the categories of pain, swallowing, teeth problems, problems with opening mouth, mouth dryness, sticky saliva, loss of senses, coughing, speech problems, feeling ill, social eating, social contact, sexuality, use of pain killers, use of oral supplements or a feeding tube, as well as weight loss and weight gain. A symptom score between 0 (= no symptoms) and 100 was calculated for each category.

2.8. Statistical Analysis

Statistical analysis of the data obtained was performed with the Statistical Package for the Social Sciences (SPSS Inc., Chicago, IL, USA). Continuous variables were represented by the arithmetic mean and the corresponding standard deviation. Categorical variables were represented by absolute and relative frequencies. Group comparisons between reconstructed and none-reconstructed patients were performed for all retrospectively gathered data as well as for all prospectively assessed functional results, with the WST being the primary study endpoint. Group comparisons of categorical variables were performed using the chi-square test or, for small data sets, the Fisher exact test. For continuous variables, the unpaired Student's t-test was applied. Survival rates were defined from the date of surgical intervention and were calculated and illustrated using the Kaplan–Meier method. Differences between survival rates were assessed using the log-rank test. A p-value of <0.05 was defined as significant in all statistical tests.

3. Results
3.1. Retrospective Analysis

From a total of 384 surgically treated T1–4 tongue carcinoma patients, 226 patients received primary closure and 158 underwent flap reconstruction. One hundred and four patients received reconstruction using a radial-forearm flap. Regarding T-status, the none-reconstruction and reconstruction groups showed a distribution of 51% vs. 32% of T1, 39% vs. 38% of T2, 6% vs. 22% of T3, and 4% vs. 8% of T4 cases. Both groups were compared, and there were significantly more cases of advanced T-status in the reconstruction group ($p < 0.0001$). Subsequently, we depicted significantly more cases of advanced N-status and positive R-status in the reconstruction group ($p = 0.03$; $p = 0.02$). The TNM status is summarized in Table 2. Adjuvant C/RT was significantly more often performed in the reconstruction group ($p < 0.0001$). Interestingly, we found a significantly higher female ratio (26% vs. 38%) in the reconstruction group ($p = 0.02$). Survival analysis was performed on T1 and T2 cases. Analyses showed a mean overall survival (OS) of 116 months in the none-reconstruction group and 118 months in the reconstruction group. There was no significant advantage regarding OS from performing flap reconstruction ($p = 0.47$, Figure 2).

Table 2. Retrospective data.

	No Reconstruction	Reconstruction	p-Value
N	226	158	
Gender, n (%)			0.02
Male: Female	167 (74)/59 (26)	98 (62)/60 (38)	
Age at initial diagnosis (years)			0.99
Mean ± SD (median)	57 ± 14 (56)	57 ± 13 (59)	
Grading, n (%)			0.82
G0	1 (0.4)	0	
G1	34 (15)	19 (12)	
G2	143 (63)	113 (72)	
G3	47 (21)	26 (17)	
G4	1 (0.4)	0	
T status, n (%)			<0.0001
T1	116 (51)	51 (32)	
T2	88 (39)	60 (38)	
T3	14 (6)	34 (22)	
T4	8 (4)	13 (8)	
N status, n (%)			0.03
N0	149 (66)	89 (56)	
N1	37 (16)	23 (15)	
N2a	5 (2)	3 (2)	
N2b	7 (3)	19 (12)	
N2c	12 (5)	10 (6)	
N3	16 (7)	14 (9)	
M status, n (%)			0.32
M0	226 (100)	157 (99)	
M1	0	1 (0.6)	
R status, n (%)			0.02
R0	219 (97)	146 (92)	
R1	7 (3)	6 (4)	
R2	0	1 (0.6)	
Rx	0	5 (3)	
Therapy			<0.0001
Surgery	152 (67)	78 (49)	
Surgery + aRT	59 (26)	52 (33)	
Surgery + aCRT	15 (7)	28 (18)	
Reconstruction			
RFF	-	104 (66)	
ALT	-	18 (11)	
Perforator	-	8 (5)	
Other	-	24 (15)	
Peroneus	-	4 (3)	

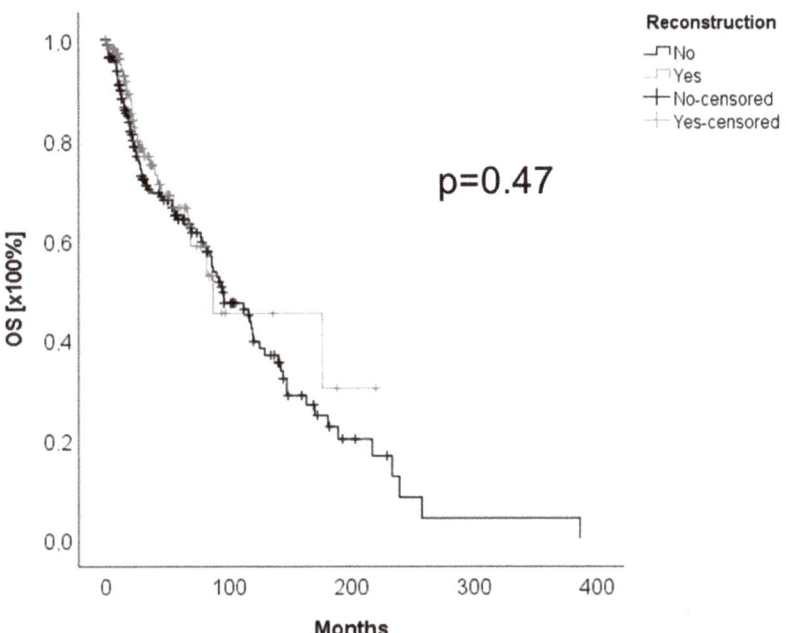

Figure 2. Overall survival (OS) for T1/2 carcinoma comparing primary closure and flap reconstruction.

To identify whether the significantly higher female ratio in the reconstruction group was due to an also advanced T-status in women, we analyzed the distribution of T status among men and women in the reconstructed patients. Analyses showed a significantly higher proportion of T3–4 status in men (34% vs. 21%; $p = 0.005$) among all reconstructed patients (Table 3).

Table 3. T status distribution among men and women in reconstructed patients ($n = 158$).

	Male	Female	*p*-Value
N	98	60	
T status, *n* (%)			0.005
T1	25 (26)	26 (43)	
T2	39 (40)	21 (35)	
T3	23 (23)	11 (18)	
T4	11 (11)	2 (3)	

In order to specify the results for early tumor stages, we performed an additional data analysis for T1 and T2 stages only. Here, there was no statistically significant difference for N, M, and R stages between the reconstructed and non-reconstructed tongue carcinomas. Regarding therapy regimens, adjuvant therapy was used more frequently in the reconstruction group, which can be attributed to the correspondingly higher presence of N+ in this group (Table 4).

Table 4. Calculation of N, M, R stages, therapy, and reconstruction method for T1/2 cases only.

	No Reconstruction	Reconstruction	p-Value
N	204	111	
N status, n (%)			0.61
N0	143 (70)	74 (67)	
N1	30 (15)	16 (14)	
N2a	4 (2)	-	
N2b	7 (3)	12 (11)	
N2c	6 (3)	4 (4)	
N3	14 (7)	5 (5)	
M status, n (%)			0.32
M0	204 (100)	110 (99)	
M1	-	1 (1)	
R status, n (%)			0.28
R0	197 (97)	106 (96)	
R1	7 (3)	3 (3)	
Rx	-	2 (2)	
Therapy			0.07
Surgery	144 (71)	68 (61)	
Surgery + aRT	48 (24)	31 (28)	
Surgery + aCRT	12 (6)	12 (11)	
Reconstruction			
RFF	-	66 (60)	
ALT	-	12 (11)	
Perforator	-	8 (7)	
Other	-	21 (19)	
Peroneus	-	4 (4)	

3.2. Epidemiology of the Prospective Functionally Analyzed Cohort

To form comparable groups for the assessment of functional outcomes in early-stage tongue cancer, we excluded all patients who received different flaps than the RFF. Finally, a total of 55 patients diagnosed with tongue cancer in tumor stages T1 and T2 participated in this study, comprising 33 patients who underwent partial glossectomy without reconstruction and 22 patients who underwent partial glossectomy with RFF reconstruction. At this point, it should be taken into account that biases with regard to patient selection are possible due to the small number of cases. Patients' treatment decision was made after the tumor board consensus and recommendation of head and neck surgeons. The mean duration between surgery and functional analysis was 78 months and 66 months, respectively, without statistically significant differences between the groups ($p = 0.49$, Table 5). The mean age of patients at initial diagnosis was 49 years and 51 years. A higher female ratio (15% vs. 36%) was found in the RFF-reconstruction group, although it could not be regarded as significant ($p = 0.09$). The height-to-weight ratio did not differ significantly between the groups ($p = 0.06$). Only one patient in the RFF-reconstruction group required a gastral tube; none required a permanent tracheostomy.

Table 5. Epidemiologic data of the functionally analyzed cohort.

	No Reconstruction	RFF Reconstruction	p-Value
N	33	22	
Delta therapy analysis (months)			0.49
Mean ± SD (median)	78 ± 66 (52)	66 ± 50 (43)	
Age at initial diagnosis (years)			0.66
Mean ± SD (median)	49 ± 13 (49)	51 ± 17 (50)	
Gender, n (%)			0.09
Male: Female	28 (85)/5 (15)	14 (64)/8 (36)	
T status, n (%)			0.91
T1	22 (67)	15 (68)	
T2	11 (33)	7 (32)	
Maximum tumor diameter (mm)			0.69
Mean ± SD (median)	16 ± 8 (18)	17 ± 7 (15)	
Maximum depth of penetration (mm)			0.77
Mean ± SD (median)	8 ± 4 (7)	9 ± 7 (6)	
N status, n (%)			0.64
N0	27 (82)	17 (77)	
N1	3 (9)	3 (14)	
N2a	1 (3)	0	
N2b	1 (3)	0	
N2c	0	1 (5)	
N3	1 (3)	1 (5)	
M status, n (%)			
M0	33 (100)	22 (100)	
M1	0	0	
Grading, n (%)			0.016
G1	4 (12)	5 (23)	
G2	20 (61)	17 (77)	
G3	9 (27)	0	
R status, n (%)			0.33
R0	33 (100)	21 (96)	
R1	0	1 (5)	
R0 on the main sample			0.45
No	11 (33)	5 (23)	
Yes	22 (67)	17 (77)	
Minimal achieved tumor-free margin (mm)			0.89
Mean ± SD (median)	4 ± 3 (4)	4 ± 2 (5)	
Neck dissection			0.09
Ipsi-lateral	23 (70)	10 (46)	
Bi-lateral	10 (30)	12 (55)	
Adjuvant therapy, n (%)			0.81
None	20 (61)	16 (73)	
aRT	11 (33)	3 (14)	
aCRT	2 (6)	3 (14)	

Table 5. Cont.

	No Reconstruction	RFF Reconstruction	p-Value
Adjuvant therapy escalation, n (%)			0.09
No	26 (79)	21 (95)	
Yes	7 (21)	1 (5)	

A distribution of T1 (67–68%) and T2 (32–33%) was evenly reported in both groups, as well as a majority of N0-status (82% and 77%). When compared to the RFF-reconstruction group, the none-reconstruction group showed a significantly advanced grading, with 89% of patients being diagnosed with G2 or G3 ($p = 0.016$). In both groups, the maximum tumor diameter ranged from 16 to 17 mm and the maximum depth of penetration from 8 to 9 mm. The minimally achieved tumor-free margin amounted to 4 mm in both groups. R0 resection on the main sample could be achieved in 67% of cases in the none-reconstruction group and in 77% of cases in the RFF-reconstruction group ($p = 0.45$). Other patients underwent R0 resection during the same surgery by follow-up resection. In this study, there was only one patient in the RFF-reconstruction group who was diagnosed with R1 resection in the final histology. The patient refused further surgical procedures and underwent adjuvant treatment.

All patients received a neck dissection. In both groups, the majority of patients did not undergo an additional adjuvant therapy, referring to nodal negativity and R0 resection. Additional radiotherapy was performed on 33% and 14%, and additional chemoradiotherapy was performed on 6% and 14%, respectively ($p = 0.81$). Subsequently, seven patients without RFF underwent adjuvant treatment escalation due to close margins, while only one patient in the RFF group underwent adjuvant treatment escalation referring to R1 status. However, this tendency did not achieve statistical significance ($p = 0.09$).

There were slightly fewer patients with prior or active use of nicotine in the none-reconstruction group, comprising 55% and 46% of none-smokers (Table 6). The average smoking time ranged from 17py in the none-reconstruction group to 15py in the RFF group. A non-significant higher consumption of alcohol could be depicted in the none-reconstruction group, showing an average daily alcohol consumption of 615 mL or 397 mL respectively ($p = 0.46$). Drinking habits, considering active, prior, or none alcohol consumption, did not differ significantly between the groups. In both groups, the patients' majority continued alcohol consumption after surgery (42% and 73%). In both groups, the most common liquid consumed was beer.

Table 6. Noxae.

	No Reconstruction	RFF Reconstruction	p-Value
Nicotine abuse (py)	17	15	0.81
None, n (%)	17 (52)	10 (46)	0.9
Prior, n (%)	11 (33)	9 (41)	
Active, n (%)	5 (15)	3 (14)	
Alcohol consumption (mL/d)	615	397	0.46
None, n (%)	9 (27)	5 (23)	0.18
Prior, n (%)	10 (30)	1 (5)	
Active, n (%)	14 (42)	16 (73)	
Liquids			0.54
None, n (%)	8 (24)	5 (23)	
Beer, n (%)	14 (42)	12 (55)	
Wine, n (%)	9 (27)	4 (18)	
Spirits, n (%)	2 (6)	1 (5)	

3.3. Swallowing

The primary endpoint of this study was swallowing function determined through the 100 mL water swallowing test (WST). The mean amount of water swallowed per second in patients with primary closure was 17.89 mL/s. Patients receiving an RFF reconstruction swallowed 15.96 mL/s. In this objective assessment of patients' swallowing function, there were no statistically significant differences between both groups ($p = 0.39$, Table 7). Additionally, no significant differences in nasal reflux (18% vs. 5%; $p = 0.1$) or in the RTOG dysphagia score (0.44 vs. 0.86; $p = 0.09$) were found. As a subjective assessment of patients swallowing function, the MD Anderson dysphagia inventory showed a remaining swallowing function range of 60–65/100 in both groups (Figure 3). No significant differences between the groups were reported in this test ($p = 0.28$).

Table 7. Functional analyses.

	No Reconstruction	RFF Reconstruction	*p*-Value
Ratio height to weight	2.30	2.58	0.06
Gastral tube, *n* (%)	0	1 (5)	0.33
Tracheostomy, *n* (%)	0	0	
Water drinking time (mL/s)			0.39
Mean ± SD (median)	17.89 ± 8.46 (18.13)	15.96 ± 7.39 (15.24)	
Nasal reflux, *n* (%)	6 (18)	1 (5)	0.10
RTOG dysphagia score	0.44	0.86	0.09
Saxon test (g/2 min)	2.07	1.87	0.53
Mallampati	2.53	2.36	0.62
Maxilla-mandible distance (mm)	60.34	61.14	0.81

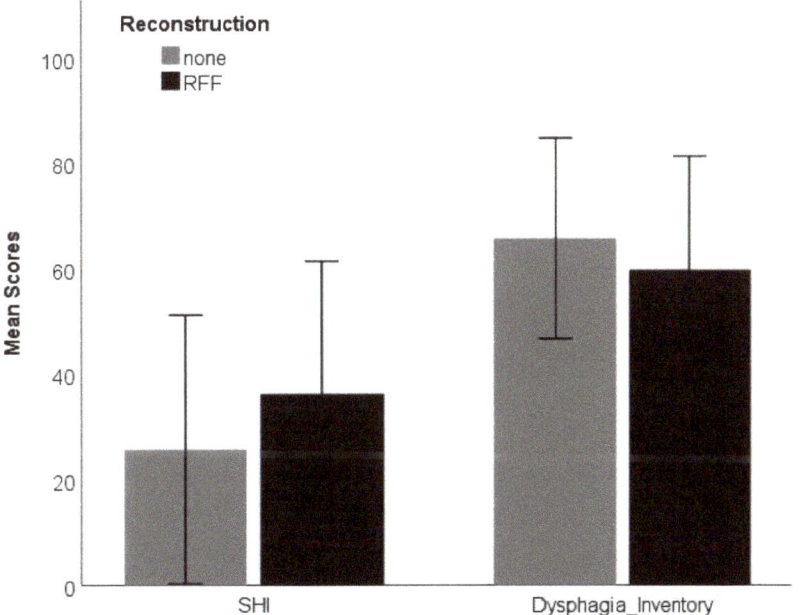

Figure 3. Results of the Speech Handicap Index (SHI) and the MD Anderson Dysphagia Inventory (MDADI) compared. A low symptom score in the SHI represents fewer problems with speech. A low score in the MDADI indicates greater difficulties in swallowing function.

3.4. Speech

The Speech Handicap Index represented the secondary endpoint of this study and depicted patients' subjective speech issues. The mean total SHI score ranged from 25 points in the none-reconstruction group to 37 points in the RFF-reconstruction group, showing fewer speaking problems in the none-reconstruction group (Figure 3). There were no significant differences between the groups ($p = 0.14$).

3.5. Xerostomia

Saliva production in the Saxon test ranged from 2.07 g/2 min in the none-reconstruction group to 1.87 g/2 min in the RFF-reconstruction group. The Sicca VAS score revealed symptom scores from 18% (Q5) to 30% (Q8) in the none-reconstruction group and 22% (Q4) to 29% (Q1) in the RFF-reconstruction group (Figure 4). In both the objective and subjective tests, no significant differences were found between the groups ($p = 0.53$; $p = 0.71$).

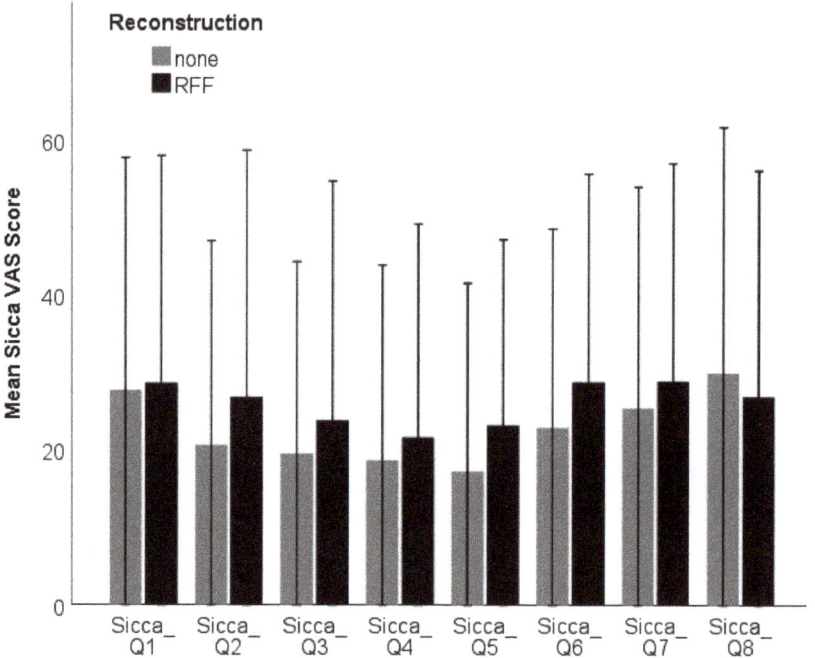

Figure 4. Results of the Sicca VAS score.

3.6. Mouth-Opening

The maxilla-mandible (gingiva-to-gingiva) distance ranged from 60.34 mm in the none-reconstruction group to 61.14 mm in the RFF-reconstruction group. The none-reconstruction group showed a Mallampati score of 2.53, and the RFF-reconstruction group had a score of 2.36, respectively. In both tests, there were no statistically significant differences between the groups ($p = 0.81$; $p = 0.62$).

3.7. Quality of Life

The most severe symptom reported in the QLQ-HN35 was mouth dryness in both groups, followed by coughing in the none-reconstruction group and social eating in the RFF-reconstruction group. On any of the symptom scales, there were no statistically significant differences found between the groups. Figure 5 illustrates all 18 symptom scales for both groups.

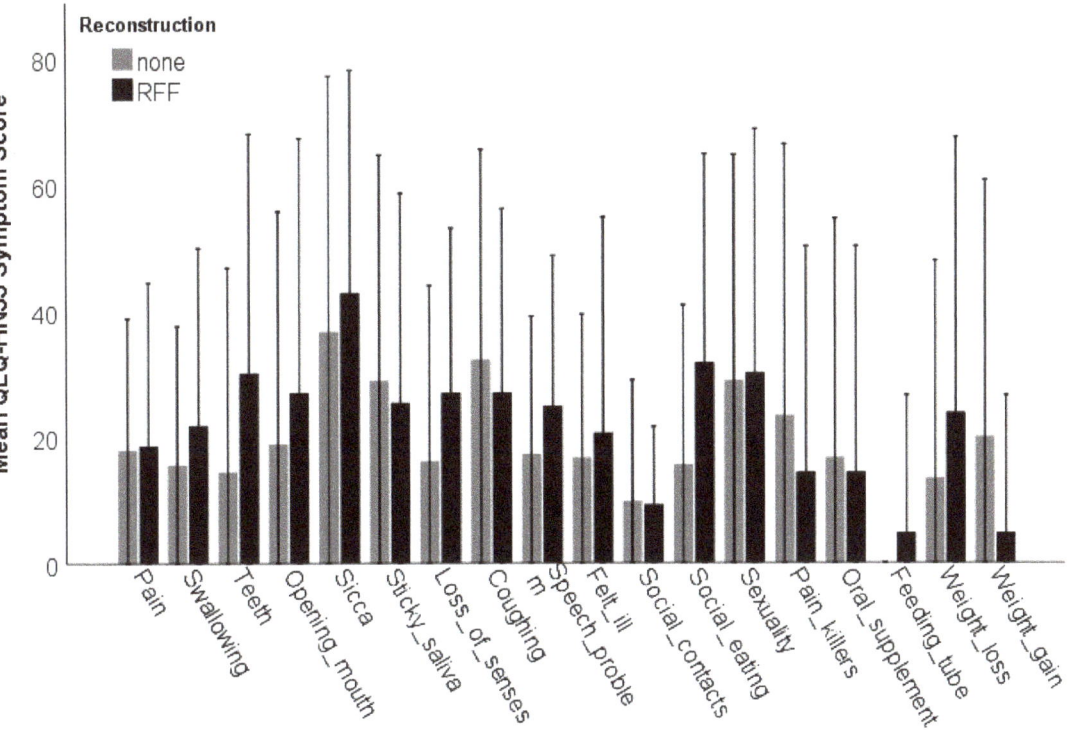

Figure 5. Results of the EORTC QLQ-HN35 for primary closure and RFF reconstruction compared.

4. Discussion

Flap reconstruction is firmly established in the advanced stages of tongue carcinomas, aiming to restore volume and preserve tongue mobility [6,21]. Our retrospective analyses of the large cohort of 384 tongue cancer patients showed significantly more cases of advanced T- and N-status as well as positive R-status in the reconstruction group when compared to the none-reconstruction group. In addition, escalation of therapy via adjuvant C/RT was depicted more often in the reconstruction group, which is coherent with advanced T-, N-, and positive R-status. These findings are consistent with the current literature [22–24]. Interestingly, our retrospective analyses also depicted a large amount of reconstructed early-stage tongue cancer. In fact, we were able to denote that the majority of reconstructed patients were diagnosed with either T1 (32%) or T2 (38%). This observation suggests either a functional or a survival benefit from performing flap reconstruction and prompted us to further investigate these parameters.

From a surgical point of view, survival can be improved by extending the distance between the tumor and the resection margin. Several studies have shown that the margin size and achieving R0 on the main sample correlate with significant improvements in recurrence-free intervals (RFI) and thus OS [25,26]. Consequently, the possibility of flap reconstruction might surgically lead to a more generous tumor resection and improve the chances of R0 on the main sample. Through this consideration, reconstruction could contribute to a survival benefit. Analyses of the histopathological data of our functionally examined patients did not show a statistically significant difference concerning R0 on the main sample between the groups. This indicates that sufficient resection can be achieved even without flap reconstruction. These results were confirmed by the analysis of overall survival in the large retrospective group. There were no statistically significant differences regarding OS in the T1 and T2 stages between the none-reconstruction and reconstruction groups (116 vs. 118 months, $p = 0.47$). In contrast, we were able to depict the more frequent use of adjuvant C/RT in the none-reconstructed group when compared to the RFF group (39% vs. 28%), despite the predominant N0 status in both groups (82% and 77%). Indications for adjuvant radiotherapy in T1/2 oral cancer include positive resection margins (R1) or the presence of lymph node metastases (N+) [27]. Lymph node metastases with extracapsular extension (ECE) are an indication of adjuvant chemo-radiotherapy [28]. In the case of close margins, adjuvant radiotherapy is also frequently applied [27]. Since the none-reconstructed group showed fewer R0 resections on the main sample, there are higher chances of close margins in these cases. The higher presence of close margins consequently led to the more frequent use of adjuvant C/RT escalation in the none-reconstruction group, comprising 21% and 5%, respectively. In turn, these results suggest that, due to the possibility of flap reconstruction, a more generous tumor resection was possible in the RFF group, with lower chances of close margins and therefore a less frequent need for adjuvant C/RT and its respective concomitant toxicities. However, this tendency failed to achieve statistical significance in our study ($p = 0.09$). Lu et al. compared margin size and recurrence rate in a large cohort of 347 early-stage tongue carcinoma patients and found that the utilization of flap reconstruction achieved a significantly larger pathologic free margin and had significantly lower recurrence rates [29].

The surgical objective after partial tongue resection should not only include the best oncological outcome but also consider functional aspects. Essential functions such as airway protection, swallowing, and speaking should be safely practicable and maintain an optimal quality of life for the patient. Regarding functionality in advanced tumor stages, Canis et al. compared microvascular flap reconstruction and primary closure in T3 tongue carcinomas and showed significant functional impairments in patients who did not receive flap reconstruction [30]. Our study assessed functionality in T1 and T2 tongue carcinomas in both subjective and objective test batteries. Our results show that there is no significant functional advantage in any field examined. Regarding swallowing, the none-reconstruction group even showed a slightly better mean of water-drinking time, a lower symptom score in the QLQ-HN35, a lower RTOG dysphagia score, and better results in the MD Anderson dysphagia inventory, despite not being statistically significant. Only the presence of nasal reflux was observed to be less frequent in the RFF reconstruction group. A similar trend could be observed in the subjective speech questionnaires: both the QLQ-HN35 symptom score for speech problems and the SHI portrayed slightly more problems with speech in the RFF-reconstruction group, although this could not be regarded as statistically significant. These findings demonstrate that the flap not only serves to provide bulk and improve mobility but can also interfere with processes such as articulation or swallowing and necessitates training. Similar results were obtained in a study by Ji et al. showing significantly worse functional outcomes in articulation, tongue mobility, and speech intelligibility in flap-reconstructed tongue carcinoma patients [6]. A study by Kaur et al. placed the main emphasis on subjective patient satisfaction and found that higher levels were achieved for the primary closure of smaller defects and for flap reconstruction of larger tongue defects [31]. Interestingly, the most important factor regarding the QLQ-HN35 with the highest symptom scores for both groups was mouth dryness, which was also demonstrated to be relevant in the Sicca VAS score. This subjectively present mouth dryness was objectively confirmed in the Saxon test, demonstrating a mean saliva production of <2.75 g/2 min in both groups, which was defined as pathological [17]. A major factor that can cause dry mouth is the use of adjuvant C/RT.

The time range between the end of therapy and functional assessment was 78 months and 66 months, respectively; therefore, this study mainly depicts long-term functional outcomes. In this period of time, other factors might have impacted speech and swallowing function, which must be considered when applying the results for clinical purposes. Still, a comparison considering long-term functional outcomes was possible since the period between therapy and functional assessment did not differ significantly between the groups ($p = 0.49$).

When analyzing our retrospective cohort, we saw a statistically significant higher distribution of women receiving flap reconstruction ($p = 0.02$). To identify whether this was due to an also advanced T-status in women, we analyzed the T-status distribution among reconstructed male and female patients. Surprisingly, analyses showed significantly smaller T status in reconstructed women when compared to men ($p = 0.005$). In conclusion, this shows that women received flap reconstruction despite having a smaller T-status. Anatomically, women tend to have smaller oral cavities and less tongue tissue, which indicates that T1 or T2 tongue carcinomas in women are proportionally larger than in men. Therefore, the more frequent usage of flap reconstruction is conclusive. Generally, these findings suggest that not only the tumor size should be taken into consideration but also its proportion to the remaining tongue tissue and protection of the mandible. A uniform classification system for tongue reconstruction does not yet exist. However, possible solutions have been pointed out in various studies so far. Mannelli et al. proposed a strategic approach for surgery of different types of tongue defects where a specific reconstruction algorithm is available for each type of defined tongue defect [23]. Ansarin et al. proposed a similar classification system that is based on the anatomical and functional components of the tongue and the spread routes of tongue cancer [32]. A proportional concept with consideration of the actual size of the tongue and oral cavity is missing in both studies. Given our results, the distance between the tumor and the tongue midline, for instance, could serve as an indicator of the relative volume loss and consequently be used as a criterion for flap reconstruction. Our research revealed no other previous study describing differences in tongue reconstruction in women.

To further determine whether N or R status exerted an influence on the decision to perform flap reconstruction, we specifically analyzed their distribution in early tumor stages of tongue carcinoma in the retrospective cohort. Again, there was no significant difference between the groups. This underlines the fact that the decision to perform flap reconstruction depends individually on the local expertise of the surgeon.

Apart from fitting the proportionally perfect flap, performing microvascular flap reconstruction also involves the management and training of non-innervated tissue, which is crucial for abilities such as speaking and eating. Furthermore, RFF reconstruction involves the loss of the radial artery at the donor site and possible complications such as necrosis of the flap due to vascular anastomosis insufficiency [33,34]. A major advantage when performing primary closure of the tongue is the shorter operative time and thus lower risk of delirium, more likely avoidance of tracheostomy, and no or short intensive care duration.

To our knowledge, this is the first study analyzing objective and subjective parameters in surgically treated early-stage tongue cancer, specifically comparing none-reconstruction to RFF-reconstruction, which is one of the strengths of this study. TNM stages, age, and gender were also evenly distributed between the functionally studied groups, which supports the results from the group comparison. At the same time, the small case number of the functionally examined cohort must be taken into account, as must the possible bias in patient selection. Moreover, the long time range between the end of therapy and functional assessment must be considered when applying the results for clinical purposes, as other factors might have impacted speech and swallowing functions during this period. In contrast, the retrospective analysis of 384 surgically treated tongue carcinoma patients provides a broad overview regarding epidemiological differences and treatment regimens. By including patients from the ENT and maxillofacial surgery departments, we were able to form a very heterogeneous collective, which can be well applied to actual clinical practice. In addition to overall survival, it would have been interesting to measure disease-specific survival as well. This could not be conducted because it was not evident from our existing data if death was caused by a tumor diagnosis. In summary, our findings indicate that a more restrained approach to the usage of flap reconstruction in smaller carcinomas of the tongue is favorable and that the loss of tongue tissue proportionally to the remaining tongue volume should be taken into consideration for an optimal functional outcome. For surgical therapy of T3/4 tongue carcinoma, flap reconstruction is undoubtedly recommended.

5. Conclusions

Our study demonstrated that there are no statistically significant differences regarding functional and survival outcomes between flap reconstruction and none-reconstruction in early-stage tongue carcinomas. This suggests that the implications of reconstructing T1 and T2 tongue carcinomas should be deeply evaluated beforehand, taking possible complications and necessary training into consideration. At the same time, we showed that the possibility of flap reconstruction leads to a more generous surgical resection, less frequent presence of close margin, and subsequently less frequent use of toxic adjuvant therapy regimens. Furthermore, we demonstrated for the first time that women were significantly more likely to be reconstructed by flap surgery, even when presenting a smaller T-status. This indicates that reconstruction cannot be determined by the tumor size alone but requires a proportional approach based on existing anatomical circumstances. Future research is needed to identify and develop clear guidelines for the usage of flap reconstruction in early-stage carcinomas of the tongue.

Author Contributions: Conceptualization, K.E.-S. and A.K.; methodology, K.E.-S., A.K., K.S., J.W. and K.-D.W.; software, K.E.-S., A.K., J.W. and K.S.; validation, K.E.-S., A.K., K.S., J.W. and K.-D.W.; formal analysis, K.E.-S., A.K., K.S., J.W. and K.-D.W.; resources, K.E.-S., A.K., K.S., J.W. and K.-D.W.; data curation, K.E.-S., A.K., K.S., J.W. and K.-D.W.; writing—original draft preparation, K.E.-S., A.K., K.S., J.W. and K.-D.W.; writing—review and editing, K.E.-S., A.K., K.S., J.W. and K.-D.W.; visualization, K.E.-S. and A.K.; supervision, K.E.-S., A.K., K.S., J.W. and K.-D.W.; project administration, K.E.-S., A.K. and K.S.; funding acquisition, A.K. All authors have read and agreed to the published version of the manuscript.

Funding: This research received no external funding.

Institutional Review Board Statement: The study was conducted in accordance with the Declaration of Helsinki, and ap-proved by the Institutional Ethics Committee (Ethikkommission Klinikum rechts der Isar, Technische Universität München (289/16S)).

Informed Consent Statement: Informed consent was obtained from all subjects involved in the study.

Data Availability Statement: The data can be shared up on request.

Conflicts of Interest: The authors declare no conflict of interest.

References

1. Karatas, O.F.; Oner, M.; Abay, A.; Diyapoglu, A. MicroRNAs in human tongue squamous cell carcinoma: From pathogenesis to therapeutic implications. *Oral Oncol.* **2017**, *67*, 124–130. [CrossRef] [PubMed]
2. Ferlay, J.; Colombet, M.; Soerjomataram, I.; Mathers, C.; Parkin, D.M.; Pineros, M.; Znaor, A.; Bray, F. Estimating the global cancer incidence and mortality in 2018: GLOBOCAN sources and methods. *Int. J. Cancer* **2019**, *144*, 1941–1953. [CrossRef] [PubMed]
3. Tota, J.E.; Anderson, W.F.; Coffey, C.; Califano, J.; Cozen, W.; Ferris, R.L.; St John, M.; Cohen, E.E.; Chaturvedi, A.K. Rising incidence of oral tongue cancer among white men and women in the United States, 1973–2012. *Oral Oncol.* **2017**, *67*, 146–152. [CrossRef] [PubMed]
4. Dahlgren, L.; Dahlstrand, H.M.; Lindquist, D.; Hogmo, A.; Bjornestal, L.; Lindholm, J.; Lundberg, B.; Dalianis, T.; Munck-Wikland, E. Human papillomavirus is more common in base of tongue than in mobile tongue cancer and is a favorable prognostic factor in base of tongue cancer patients. *Int. J. Cancer* **2004**, *112*, 1015–1019. [CrossRef] [PubMed]
5. Iyer, N.G.; Tan, D.S.; Tan, V.K.; Wang, W.; Hwang, J.; Tan, N.C.; Sivanandan, R.; Tan, H.K.; Lim, W.T.; Ang, M.K.; et al. Randomized trial comparing surgery and adjuvant radiotherapy versus concurrent chemoradiotherapy in patients with advanced, nonmetastatic squamous cell carcinoma of the head and neck: 10-year update and subset analysis. *Cancer* **2015**, *121*, 1599–1607. [CrossRef]
6. Ji, Y.B.; Cho, Y.H.; Song, C.M.; Kim, Y.H.; Kim, J.T.; Ahn, H.C.; Tae, K. Long-term functional outcomes after resection of tongue cancer: Determining the optimal reconstruction method. *Eur. Arch. Oto-Rhino-Laryngol.* **2017**, *274*, 3751–3756. [CrossRef]
7. Kazi, R.; Johnson, C.; Prasad, V.; De Cordova, J.; Venkitaraman, R.; Nutting, C.; Clarke, P.; Evans, P.R.; Harrington, K. Quality of life outcome measures following partial glossectomy: Assessment using the UW-QOL scale. *J. Cancer Res. Ther.* **2008**, *4*, 116. [CrossRef]

8. Chuanjun, C.; Zhiyuan, Z.; Shaopu, G.; Xinquan, J.; Zhihong, Z. Speech after partial glossectomy: A comparison between reconstruction and nonreconstruction patients. *J. Oral Maxillofac. Surg.* **2002**, *60*, 404–407. [CrossRef]
9. Kansy, K.; Mueller, A.A.; Mücke, T.; Koersgen, F.; Wolff, K.D.; Zeilhofer, H.F.; Hölzle, F.; Pradel, W.; Schneider, M.; Kolk, A.; et al. A worldwide comparison of the management of T1 and T2 anterior floor of the mouth and tongue squamous cell carcinoma—Extent of surgical resection and reconstructive measures. *J. Cranio-Maxillo-Facial Surg.* **2017**, *45*, 2097–2104. [CrossRef]
10. Huang, C.H.; Chen, H.C.; Huang, Y.L.; Mardini, S.; Feng, G.M. Comparison of the radial forearm flap and the thinned anterolateral thigh cutaneous flap for reconstruction of tongue defects: An evaluation of donor-site morbidity. *Plast. Reconstr. Surg.* **2004**, *114*, 1704–1710. [CrossRef]
11. Wu, M.C.; Chang, Y.C.; Wang, T.G.; Lin, L.C. Evaluating swallowing dysfunction using a 100-ml water swallowing test. *Dysphagia* **2004**, *19*, 43–47. [CrossRef] [PubMed]
12. Patterson, J.M.; Hildreth, A.; McColl, E.; Carding, P.N.; Hamilton, D.; Wilson, J.A. The clinical application of the 100 mL water swallow test in head and neck cancer. *Oral Oncol.* **2011**, *47*, 180–184. [CrossRef] [PubMed]
13. Vermaire, J.A.; Terhaard, C.H.; Verdonck-de Leeuw, I.M.; Raaijmakers, C.P.; Speksnijder, C.M.J.H. Reliability of the 100 mL water swallow test in patients with head and neck cancer and healthy subjects. *Head Neck* **2021**, *43*, 2468–2476. [CrossRef] [PubMed]
14. Chen, A.Y.; Frankowski, R.; Bishop-Leone, J.; Hebert, T.; Leyk, S.; Lewin, J.; Goepfert, H. The development and validation of a dysphagia-specific quality-of-life questionnaire for patients with head and neck cancer: The M. D. Anderson dysphagia inventory. *Arch. Otolaryngol.—Head Neck Surg.* **2001**, *127*, 870–876. [PubMed]
15. Cox, J.D.; Stetz, J.; Pajak, T.F. Toxicity criteria of the Radiation Therapy Oncology Group (RTOG) and the European Organization for Research and Treatment of Cancer (EORTC). *Int. J. Radiat. Oncol. Biol. Phys.* **1995**, *31*, 1341–1346. [CrossRef] [PubMed]
16. Rinkel, R.N.; Verdonck-de Leeuw, I.M.; van Reij, E.J.; Aaronson, N.K.; Leemans, C.R. Speech Handicap Index in patients with oral and pharyngeal cancer: Better understanding of patients' complaints. *Head Neck* **2008**, *30*, 868–874. [CrossRef]
17. Kohler, P.F.; Winter, M.E. A quantitative test for xerostomia. The Saxon test, an oral equivalent of the Schirmer test. *Arthritis Rheum.* **1985**, *28*, 1128–1132. [CrossRef]
18. Pai, S.; Ghezzi, E.M.; Ship, J.A. Development of a Visual Analogue Scale questionnaire for subjective assessment of salivary dysfunction. *Oral Surg. Oral Med. Oral Pathol. Oral Radiol. Endod.* **2001**, *91*, 311–316. [CrossRef]
19. Kamstra, J.I.; Dijkstra, P.U.; van Leeuwen, M.; Roodenburg, J.L.; Langendijk, J.A. Mouth opening in patients irradiated for head and neck cancer: A prospective repeated measures study. *Oral Oncol.* **2015**, *51*, 548–555. [CrossRef]
20. Bjordal, K.; de Graeff, A.; Fayers, P.M.; Hammerlid, E.; van Pottelsberghe, C.; Curran, D.; Ahlner-Elmqvist, M.; Maher, E.J.; Meyza, J.W.; Bredart, A.; et al. A 12 country field study of the EORTC QLQ-C30 (version 3.0) and the head and neck cancer specific module (EORTC QLQ-H&N35) in head and neck patients. EORTC Quality of Life Group. *Eur. J. Cancer* **2000**, *36*, 1796–1807. [CrossRef]
21. Hsiao, H.T.; Leu, Y.S.; Liu, C.J.; Tung, K.Y.; Lin, C.C. Radial forearm versus anterolateral thigh flap reconstruction after hemiglossectomy: Functional assessment of swallowing and speech. *J. Reconstr. Microsurg.* **2008**, *24*, 85–88. [CrossRef] [PubMed]
22. Kansy, K.; Mueller, A.A.; Mücke, T.; Koersgen, F.; Wolff, K.D.; Zeilhofer, H.F.; Hölzle, F.; Pradel, W.; Schneider, M.; Kolk, A.; et al. A worldwide comparison of the management of surgical treatment of advanced oral cancer. *J. Cranio-Maxillo-Facial Surg.* **2018**, *46*, 511–520. [CrossRef] [PubMed]
23. Mannelli, G.; Arcuri, F.; Agostini, T.; Innocenti, M.; Raffaini, M.; Spinelli, G. Classification of tongue cancer resection and treatment algorithm. *J. Surg. Oncol.* **2018**, *117*, 1092–1099. [CrossRef]
24. Vincent, A.; Kohlert, S.; Lee, T.S.; Inman, J.; Ducic, Y. Free-Flap Reconstruction of the Tongue. *Semin. Plast. Surg.* **2019**, *33*, 38–45. [CrossRef] [PubMed]
25. Backes, C.; Bier, H.; Knopf, A. Therapeutic implications of tumor free margins in head and neck squamous cell carcinoma. *Oncotarget* **2017**, *8*, 84320–84328. [CrossRef] [PubMed]
26. Eldeeb, H.; Macmillan, C.; Elwell, C.; Hammod, A. The effect of the surgical margins on the outcome of patients with head and neck squamous cell carcinoma: Single institution experience. *Cancer Biol. Med.* **2012**, *9*, 29–33. [CrossRef]
27. Dik, E.A.; Willems, S.M.; Ipenburg, N.A.; Adriaansens, S.O.; Rosenberg, A.J.; van Es, R.J. Resection of early oral squamous cell carcinoma with positive or close margins: Relevance of adjuvant treatment in relation to local recurrence: Margins of 3 mm as safe as 5 mm. *Oral Oncol.* **2014**, *50*, 611–615. [CrossRef]
28. Bernier, J.; Cooper, J.S.; Pajak, T.F.; van Glabbeke, M.; Bourhis, J.; Forastiere, A.; Ozsahin, E.M.; Jacobs, J.R.; Jassem, J.; Ang, K.K.; et al. Defining risk levels in locally advanced head and neck cancers: A comparative analysis of concurrent postoperative radiation plus chemotherapy trials of the EORTC (#22931) and RTOG (#9501). *Head Neck* **2005**, *27*, 843–850. [CrossRef]
29. Lu, C.C.; Tsou, Y.A.; Hua, C.H.; Tsai, M.H. Free flap reconstruction for early stage tongue squamous cell carcinoma: Surgical margin and recurrence. *Acta Oto-Laryngol.* **2018**, *138*, 945–950. [CrossRef]
30. Canis, M.; Weiss, B.G.; Ihler, F.; Hummers-Pradier, E.; Matthias, C.; Wolff, H.A. Quality of life in patients after resection of pT3 lateral tongue carcinoma: Microvascular reconstruction versus primary closure. *Head Neck* **2016**, *38*, 89–94. [CrossRef]
31. Kaur, R.; Sahni, V.R.; Choudhary, S.; Bharthuar, A.; Chopra, S. Functional outcomes of oral tongue reconstruction: A subjective analysis. *Head Neck* **2019**, *7*, 26.
32. Ansarin, M.; Bruschini, R.; Navach, V.; Giugliano, G.; Calabrese, L.; Chiesa, F.; Medina, J.E.; Kowalski, L.P.; Shah, J.P. Classification of GLOSSECTOMIES: Proposal for tongue cancer resections. *Head Neck* **2019**, *41*, 821–827. [CrossRef] [PubMed]

33. Jeremić, J.V.; Nikolić, Ž.S. Versatility of radial forearm free flap for intraoral reconstruction. *Srp. Arh. Celok. Lek.* **2015**, *143*, 256–260. [CrossRef] [PubMed]
34. Lutz, B.S.; Wei, F.-C.; Chang, S.C.; Yang, K.-H.; Chen, I.-H. Donor site morbidity after suprafascial elevation of the radial forearm flap: A prospective study in 95 consecutive cases. *Plast. Reconstr. Surg.* **1999**, *103*, 132–137. [CrossRef]

Disclaimer/Publisher's Note: The statements, opinions and data contained in all publications are solely those of the individual author(s) and contributor(s) and not of MDPI and/or the editor(s). MDPI and/or the editor(s) disclaim responsibility for any injury to people or property resulting from any ideas, methods, instructions or products referred to in the content.

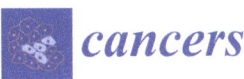

Article

Patterns of Postoperative Trismus Following Mandibulectomy and Fibula Free Flap Reconstruction

Rex H. Lee [1], Cara Evans [1], Joey Laus [1], Cristina Sanchez [2], Katherine C. Wai [1], P. Daniel Knott [1], Rahul Seth [1], Ivan H. El-Sayed [1], Jonathan R. George [1], William R. Ryan [1], Chase M. Heaton [1], Andrea M. Park [1] and Patrick K. Ha [1,*]

[1] Department of Otolaryngology–Head and Neck Surgery, University of California San Francisco, San Francisco, CA 94158, USA
[2] Department of Oral and Maxillofacial Surgery, University of California San Francisco, San Francisco, CA 94143, USA
* Correspondence: patrick.ha@ucsf.edu

Simple Summary: Trismus is a serious sequela of head and neck cancer (HNC) treatment that can profoundly affect quality of life. While the relationship between radiotherapy and trismus in HNC has been established, the surgical risk factors for trismus in HNC patients are largely unclear. This study reports the prevalence of postoperative trismus in a large cohort of patients who underwent mandibulectomy and fibula free flap reconstruction. Patients with a posterior mandibulotomy that involved or removed the ramus had significantly higher rates of persistent trismus >6 months after surgery, which was also demonstrated in a multivariable logistic regression. These findings may inform future surgical planning and potentially optimize functional outcomes in patients undergoing significant mandibular resection.

Abstract: The factors that contribute to postoperative trismus after mandibulectomy and fibula free flap reconstruction (FFFR) are undefined. We retrospectively assessed postoperative trismus (defined as a maximum interincisal opening ≤35 mm) in 106 patients undergoing mandibulectomy with FFFR, employing logistic regression to identify risk factors associated with this sequela. The surgical indication was primary ablation in 64%, salvage for recurrence in 24%, and osteonecrosis in 12%. Forty-five percent of patients had existing preoperative trismus, and 58% of patients received adjuvant radiation/chemoradiation following surgery. The overall rates of postoperative trismus were 76% in the early postoperative period (≤3 months after surgery) and 67% in the late postoperative period (>6 months after surgery). Late postoperative trismus occurred more frequently in patients with ramus-involving vs. ramus-preserving posterior mandibulotomies (82% vs. 46%, $p = 0.004$). A ramus-involving mandibulotomy was the only variable significantly associated with trismus >6 months postoperatively on multivariable logistic regression (OR, 7.94; 95% CI, 1.85–33.97; $p = 0.005$). This work demonstrates that trismus is common after mandibulectomy and FFFR, and suggests that posterior mandibulotomies that involve or remove the ramus may predispose to a higher risk of persistent postoperative trismus.

Keywords: trismus; mouth opening; mandibulectomy; fibula free flap; postoperative; ramus; MIO; interincisal opening; head and neck; survivorship

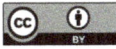

1. Introduction

Trismus, or restricted mouth opening, is an increasingly recognized condition among patients with head and neck cancer (HNC). The impact of trismus on quality of life can be devastating, including marked limitations in communication, inadequate nutrition, and chronic pain, which predispose to social isolation and depression [1–3]. Difficulty performing adequate dental care with decreased mouth opening also frequently leads to poor oral hygiene and caries, which is especially concerning in irradiated patients given the risk of osteoradionecrosis if dental extraction is required [4]. The prevalence of trismus in HNC patients varies widely by study, from less than 10% to greater than 50% [5–8]. This broad range suggests that trismus development is influenced by many overlapping demographic and treatment parameters, which are challenging to individually delineate in varied patient cohorts. Furthermore, there is inconsistency in the definition of trismus between HNC care providers, such as the use of subjective jaw mobility assessments rather than quantitative measurements and disagreement over the numerical cutoffs for mouth opening that constitute trismus [6]. These limitations in the literature create barriers to comparing the scope of this problem across patients and institutions.

While radiotherapy (RT) has a well-recognized and dose-dependent relationship with trismus in HNC patients, the influence of surgical interventions on trismus is less clear [8–10]. Previous work has demonstrated that certain intraoperative actions may decrease trismus risk, such as prophylactic coronoidectomy, division of the ipsilateral masseter and/or medial pterygoid muscles, and immediate rather than delayed reconstruction of surgical defects [8,11–13]. It is essential to identify the surgical factors that predispose to trismus, and understand how these operative features are affected by preoperative clinical characteristics, so that surgical resections may be modified to optimize functional outcomes.

One surgical cohort that may be especially susceptible to postoperative trismus are patients undergoing mandibulectomy with fibula free flap reconstruction (FFFR). These patients represent a unique challenge in the early postoperative period, as physicians may be reticent to initiate early jaw stretching exercises out of concern for stressing the newly placed bone graft. There is little data on the prevalence and severity of trismus in patients with significant mandibular resection (i.e., segmental mandibulectomy resulting in a bony continuity defect). A previous study in HNC patients receiving free flap reconstruction of lateral segmental mandibular defects found that 94% of patients demonstrated "little to no trismus" postoperatively, with a mean follow-up time of 17 months after surgery [14]. In stark contrast, another group reported that approximately 30% of patients experienced trismus following flap reconstruction of posterior mandibular defects at the most recent follow-up (average of 42 months) [15].

Multiple key questions remain unanswered with respect to trismus after mandibulectomy and FFFR. The lack of quantitative mouth opening measurements over time, including change from preoperative baseline to postoperative follow-ups, is a major limitation in determining the natural course and trajectory of this complication. Furthermore, key modifying characteristics that predispose to postoperative trismus following mandibulectomy and FFFR have not been explored, including patients' preoperative mouth opening, indication for surgery, and anatomy of the bony resection. Identifying these factors may have actionable implications for clinical practice. In this study, we sought to define the scope of trismus in patients after mandibulectomy and FFFR, including factors predictive of worse trismus outcomes.

2. Materials and Methods

2.1. Patient Selection

The study subjects were identified from a database composed of 277 patients who underwent fibula free flap reconstruction (FFFR) from August 2011 to March 2022. A retrospective chart review of all patients in the database was first performed to determine the patients' baseline (preoperative) mouth opening status. The patients with a documented preoperative quantitative measurement, most commonly maximum interincisal opening (MIO), were advanced to the next step of the workflow. Aside from MIO, the charts were also queried for multiple related terms indicative of this metric, including "maximum jaw opening" (MJO) and "mouth opening", as well as units of measurement ("mm" and "cm"). For patients without any quantitative indication of preoperative mouth opening, the otolaryngology provider notes were then searched for a qualitative description of whether the patient had "trismus" or "no trismus" prior to surgery. If available, the degree of mouth opening described in our institution's preoperative anesthesia note was also used to confirm the trismus status in these patients, with "poor" mouth opening indicating trismus and "good" or "excellent" indicating lack of trismus. An anesthesia mouth opening descriptor of "fair" was considered ambiguous, and such patients were not advanced further if this was the only indication of preoperative trismus status. The patients with neither a preoperative quantitative measurement (referred to collectively as "MIO" from this point forward) nor qualitative description of mouth opening were not included in subsequent steps.

Next, the patient charts that met the above criteria for indication of preoperative mouth opening were searched for quantitative postoperative mouth opening measurements using the same search strategy described above. All documented postoperative MIO measurements were recorded, often from multiple sources, including progress notes from speech–language pathologists and dental oncology colleagues, who work closely with the Head and Neck Surgery program at our institution. All patients with preoperative mouth opening status (either MIO or qualitative) and at least one documented postoperative MIO ($n = 131$) were advanced to the next step of the workflow. For patients without any documented postoperative MIO, the date of the last follow-up with our department was recorded. Those patients without any postoperative MIO and a last follow-up of more than three years prior to the chart review were excluded from further analysis.

The 131 patients meeting the aforementioned preoperative and postoperative measurement criteria then underwent chart abstraction for demographic, clinical, and treatment-related variables. Only the patients who underwent FFFR for segmental mandibulectomy defects (including hemimandibulectomy) were analyzed; 22 patients who had received a maxillectomy prior to FFFR were excluded, as well as 3 patients who received reconstruction only for a remote ablative surgery. This led to a final study size of 106, 52 of whom had both preoperative and postoperative MIO and 54 who had postoperative MIO and only qualitative preoperative mouth opening descriptors.

2.2. Defining Trismus and Postoperative Analysis Intervals

We defined trismus as an MIO ≤ 35 mm and the lack of trismus as an MIO > 35 mm, based on multiple prior studies assessing functional and quality of life outcomes [16,17]. The presence or absence of trismus was analyzed at two main intervals: an early postoperative period (≤ 3 months after surgery) and a late postoperative period (>6 months after surgery). The ≤ 3 month timepoint was chosen to maximize the number of patients with an early postoperative measurement, as the majority of patients (76/106) had one or two MIOs within this time interval. The late timepoint was intended to encompass persistent postoperative trismus with a higher likelihood of representing a chronic condition; a period of >6 months postoperatively captured at least one MIO in 58/106 patients. In contrast to these early and late timepoints, relatively fewer patients (38/106) had MIOs in the intermediate timepoint between 3 and 6 months after surgery, which also plausibly represents a transition period between acute and chronic trismus in which patients may experience resolution. For patients with multiple MIO measurements within the early or late time periods, the most recent MIO was used. We defined ΔMIO as the difference between a patient's preoperative MIO and the MIO measured at the most recent follow-up.

2.3. Categorizing Mandibulotomy Anatomy

For all patients, the sites of the anterior and posterior mandibulotomies were recorded and broadly divided into "ramus-involving" and "ramus-preserving" cuts. "Ramus-involving" cuts were defined as mandibulotomies that removed any part of the ascending ramus; these cuts were either entirely superior and posterior to the mandibular angle, or they began at the angle and traversed superiorly/posteriorly to involve a portion of the ascending ramus (e.g., spanning from the angle to the sigmoid notch or coronoid process). In contrast, "ramus-preserving" mandibulotomies involved only the angle region itself or were positioned anterior to the angle.

2.4. Statistical Analysis

The rates of postoperative trismus at early and late timepoints were compared using the Pearson chi-square test. The proportion of patients with postoperative trismus were compared by surgical indication, presence vs. absence of preoperative trismus, receipt of adjuvant RT/CRT vs. no adjuvant therapy, and ramus-involving vs. ramus-preserving posterior mandibulotomy. We used the Bonferroni correction method to account for multiple comparisons of the preoperative and postoperative trismus rates, with a corrected significance threshold of $\alpha < 0.005$ ($\alpha_{original}$ of 0.05/11 total comparisons).

Logistic regression was performed with the binary outcome of yes/no trismus >6 months postoperatively, using the most recent MIO available. Univariate logistic regressions were conducted for age, preoperative trismus status, surgical indication, adjuvant therapy, and posterior mandibulotomy location. A multivariable analysis was also conducted with the same variables. Tumor T stage was not included as a variable in the final model, as staging information was available only for patients undergoing primary ablation and not surgery for recurrent disease or osteonecrosis.

The distribution of ΔMIO between groups was visualized with a waterfall plot for all patients with a measurement at >6 months, separated by the same variables used in the regression analyses. To compare the magnitude of ΔMIO change between these variables, the mean ΔMIO between groups were compared via two-tailed student's t-test. Statistical analyses were performed using Stata software version 17.0 (StataCorp LLC; College Station, TX, USA), and the figures were generated via GraphPad Prism 9.3.1.

3. Results

3.1. Demographic and Treatment Characteristics of the Patient Cohort

A total of 106 patients who underwent mandibulectomy and FFFR met the study criteria. The preoperative demographic and clinical characteristics are presented in Table 1. The cohort was 58% male and 42% female, with an average age of 62.1 years (SD 14.3). The indication for surgery was primary ablation with curative intent in 64% (68/106), salvage resection for recurrent disease in 24% (25/106), and mandibular osteonecrosis in 12% (13/106, including 11 patients with osteoradionecrosis and 2 patients with bisphosphonate-related osteonecrosis of the jaw). Overall, 27% (29/106) of the cohort had a history of prior head and neck irradiation, either for a tumor that subsequently recurred or for a distinct primary tumor prior to developing a second malignancy. Of the patients undergoing surgery for primary ablation with tumor staging available (63/68), the T stage was 11% T1 (7/63), 8% T2 (5/63), 2% T3 (1/63), and 79% T4 (50/63); the N stage was N0 in 49% (31/63) and N+ in 51% (32/63).

Prior to surgery, 45% (48/106) of patients had preoperative trismus, while 55% (58/106) did not have preoperative trismus (Table 1). The posterior mandibulotomy was ramus-involving in 56% (59/106) and ramus-preserving in 44% (47/106). Following mandibulectomy and FFFR, 36% (38/106) received adjuvant radiation (RT), 23% (24/106) received adjuvant chemoradiation (CRT), and 42% (44/106) were not administered adjuvant therapy (Table 1). The proportion of patients administered adjuvant therapy was higher in those without preoperative trismus compared to patients with preoperative trismus (68% vs. 32%, $p = 0.001$) (Table 2). Of those who underwent adjuvant RT/CRT with precise start and end dates available, the median time from surgery to completion of the adjuvant therapy was 112 days ($Q_1 = 99$ days, $Q_3 = 131$ days). Among all patients, the median time from surgery to the most recent follow-up with our department was 687 days ($Q_1 = 241$ days, $Q_3 = 1274$ days).

Table 1. Baseline demographic characteristics and treatment variables for the study cohort.

		n (%)
Age	Mean (SD)	62.1 (14.3)
Sex	Male	62 (58)
	Female	44 (42)
Surgical Indication	Primary Ablation	68 (64)
	Salvage	25 (24)
	Osteonecrosis	13 (12)
Stage (primary tumors)	T1/T2	12 (11)
	T3/T4	51 (48)
	N0	31 (29)
	N+	32 (30)
	Stage NA/NR	43 (41)
Preoperative Trismus	Present	48 (45)
	Absent	58 (55)
Adjuvant Therapy	Adjuvant RT/CRT	62 (58)
	None	44 (42)
Posterior Mandibulotomy	Ramus-Involving	59 (56)
	Ramus-Preserving	47 (44)

SD, standard deviation; RT, radiation; CRT, chemoradiation; NA, not available; NR, not relevant (for indications of salvage or osteonecrosis).

Table 2. Proportion of patients experiencing trismus at three timepoints: preoperative baseline, early postoperative period (≤3 months after surgery), and late postoperative period (>6 months after surgery).

		Preop. Baseline (N = 106)			≤3 Months Postop. (N = 76)			>6 Months Postop. (N = 58)		
		Trismus n (%) (N = 48)	No Trismus n (%) (N = 58)	p-Value	Trismus n (%) (N = 58)	No Trismus n (%) (N = 18)	p-Value	Trismus n (%) (N = 39)	No Trismus n (%) (N = 19)	p-Value
Surgical Indication	Primary Ablation	24 (35)	44 (65)	0.003 *	34 (71)	14 (29)	0.313	21 (58)	15 (42)	0.070
	Salvage	13 (52)	12 (48)		15 (83)	3 (17)		10 (71)	4 (29)	
	Osteonecrosis	11 (85)	2 (15)		9 (90)	1 (10)		8 (100)	0 (0)	
Preoperative Trismus	Present	48 (100)	-	-	32 (89)	4 (11)	0.014	20 (80)	5 (20)	0.072
	Absent	-	58 (100)		26 (65)	14 (35)		19 (58)	14 (42)	
Adjuvant Therapy	Adjuvant RT/CRT	20 (32)	42 (68)	0.001 *	31 (74)	11 (26)	0.568	24 (62)	15 (38)	0.185
	None	28 (64)	16 (36)		27 (79)	7 (21)		15 (79)	4 (21)	
Posterior Mandibulotomy	Ramus-Involving	33 (56)	26 (44)	0.014	34 (81)	8 (19)	0.291	28 (82)	6 (18)	0.004 *
	Ramus-Preserving	15 (32)	32 (68)		24 (71)	10 (29)		11 (46)	13 (54)	

Preop., preoperative; Postop., postoperative; RT, radiation; CRT, chemoradiation. Asterisks (*) designate significance with α < 0.005 (Bonferroni correction for multiple comparisons).

3.2. Trismus Prevalence at Early and Late Postoperative Timepoints

In the early postoperative period (≤3 months after surgery), a total of 76 patients had at least one MIO measurement, and the majority experienced trismus (58/76, 76%). Eighty-nine percent of the patients with preoperative trismus demonstrated early postoperative trismus, and 65% of the patients without preoperative trismus demonstrated early postoperative trismus ($p = 0.014$). There were no significant differences in the rates of early postoperative trismus by surgical indication, receipt of adjuvant RT/CRT, or between patients with ramus-involving and ramus-preserving posterior mandibulotomies (Table 2).

In the late postoperative period (>6 months after surgery), a total of 58 patients had at least one MIO measurement. Overall, 67% of patients (39/58) had trismus at this time point. The rates of late postoperative trismus for patients with preoperative trismus and patients without preoperative trismus were 80% and 58%, respectively ($p = 0.072$). Trismus prevalence was again not significantly different when compared by surgical indication or receipt of adjuvant RT/CRT. However, patients with ramus-involving mandibulotomies had significantly higher rates of long-term trismus when compared to ramus-preserving mandibulotomies (82% vs. 46%, $p = 0.004$) (Table 2).

3.3. Exploring Variables Associated with Persistent Postoperative Trismus

To delineate the patient-level and treatment-level factors associated with persistent trismus, we employed logistic regression for patients with at least one MIO measurement >6 months postoperatively. For the univariate analysis, the location of the posterior mandibulotomy was the only variable significantly associated with the presence of postoperative trismus at >6 months, with ramus-involving mandibulotomies demonstrating an odds ratio (OR) of 5.52 (95% CI, 1.67–18.17) compared to ramus-preserving mandibulotomies ($p = 0.005$). The presence of existing preoperative trismus approached significance (OR, 2.95; 95% CI, 0.89–9.77; $p = 0.077$). Patients who underwent surgery for osteonecrosis could not be included in the regression model, as all eight osteonecrosis patients with MIO measurements taken >6 months had postoperative trismus (i.e., an indication of osteonecrosis perfectly predicted the regression outcome). This necessitated the reduction of the surgical indication variable from three categories to two (primary ablation vs. salvage for recurrence). Surgical indication, age, and receipt of adjuvant therapy were not significantly associated with persistent postoperative trismus in the univariate analysis (Table 3).

Table 3. Univariate and multivariable logistic regressions for the presence of persistent late postoperative trismus (>6 months postoperatively).

		Univariate Model		Multivariable Model	
		OR (95% CI)	p-Value	OR (95% CI)	p-Value
	Age	1.00 (0.96–1.05)	0.876	1.00 (0.95–1.04)	0.906
Preoperative Trismus	Absent	Ref.		Ref.	
	Present	2.95 (0.89–9.77)	0.077	0.81 (0.16–4.17)	0.799
Surgical Indication	Primary Ablation	Ref.		Ref.	
	Salvage	1.79 (0.47–6.79)	0.395	2.00 (0.29–13.59)	0.478
	Osteonecrosis	-	-	-	-
Adjuvant Therapy	None	Ref.		Ref.	
	Adjuvant RT/CRT	0.43 (0.12–1.53)	0.191	1.10 (0.13–9.58)	0.933
Posterior Mandibulotomy	Ramus-Preserving	Ref.		Ref.	
	Ramus-Involving	5.52 (1.67–18.17)	0.005	7.94 (1.85–33.97)	0.005

RT, radiation; CRT, chemoradiation.

In the multivariable logistic regression with the same variables, posterior mandibulotomy location remained the only variable significantly associated with trismus >6 months postoperatively, with an OR of 7.94 for ramus-involving vs. ramus-preserving cuts (95% CI, 1.85–33.97; $p = 0.005$). As with the univariate analysis, age, surgical indication, and adjuvant therapy were not significantly associated with persistent postoperative trismus in the multivariable regression (Table 3).

3.4. Comparing ΔMIO at the Late Postoperative Timepoint

Of the 58 total patients with postoperative MIO measurements taken >6 months postoperatively, 27 patients also had a preoperative MIO available. The overall distribution of ΔMIOs from the preoperative visit to the most recent visit's MIO measurement >6 months postoperatively for these 27 patients is shown in Figure 1A, separately stratified by preoperative trismus status, receipt of adjuvant therapy, surgical indication, and ramus involvement of the posterior mandibulotomy. The mean ΔMIOs between these groups at the same timepoint are displayed in Figure 1B. On average, patients without preoperative trismus had a decline in ΔMIO, while those with existing preoperative trismus had a mean positive change in ΔMIO (−7.07 vs. +1.83 mm, $p = 0.038$). The mean ΔMIO for patients who received adjuvant RT/CRT was −5.11 mm and +1.63 mm in those without adjuvant therapy ($p = 0.159$). By indication, the mean ΔMIOs for primary ablation, salvage, and osteonecrosis were −4.72, +0.50, and −0.67 mm, respectively ($p = 0.362$ for a comparison between primary ablation and salvage surgery). The mean ΔMIO for the ramus-involving vs. ramus preserving mandibulectomies were −3.18 and −3.00 mm, respectively ($p = 0.970$).

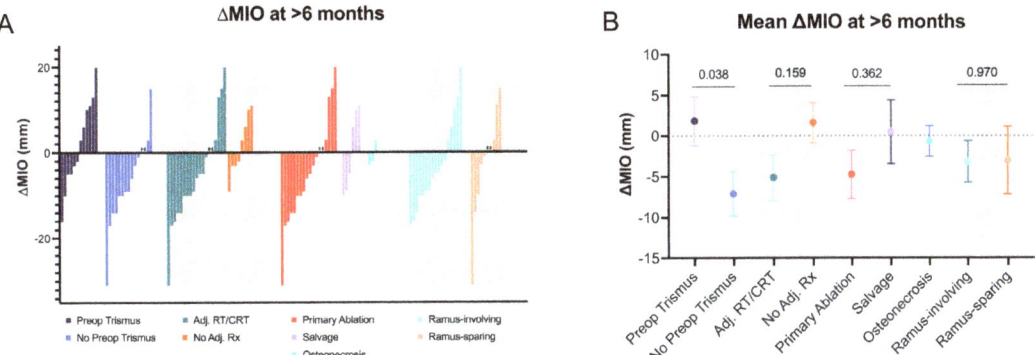

Figure 1. (**A**) Waterfall plot of ΔMIO for all patients with preoperative MIO and MIO measurement taken >6 months postoperatively ($n = 27$), separated by preoperative trismus status, receipt of adjuvant therapy, surgical indication, and ramus involvement of the posterior mandibulotomy; (**B**) mean ΔMIO > 6 months postoperatively for the same 27 patients when compared by preoperative trismus status, receipt of adjuvant therapy, surgical indication, and ramus involvement of the posterior mandibulotomy.

4. Discussion

Trismus is a complex, multifactorial condition that represents a formidable challenge in patients with HNC. In surgically treated patients, data on trismus outcomes are limited, especially when compared to the preponderance of work assessing the relationship between trismus and RT. Many previous studies utilize heterogenous HNC patient cohorts receiving a variety of treatment approaches, which makes it difficult to disentangle the individual demographic and treatment-related characteristics that contribute to this sequela. In this study, we focused specifically on one unique surgical population—those undergoing mandibulectomy and FFFR.

The first step towards conducting meaningful trismus studies that are generalizable across patients and institutions is specifying an appropriate definition of trismus. The current evidence suggests that a mouth opening of ≤35 mm is a suitable and clinically meaningful demarcation of trismus that predicts health-related quality of life [16,17]. However, even in the presence of an appropriate trismus metric, obtaining consistent post-treatment jaw opening measurements is a significant challenge. By far, the largest obstacle in this study was a lack of regular MIO measurements taken at both preoperative and postoperative visits. From a database of 277 fibula free flap patients, fewer than half (131/277) had postoperative MIO measurements and either a quantitative or qualitative indication of preoperative mouth opening. Furthermore, of the 106 patients who met the final study criteria, only 52 had a quantitative mouth opening measurement (MIO) taken preoperatively.

Because most patients in this cohort did not have both baseline preoperative MIOs and regular postoperative MIOs, our ability to compare the magnitude of change in mouth opening over time was limited (only 27 total patients with follow-up >6 months after surgery had both preoperative and postoperative MIOs). Nonetheless, the comparison between the mean ΔMIO at >6 months was significant between the patients with preoperative trismus compared to the patients without preoperative trismus (ΔMIO_{avg} of +1.83 vs. −7.07 mm, respectively; $p = 0.038$). Indeed, while half (6/12) of the patients with preoperative trismus experienced increased MIO at >6 months, only 13% (2/15) of patients without preoperative trismus demonstrated an increase in MIO at this late time point. This suggests that while patients who are trismus-free preoperatively will generally experience a decline in postoperative MIO, patients with existing preoperative trismus may exhibit a marginal improvement in postoperative MIO. However, it is important to recognize that the majority of patients with preoperative trismus continued to have chronic trismus (i.e., MIO $\leq$ 35 mm) postoperatively. In addition, because MIO measurements were taken at different intervals for different patients, it was not feasible to infer a general timeline of the trajectory of MIO decline following mandibulectomy and FFFR. Future work that incorporates consistent mouth opening measurements at defined and frequent postoperative intervals may allow for the construction of a generalizable timeline for the development of (and recovery from) trismus in this population.

A key limitation of this study was our inability to assess the impact of jaw stretching interventions on the risk of trismus development in this cohort of mandibulectomy and FFFR patients. At our institution, home jaw stretching and neck stretching exercises are routinely taught and implemented with postsurgical patients by our team of speech–language pathologists (SLPs). However, details on the adherence to these regimens and the time periods over which stretching is practiced are often unable to be accurately extrapolated from retrospective chart review. The limitations of the documentation also precluded the analysis of the benefit of active device-based intervention (using products such as the TheraBite® or OraStretch®) in this study. Given the high out-of-pocket cost of these devices coupled with inconsistent clearance by insurance providers, it is often unclear if patients even received the stretching device recommended to them, let alone the adherence to the stretching exercises with the device itself. In patients with mandibulectomy and FFFR, concern for imparting excessive stress on the newly placed vascularized bone graft may generate reticence over initiating early jaw stretching exercises postoperatively. There have been reports of serious complications while using the TheraBite® in the post-treatment setting, including a mandibular fracture in an HNC patient with undiagnosed mandibular osteoradionecrosis (ORN) [18], and fracture of titanium mandibular reconstruction plates in the setting of mandibular recurrence following mandibulectomy and FFFR [19]. However, it is notable that both complications occurred in patients with bone that was ostensibly already structurally compromised (due to ORN or recurrent cancer). The true risk of trismus devices in mandibulectomy and FFFR patients with a healthy flap and expected postoperative healing has not been studied. Additional work will help to clarify the earliest time period following surgery that is safe for device-assisted jaw stretching, and the optimal timing for trismus interventions in these patients.

Our work suggests that the location of the posterior mandibulotomy may affect the risk of postoperative trismus after mandibulectomy and FFFR. At >6 months, patients with ramus-involving posterior mandibulotomies experienced trismus at nearly twice the rate of patients with ramus-preserving cuts (82% vs. 46%), the most robust difference in magnitude among any variables compared in this study. Multivariable logistic regression revealed a nearly eight-fold greater odds of persistent postoperative trismus for patients with ramus-involving posterior mandibulotomies, when adjusted for age, preoperative trismus status, surgical indication, and receipt of adjuvant therapy. However, we could not demonstrate a significant difference in ΔMIO between these groups, most likely due to the very small number of patients with paired preoperative and postoperative MIO measurements, as discussed above. There are multiple possible explanations for the observation of marked differences in late postoperative trismus rates by mandibulotomy location. Acute or chronic inflammation of structures surrounding the mandibular ramus, condyle, or coronoid can either directly limit movement around the temporomandibular joint and/or induce pain resulting in a reflex trismus (as is often also seen in non-neoplastic conditions such as peritonsillar abscesses or lateral pharyngeal space infections) [20]. Violation of the region surrounding the ramus during surgery may also result in the fibrotic shortening of the pterygoids or pterygomandibular ligament during healing, thereby further contracting mouth opening. While the extent of disease is the largest factor dictating whether the ramus can be spared during resection, our data identify patients at a particularly high risk of late postoperative trismus, who may especially benefit from vigilant surveillance of mouth opening and early trismus interventions. It is also critical to note that a large portion of

HNC patients undergoing mandibulectomy and FFFR will demonstrate adverse features on surgical pathology, necessitating adjuvant RT/CRT for optimal oncologic control. Radiation itself has a well-known, dose-dependent relationship with trismus secondary to fibrosis of the masticatory apparatus, especially with large doses to the masseter and medial pterygoid muscles [21–23]. It will be important to determine how radiation interacts with postoperative anatomy in mandibulectomy and FFFR patients, and how irradiation of the retained masticatory musculature contributes to trismus severity specifically following surgical disruption of the ramus.

5. Conclusions

In summary, this study described the scope of postoperative trismus following mandibulectomy and FFFR, including potential contributing factors to this sequela. We demonstrated that most patients (76%) experienced trismus in the early (≤3 months) postoperative period and persistent trismus remained common in the late (>6 months) postoperative period (occurring in 67% of patients in this study). Using logistic regression, we found that a posterior mandibulotomy involving or removing the ramus was associated with a substantially higher odds of persistent trismus after surgery. To our knowledge, this is the first study that implicates mandibulotomy location as a surgical risk factor for postoperative trismus. Larger-scale studies are critical for identifying patients at the highest risk of trismus after mandibulectomy with FFFR, and delineating precise temporal changes in mouth opening may inform key postoperative intervals for active trismus intervention.

Author Contributions: Conceptualization, R.H.L., C.E., C.S., P.D.K., R.S., I.H.E.-S., J.R.G., W.R.R., C.M.H., A.M.P. and P.K.H.; Methodology, R.H.L., C.E., J.L., C.S., K.C.W. and P.K.H.; Formal analysis, R.H.L. and K.C.W.; Investigation, R.H.L.; Writing—original draft, R.H.L. and P.K.H.; Writing—review & editing, R.H.L., C.E., J.L., C.S., K.C.W., P.D.K., R.S., I.H.E.-S., J.R.G., W.R.R., C.M.H., A.M.P. and P.K.H.; Visualization, R.H.L.; Supervision, A.M.P. and P.K.H. All authors have read and agreed to the published version of the manuscript.

Funding: This research received no external funding.

Institutional Review Board Statement: The study was conducted in accordance with the guidelines of the Declaration of Helsinki and approved by the Institutional Review Board of the University of California, San Francisco (UCSF).

Informed Consent Statement: Informed consent was obtained from all subjects involved in the study.

Data Availability Statement: De-identified data presented in this study are available upon reasonable request from the corresponding author.

Conflicts of Interest: W.R.R. is a member of the Scientific Advisory Boards for Olympus and Rakuten Medical and was briefly a consultant for Intuitive Surgical in 2021. P.K.H. has received educational funding from Stryker and Medtronic and is a consultant for Privo Technologies and Checkpoint Surgical.

Abbreviations

FFFR	Fibula free flap reconstruction
HNC	Head and neck cancer
MIO	Maximum interincisal opening
OR	Odds radio
Q_1	First quartile
Q_3	Third quartile
RT/CRT	Radiation/chemoradiation
SD	Standard deviation
SLP	Speech–language pathologist

References

1. Lydiatt, W. Trismus: A sequela of head and neck cancer and its treatment. *JCO Oncol. Pract.* **2020**, *16*, 654–655. [CrossRef] [PubMed]

2. Johnson, J.; Johansson, M.; Rydén, A.; Houltz, E.; Finizia, C. Impact of trismus on health-related quality of life and mental health. *Head Neck* **2015**, *37*, 1672–1679. [CrossRef] [PubMed]
3. Lee, L.Y.; Chen, S.C.; Chen, W.C.; Huang, B.S.; Lin, C.Y. Postradiation trismus and its impact on quality of life in patients with head and neck cancer. *Oral Surg. Oral Med. Oral Pathol. Oral Radiol.* **2015**, *119*, 187–195. [CrossRef]
4. Sroussi, H.Y.; Epstein, J.B.; Bensadoun, R.J.; Saunders, D.P.; Lalla, R.V.; Migliorati, C.A.; Heaivilin, N.; Zumsteg, Z.S. Common oral complications of head and neck cancer radiation therapy: Mucositis, infections, saliva change, fibrosis, sensory dysfunctions, dental caries, periodontal disease, and osteoradionecrosis. *Cancer Med.* **2017**, *6*, 2918–2931. [CrossRef] [PubMed]
5. Thomas, F.; Ozanne, F.; Mamelle, G.; Wibault, P.; Eschwege, F. Radiotherapy alone for oropharyngeal carcinomas: The role of fraction size (2 Gy vs 2.5 Gy) on local control and early and late complications. *Int. J. Radiat. Oncol. Biol. Phys.* **1988**, *15*, 1097–1102. [CrossRef] [PubMed]
6. Dijkstra, P.U.; Kalk, W.W.I.; Roodenburg, J.L.N. Trismus in head and neck oncology: A systematic review. *Oral Oncol.* **2004**, *40*, 879–889. [CrossRef] [PubMed]
7. Kraaijenga, S.A.C.; Oskam, I.M.; van der Molen, L.; Hamming-Vrieze, O.; Hilgers, F.J.M.; van den Brekel, M.W.M. Evaluation of long term (10-Years+) dysphagia and trismus in patients treated with concurrent chemo-radiotherapy for advanced head and neck cancer. *Oral Oncol.* **2015**, *51*, 787–794. [CrossRef]
8. Abboud, W.A.; Hassin-Baer, S.; Alon, E.E.; Gluck, I.; Dobriyan, A.; Amit, U.; Yahalom, R.; Yarom, N. Restricted mouth opening in head and neck cancer: Etiology, prevention, and treatment. *JCO Oncol. Pract.* **2020**, *16*, 643–653. [CrossRef]
9. Ichimura, K.; Tanaka, T. Trismus in patients with malignant tumours in the head and neck. *J. Laryngol. Otol.* **1993**, *107*, 1017–1020. [CrossRef]
10. Goldstein, M.; Maxymiw, W.G.; Cummings, B.J.; Wood, R.E. The effects of antitumor irradiation on mandibular opening and mobility: A prospective study of 58 patients. *Oral Surg. Oral Med. Oral Pathol. Oral Radiol. Endod.* **1999**, *88*, 365–373. [CrossRef]
11. Tsai, C.C.; Wu, S.L.; Lin, S.L.; Ko, S.Y.; Chiang, W.F.; Yang, J.W. Reducing trismus after surgery and radiotherapy in oral cancer patients: Results of alternative operation versus traditional operation. *J. Oral Maxillofac. Surg.* **2016**, *74*, 1072–1083. [CrossRef] [PubMed]
12. Chang, Y.M.; Deek, N.F.A.; Wei, F.C. Trismus secondary release surgery and microsurgical free flap reconstruction after surgical treatment of head and neck cancer. *Clin. Plast. Surg.* **2016**, *43*, 747–752. [CrossRef] [PubMed]
13. Qing-Gong, M.; Si, C.; Xing, L. Conservative treatment of severe limited mouth opening after transtemporal craniotomy. *J. Craniofac. Surg.* **2011**, *22*, 1746–1750. [CrossRef]
14. Dean, N.R.; Wax, M.K.; Virgin, F.W.; Magnuson, J.S.; Carroll, W.R.; Rosenthal, E.L. Free flap reconstruction of lateral mandibular defects: Indications and outcomes. *Otolaryngol. Head Neck Surg.* **2012**, *146*, 547–552. [CrossRef]
15. Chang, E.I.; Boukovalas, S.; Liu, J.; Largo, R.D.; Hanasono, M.M.; Garvey, P.B. Reconstruction of posterior mandibulectomy defects in the modern era of virtual planning and three-dimensional modeling. *Plast. Reconstr. Surg.* **2019**, *144*, 453e–462e. [CrossRef] [PubMed]
16. Dijkstra, P.U.; Huisman, P.M.; Roodenburg, J.L.N. Criteria for trismus in head and neck oncology. *Int. J. Oral Maxillofac. Surg.* **2006**, *35*, 337–342. [CrossRef]
17. Scott, B.; Butterworth, C.; Lowe, D.; Rogers, S.N. Factors associated with restricted mouth opening and its relationship to health-related quality of life in patients attending a maxillofacial oncology clinic. *Oral Oncol.* **2008**, *44*, 430–438. [CrossRef]
18. Marunick, M.T.; Garcia-Gazaui, S.; Hildebrand, J.M. Mandibular pathological fracture during treatment with a dynamic mouth opening device: A clinical report. *J. Prosthet. Dent.* **2016**, *116*, 488–491. [CrossRef] [PubMed]
19. Kamstra, J.I.; Roodenburg, J.L.N.; Beurskens, C.H.G.; Reintsema, H.; Dijkstra, P.U. TheraBite exercises to treat trismus secondary to head and neck cancer. *Support. Care Cancer* **2013**, *21*, 951–957. [CrossRef]
20. Beekhuis, J.G.; Harrington, E.B. Trismus. Etiology and management of inability to open the mouth. *Laryngoscope* **1965**, *75*, 1234–1258. [CrossRef]
21. Rao, S.D.; Saleh, Z.H.; Setton, J.; Tam, M.; McBride, S.M.; Riaz, N.; Deasy, J.O.; Lee, N.Y. Dose-volume factors correlating with trismus following chemoradiation for head and neck cancer. *Acta Oncol.* **2016**, *55*, 99–104. [CrossRef] [PubMed]
22. Kraaijenga, S.A.; Hamming-Vrieze, O.; Verheijen, S.; Lamers, E.; van der Molen, L.; Hilgers, F.J.; van den Brekel, M.W.; Heemsbergen, W.D. Radiation dose to the masseter and medial pterygoid muscle in relation to trismus after chemoradiotherapy for advanced head and neck cancer. *Head Neck* **2019**, *41*, 1387–1394. [CrossRef] [PubMed]
23. Teguh, D.N.; Levendag, P.C.; Voet, P.; van der Est, H.; Noever, I.; de Kruijf, W.; van Rooij, P.; Schmitz, P.I.M.; Heijmen, B.J. Trismus in patients with oropharyngeal cancer: Relationship with dose in structures of mastication apparatus. *Head Neck* **2008**, *30*, 622–630. [CrossRef] [PubMed]

Disclaimer/Publisher's Note: The statements, opinions and data contained in all publications are solely those of the individual author(s) and contributor(s) and not of MDPI and/or the editor(s). MDPI and/or the editor(s) disclaim responsibility for any injury to people or property resulting from any ideas, methods, instructions or products referred to in the content.

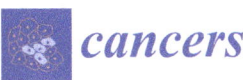

Article

Exploring Precise Medication Strategies for OSCC Based on Single-Cell Transcriptome Analysis from a Dynamic Perspective

Qingkang Meng [1,†], Feng Wu [2,†], Guoqi Li [1], Fei Xu [1], Lei Liu [1], Denan Zhang [1], Yangxu Lu [1], Hongbo Xie [1] and Xiujie Chen [1,*]

[1] Department of Pharmacogenomics, College of Bioinformatics Science and Technology, Harbin Medical University, Harbin 150081, China
[2] Department of Orthopedics, The Second Affiliated Hospital of Harbin Medical University, Harbin 150086, China
* Correspondence: chenxiujie@ems.hrbmu.edu.cn
† These authors contributed equally to this work.

Simple Summary: At the time of diagnosis, most oral squamous cell carcinoma (OSCC) patients are in the middle or advanced stages, and advanced patients usually have poor prognosis after traditional therapy. One of the primary causes has been demonstrated to be heterogeneity. However, most of the current studies on tumor heterogeneity are static, while the development of cancer is dynamic. Thus, understanding the tumor development process from a dynamic perspective is deeply necessary. Here, we combined static and dynamic analysis based on single-cell RNA-Seq data to comprehensively dissect the complex heterogeneity and evolutionary process of OSCC. We pioneered the concept of pseudo-time score, which is closely related to patient's prognosis. Finally, we identified candidate drugs and proposed precision medication strategies to control OSCC in two respects: treatment and blocking. Our findings offer new insights for clinical practice and could help improve the treatment of advanced OSCC.

Abstract: At present, most patients with oral squamous cell carcinoma (OSCC) are in the middle or advanced stages at the time of diagnosis. Advanced OSCC patients have a poor prognosis after traditional therapy, and the complex heterogeneity of OSCC has been proven to be one of the main reasons. Single-cell sequencing technology provides a powerful tool for dissecting the heterogeneity of cancer. However, most of the current studies at the single-cell level are static, while the development of cancer is a dynamic process. Thus, understanding the development of cancer from a dynamic perspective and formulating corresponding therapeutic measures for achieving precise treatment are highly necessary, and this is also one of the main study directions in the field of oncology. In this study, we combined the static and dynamic analysis methods based on single-cell RNA-Seq data to comprehensively dissect the complex heterogeneity and evolutionary process of OSCC. Subsequently, for clinical practice, we revealed the association between cancer heterogeneity and the prognosis of patients. More importantly, we pioneered the concept of pseudo-time score of patients, and we quantified the levels of heterogeneity based on the dynamic development process to evaluate the relationship between the score and the survival status at the same stage, finding that it is closely related to the prognostic status. The pseudo-time score of patients could not only reflect the tumor status of patients but also be used as an indicator of the effects of drugs on the patients so that the medication strategy can be adjusted on time. Finally, we identified candidate drugs and proposed precision medication strategies to control the condition of OSCC in two respects: treatment and blocking.

Keywords: single-cell RNA-Seq; oral squamous cell carcinoma; cell trajectory inference; precise medication; drug discovery

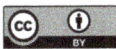

1. Introduction

Oral squamous cell carcinoma (OSCC) is the most common type of head and neck squamous cell carcinoma (HNSC), accounting for approximately 95% of cases [1]. At present, the clinical classification and treatment of OSCC are mainly based on the TNM staging system of the American Joint Committee on Cancer (AJCC) and the International Union for Cancer Control (UICC). In general, patients in the early stages (i.e., stages I and II)—approximately 30–40% of the patients diagnosed—have small tumors without significant lymph node involvement. Surgery and radiation therapy can provide effective tumor control and improve long-term survival in approximately 70–90% of early stage patients [2]. For patients with advanced stages (i.e., stages III and IV), which are characterized by varying degrees of surrounding tissue invasion, lymph node involvement, and metastatic spread, it is difficult to eliminate or kill tumors completely via surgery or radiotherapy. Although systematic treatment with drugs (e.g., platinum, taxanes, antifolates, cetuximab, etc.) can be conducted for the remission of recurrence and metastasis [2], more than 65% of these patients have a poor prognosis due to the significant heterogeneity, which appears not only between individuals but also within the same individual or even the same tissue—that is, intratumoral heterogeneity [3]. Therefore, conquering advanced OSCC has become an urgent problem to be solved in the field of HNSC treatment. Although many studies have been carried out successively, and some progress has been made in the diagnosis and treatment of OSCC, most advanced patients will still experience recurrence or metastasis (or both) [2]. Further study of the heterogeneity of advanced OSCC and, accordingly, exploration of improved therapeutic strategies to perform more precise treatment and increase the cure rate is highly necessary.

In recent years, the rapid development of single-cell sequencing technology has provided a powerful tool for basic cancer research. Relative to traditional bulk sequencing methods, single-cell sequencing takes a single cell as the basic unit and, therefore, provides much better insight into the heterogeneity between cells. The methods based on single-cell sequencing bring new opportunities to dissect the intratumoral heterogeneity of tumors at high resolution. However, in addition to this, there is asynchrony in the development process of tumor cells in organisms—that is, the cycle states of different cells are not the same [4]. Bulk-based sequencing is performed on the whole tissue, in which cells with different cycle states are contained, thus also masking temporal heterogeneity between cells. Hence, at present, a large number of methods have emerged for single-cell trajectory inference, which can infer the position of each cell on the pseudo-time axis through algorithms based on expression profiles, so as to reproduce the trajectory of cell differentiation over time. The traditional clinical stage can reflect the time status of the development of a tumor; therefore, single-cell pseudo-time trajectory inference combined with clinical stages can more clearly analyze the dynamic process of tumor development, so as to more accurately discover the biological factors that promote tumor evolution and, finally, to promote the development of clinical treatment.

Therefore, our study emphasized the dynamic development process of OSCC. Unsupervised clustering based on single-cell transcriptomics was first performed to analyze the heterogeneity of OSCC. Pseudo-time trajectory inference was subsequently performed based on the unsupervised clustering results to dissect the complex development trajectory of OSCC from the early to the late stages. Next, to validate the cell trajectory, an analysis of receptor–ligand-based cell communication was conducted. At present, the single-cell field is under the transition from descriptive biology to predictive biology [5]; therefore, in order to promote the theory in clinical applications, we used bulk RNA-Seq data from the TCGA HNSC cohort to analyze the effects of different cell cluster compositions on patients' survival time. More importantly, we proposed pseudo-time score that can combine heterogeneity with the pseudo-time occupied by cell clusters and can quantify the status of patients during cancer development. We also used the external cohort from the ICGC [6] database to validate the pseudo-time score. Finally, based on the heterogeneity and complex development trajectory of OSCC, we discovered potential targeted therapeutic drugs that can not only personalize the treatment according to the individual's cell cluster composition but also block the development and deterioration of OSCC as much as possible in order to jointly improve the current situation of clinical treatment of advanced OSCC.

2. Results

2.1. High Heterogeneity of OSCC

We first performed quality control on the data by examining the number of cells and the gene expression levels of all patients; we removed five patients, including 24 cells, which are represented in red in Figure 1A,B. Next, we extracted 12,000 highly variable genes from a total of 23,686 genes to perform feature selection and to improve the accuracy of downstream analysis. Principal component analysis (PCA), which is a widely used dimensionality-reduction method, was used to process the expression profiles of highly variant genes. The optimal number of dimensions was determined by the elbow method, as shown in Figure 1C. Finally, the top 20 principal components were selected for unsupervised clustering (Figure S1).

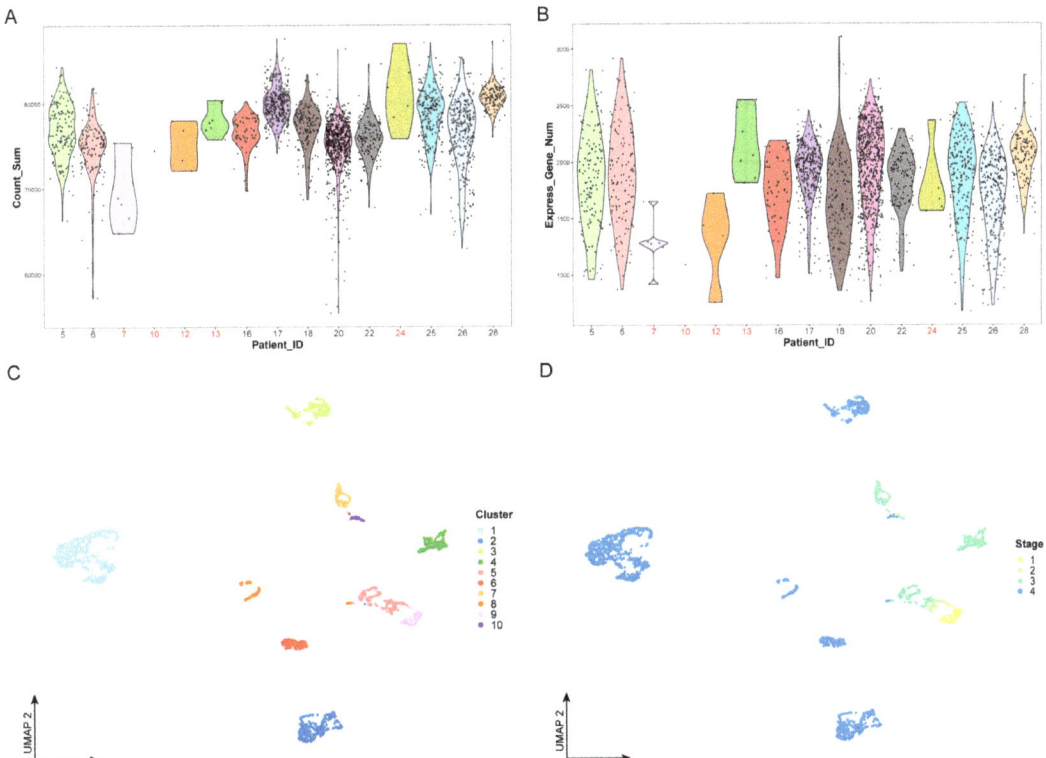

Figure 1. Data preprocessing and unsupervised clustering: (**A**) Violin plot of gene expression counts. The *x*-axis represents the patient ID, while the *y*-axis represents the sum values of gene expression counts. The dots represent the cells. Patient IDs that failed quality control are marked in red. (**B**) Violin plot of expressed gene numbers. The *x*-axis represents the patient ID, while the *y*-axis represents the number of expressed genes. The dots represent the cells. Patient IDs that failed quality control are marked in red. (**C,D**) The results of cell clustering. The dots represent the cells. The *x*- and *y*-axes represent the two dimensionalities of UMAP, respectively. Cells are colored by cluster label in panel C and by clinical stage in panel D.

Based on the top 20 principal components, we performed unsupervised clustering on 2176 cancer cells, which were divided into 10 clusters (Figure 1C,D). We found that, with the progression of the clinical stages, the number of cell clusters also gradually increased, indicating that there is greater heterogeneity in advanced OSCC (Figure 1D). This could explain the difficulty of completely curing advanced OSCC with current clinical treatments.

2.2. Different Development Fates of OSCC Cells

To reveal the developmental process of OSCC from the early to the advanced stages, we performed cell trajectory inference analysis based on pseudo-time for all cells using Monocle (Figure 2A,C). It is worth noting that the development of OSCC cells did not follow a single trajectory and was divided into two paths by a branch point. In terms of cell clusters (Figure 2A), clusters 9 and 5 appeared before the branch point, Path I developed along with the order of clusters 4, 10, 7, and 3, and Path II developed along with the order of clusters 6 (2), 8, and 1. From the perspective of clinical stages (Figure 2B), the temporal order was followed by stages I, II, III, and IV, consistent with the actual clinical development progress. Cells from stages I and II mainly appeared before the branch point, which appeared at stage III. Cells developed along the two paths and eventually deteriorated into stage IV. However, the two paths had different deterioration trends. Some cells from the branch point directly developed into stage IV (Path II), while the other cells remained in stage III (Path I) for a long time before eventually developing to stage IV. Therefore, identifying the key genes driving these two paths, with the goal of finding appropriate drugs to prevent the progression of cancer, would make significant progress in improving the current treatment of advanced OSCC.

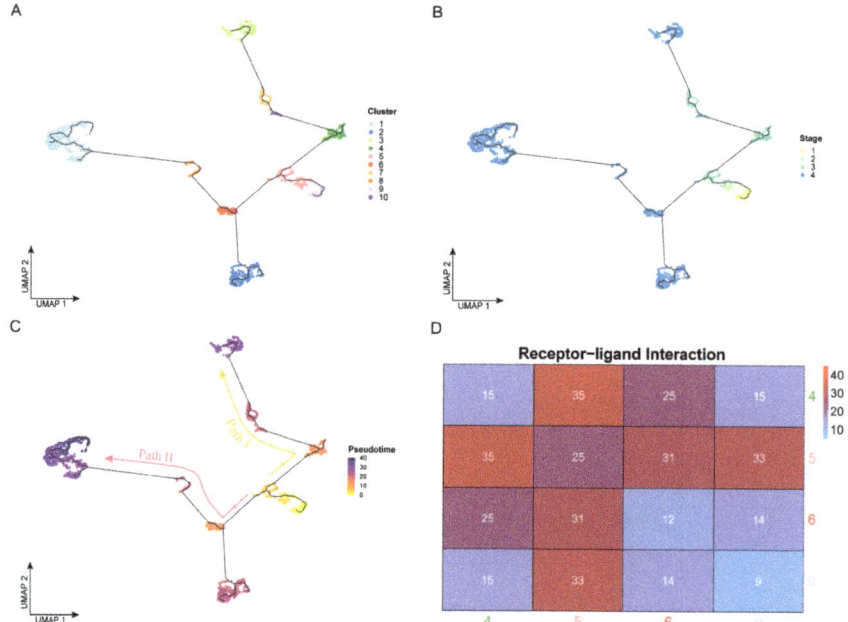

Figure 2. Cell trajectory inference: (**A–C**) Cell development trajectory. The dots represent the cells. The *x*- and *y*-axes represent the two dimensionalities of UMAP, respectively. Cells are colored by cluster label in panel A, by clinical stage in panel B, and by pseudo-time value in panel C. Based on the pseudo-time, the cell evolution direction could be determined, which was mainly divided into two paths: Path I (yellow) and Path II (red). (**D**) Results of cell communication analysis. The axis represents the four cell clusters near the branch point. The color and the number labeled by this heatmap were determined by the receptor–ligand pair number between two cell clusters.

2.3. Characteristic Analysis of Intercellular Communication

In the whole body or a specific tissue, the complex interactive relationships between cells constitute the cell communication network, which can reflect the tightness of the connection between different cells. Based on this, we hypothesized that the stronger the intercellular communication, the closer the connection, and the closer it is in the time series.

Therefore, to verify the accuracy of the cell trajectory inference, we performed receptor–ligand-based cell communication analysis. Throughout the trajectory, directly connected cells should tend to interact more tightly, while indirectly connected cells should have a weaker interaction because they require the transition of the intermediate cells—that is, there should be a tighter interaction between adjacent cell clusters in the trajectory. Here, we used CellPhoneDB to perform receptor–ligand-based analysis on cells of four clusters (4, 5, 6, and 9) near the branch point that separates the two paths in order to reveal their intercellular interaction relationships. The level of intercellular interactions was measured by the number of receptor–ligand pairs. As shown in Figure 2D, from the overall point of view, the tightness of the connection between cell clusters 5-4, 5-6, and 5-9 was much higher than that between the other cluster pairs, and as expected, these cell clusters were located adjacent to one another in the pseudo-time trajectory. In addition, we found that the interaction strength between clusters 4 and 5 was the highest. These two cell clusters not only were located close to one another in the pseudo-time trajectory but also belonged to the same stage (III), so the intercellular communication connection between them should also have been closed. The number of receptor–ligand pairs between clusters 5 and 9 was the second highest, at 33. These cells were from stages I, II, and III, but they were all located before the branch point, so the level of communication between them was higher than that of others after the branch point.

In conclusion, the analysis of intercellular communication based on receptor–ligand pairs was consistent with the results of cell trajectory based on pseudo-time and, thus, could further validate the extremely complex landscape during the development of OSCC cells from the early to the late stages.

2.4. Biological Factors Driving the Two Paths at the Branch Point in the Cell Development Trajectory

In order to further explore the driving factors of the branch point that separated Paths I and II, we used the BEAM method to perform pseudo-time-based differential gene expression analysis on four cell clusters (4, 5, 6, and 9) near the branch point. As a result, we identified 267 genes that showed significant fluctuation in their expression at the branch point (Figure 3; Table S2). Compared with traditional differential gene expression analysis, BEAM combines pseudo-time to reflect the continuous changes in gene expression. Through hierarchical clustering of these genes, all genes were divided into two gene sets. We found that the majority of these genes showed mutually exclusive expression characteristics in two directions—that is, high expression characteristics in Path I but low expression characteristics in Path II, or vice versa—indicating that these genes regulate two mutually exclusive cell fates. In addition to this, genes in a gene set of hierarchical clustering usually have co-expression characteristics that may co-regulate some biological functions.

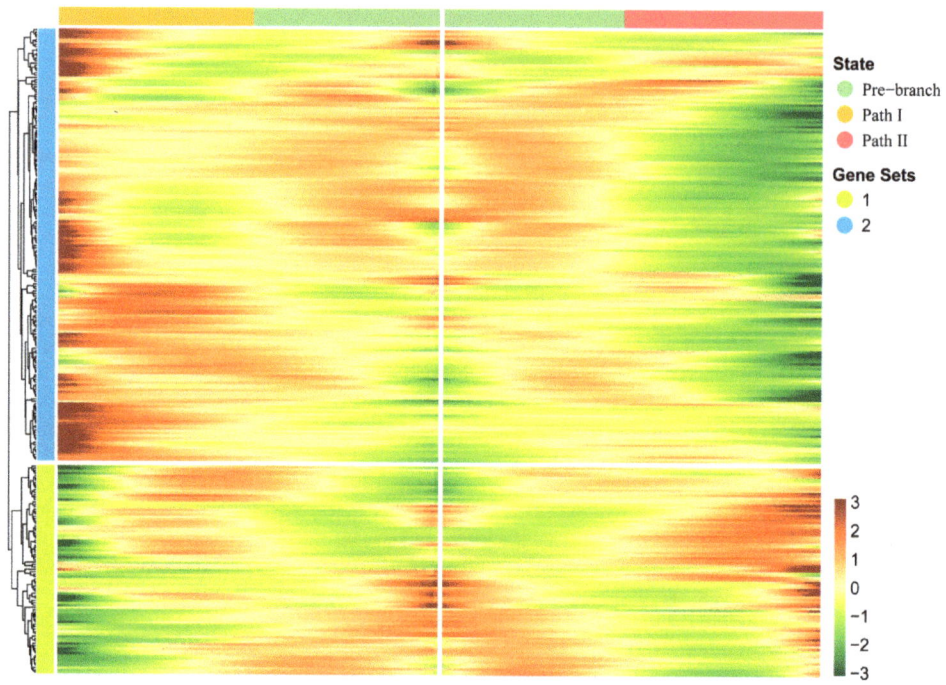

Figure 3. Key genes driving the occurrence of the branch point: The heatmap of gene expression levels during the progression of OSCC. Gene clusters were generated by hierarchical clustering.

Therefore, in order to reveal the biological functions regulated by these genes, we performed Gene Ontology (GO) enrichment analysis on two gene sets (Figure 4). The results showed that genes highly expressed in Path I (gene cluster 2) were significantly enriched mainly in biological processes, such as the cell migration and apoptosis signal regulation pathways (Figure 4B). The important role of cell migration and apoptosis in the development and progression of OSCC has been confirmed [1]. Marker genes regulating the cell cycle, apoptosis, and migration have differential expression in OSCC patients or are significantly associated with prognosis [1], such as survivin and heat shock proteins (HSPs) associated with apoptosis. Survivin is a member of the inhibitor of apoptosis proteins (IAP) family that inhibits capase 3, 7, and 9, and its expression is higher in OSCC patients than in epithelial dysplasia patients. High expression of heat shock protein 27 (HSP27) is associated with a better prognosis. The expression of urokinase plasminogen activator receptor (UPAR)—a marker gene associated with cell migration—was negatively correlated with prognosis [1]. Therefore, the genes highly expressed in Path I suggest that OSCC cells may have active metastatic characteristics in clinical stage III. The genes highly expressed in Path II (gene cluster 1) were mainly enriched in biological functions related to MHC class II in BPs (biological processes), CCs (cellular components), and MFs (molecular functions) (Figure 4A). MHC is a collective term for a group of genes encoding major histocompatibility antigens in animals, also known as HLA in humans, which is also involved in the immune process of the body as an antigen. There is literature confirming the upregulation of class II molecules of the major histocompatibility complex (MHC) by keratinocytes in oral squamous cell carcinoma [7]. However, the significance of its high expression in advanced OSCC is currently unclear. Another study confirmed that the keratinocyte line expressing MHC II has the characteristics of the absence of CD80 and CD86 in head and neck cancer, which may be a way for tumors to evade immune surveillance [8].

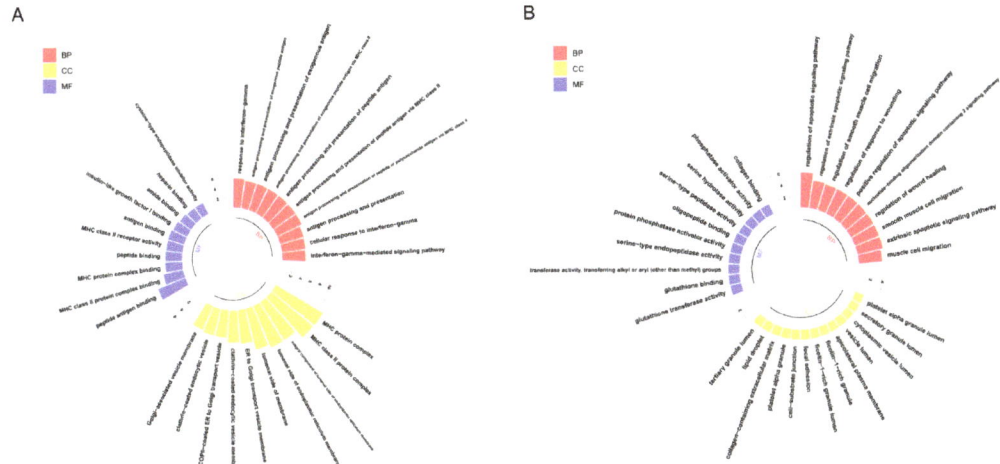

Figure 4. GO enrichment analysis of key genes: The results of GO enrichment analysis of gene clusters 1 and 2 are shown in panels (**A**,**B**), respectively. The x-axis represents GO terms, which are displayed in three colors according to the three types (BPs, CCs, and MFs), while the y-axis represents -$\log_{10}$(p.adjust). Only the 10 most significant GO terms of each type are shown here.

2.5. Relationship between Prognosis and Heterogeneity of Advanced OSCC

Our findings show that advanced OSCC has more significant heterogeneity than early OSCC, and it is difficult to characterize this heterogeneity via traditional bulk research. Therefore, to further dissect the relationship between this heterogeneity and prognosis, we integrated clinical information and expression profiles from the TCGA database to explore the prognosis of stage III and IV patients with greater heterogeneity, which would also indirectly verify the accuracy of our predicted cell clusters.

Since the data from the TCGA database are at the bulk level, we first mapped corresponding cell clusters to bulk expression profiles to infer the cell cluster composition of each patient. Based on the custom background gene sets (Table S3) derived from differential expression analysis, CIBERSORT was performed for stage III and IV patients from TCGA (Table S4). Next, in order to reveal the impact of cell cluster composition on the prognosis of patients, we performed unsupervised hierarchical clustering based on the results of CIBERSORT. The patients in stages III and IV were divided into two groups. Each patient group had similar cell cluster composition, and there were significant differences between the patient groups (Figure 5A,D). For patients in stage III, including four clusters, group 1 mainly contained cell cluster 7, while group 2 mainly contained cell clusters 5 and 10. For patients in stage IV, composed of six clusters, group 1 mainly contained cell cluster 6, while group 2 mainly contained cell cluster 2.

Survival analysis was performed for the two groups of patients in stages III and IV. The results showed differences in survival time between the two groups (Figure 5B,E), indicating that different cell compositions could impact prognosis. For patients in stage III, the survival time of patient group 1 was shorter, while for stage IV, the survival time of patient group 1 was longer.

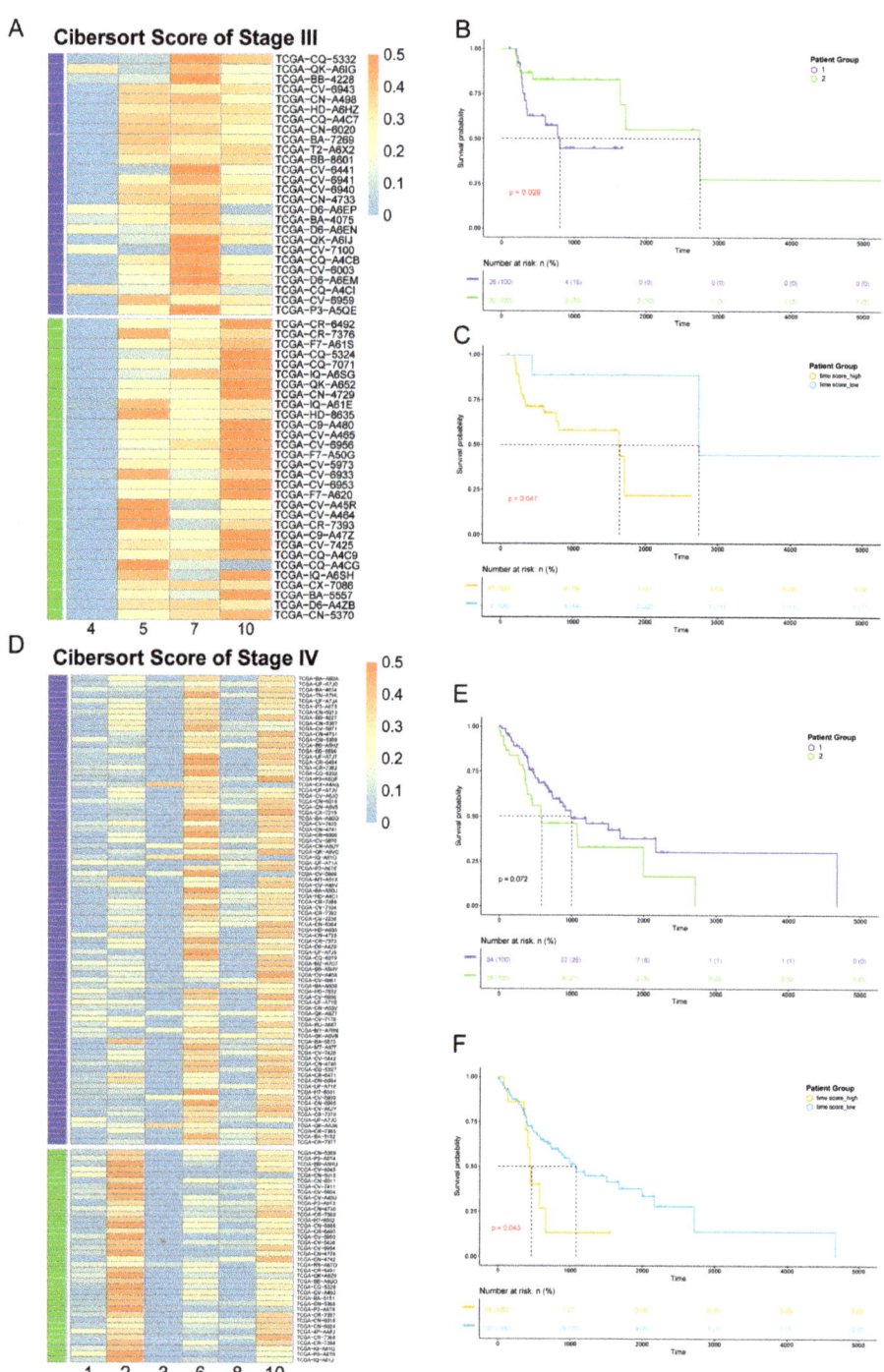

Figure 5. Association between heterogeneity and clinical prognosis. (**A,D**) The results of CIBERSORT. Patients were divided into two groups by hierarchical clustering. Patients in stage III are shown in

panel A, while patients in stage IV are shown in panel D. (**B,E**) Survival analysis. The survival curve is shown above, with the *x*-axis representing the survival time (days), the *y*-axis representing the survival probability, and the censored values indicated by "+" in the curve. The color of the curve is consistent with panel A (**D**) and represents two patient groups. Below is the risk table showing the number (or percentage) of survivors at each time point. The results of patients in stage III are shown in panel B, while those of patients in stage IV are shown in panel E. (**C,F**) Survival analysis based on pseudo-time score for grouping. The color of the curve represents the two patient groups, which are distinguished by their pseudo-time score. The result of patients in stage III is shown in panel C, while those of patients in stage IV are shown in panel F.

In order to explore the reason(s) that this heterogeneity has an impact on the survival time of patients, we constructed pseudo-time score by combining cell trajectory inference to quantify the temporal status of each patient group. The pseudo-time score considers both the cell composition of patients and the development order of each cell cluster in the same clinical stage. The higher the score, the closer the patient is to the advanced stage. The results showed that, in stage III, $S_{\text{patient group 1}} = 16.35$ and $S_{\text{patient group 2}} = 15.19$. As for stage IV, $S_{\text{patient group 1}} = 18.59$ and $S_{\text{patient group 2}} = 20.44$. According to the survival analysis, the groups with smaller pseudo-time score tended to have a better prognosis. Therefore, the difference in prognosis status between patient groups lies in the different cell compositions, which contribute to the different temporal status during the development of cancer. Our results also show that even patients at the same clinical stage would have many differences in cell composition and prognosis.

To further analyze the relationship between the pseudo-time score and patients' prognosis, we regrouped patients according to their pseudo-time score, and the results showed that the pseudo-time score could be used as the marker to distinguish survival time in both stage III and stage IV patients, with *p*-values of 0.047 and 0.043, respectively, as measured by the log-rank test. The patient groups with the higher score had the worse prognosis (Figure 5C,F).

To confirm the above results, the same methods were used to process the dataset from ICGC, and the cell cluster composition inference of patients was performed using CIBERSORT based on the same background gene sets. Then, these patients were divided into two groups based on their pseudo-time score, and survival analysis also illustrated that the two groups of patients showed significant differences in survival time ($p = 0.049$, log-rank test) (Figure S2).

In summary, the pseudo-time score that we constructed has a significant correlation with prognosis, can be used as a prognostic marker, and is robust across multiple datasets.

2.6. Identification of Candidate Drugs Based on PPI Networks

Transcriptomic analysis at the single-cell level with high resolution is a way to improve the efficacy of medication by dissecting the diverse cell clusters in the tumor and by selecting the targeted therapy strategy. In addition, it is also essential to find key genes with synchronous expression changes during the development of OSCC and to use these genes as potential targets to discover blockers to slow or even block the deterioration of OSCC in order to prolong the treatment time in clinical practice and to maximize the lifespan of patients. Therefore, we performed drug discovery in the following two respects: (1) searching for drugs to block OSCC progression and (2) searching for cell-cluster-specific drugs to achieve targeted therapy.

For the first respect, 267 key genes at the branch point revealed by the BEAM analysis were first used for protein–protein interaction (PPI) network construction using the STRING [9] database. Cytoscape software was used for network visualization (Figure S3). There were 218 nodes and 649 edges in the PPI network. We used the cytoHubba [10] plugin built in Cytoscape to identify the hub genes, and all 12 topological analysis methods were taken into account to improve the robustness. Then, the expression trends of these hub genes with pseudo-time were manually checked, and only genes showing a significant trend of upregulation in Path II and downregulation in Path I were retained as marker hub genes. As a result, 15 marker hub genes were identified (Figure 6). Except for ALDH3A1, CD40, CXCL11, HLA-DRA, and HLA-DRB have been validated by the literature to have positive relationships between expression and prognosis, so we removed them from candidate drug targets, while the others presented malignant characteristics (Table S5). Finally, using the 10 remaining genes as targets, 195 drugs were extracted from integrated drug–target relationships, including first-line antitumor drugs, such as cisplatin, fluorouracil, methotrexate, gemcitabine, p-phenylenediamine, etc. (Table S6, Sheet 1). Among them, 90 drugs were validated based on CCLE experimental data (Table S6, Sheet 2), and 77 of the remaining 105 drugs were validated based on the literature (Table S6, Sheets 2 and 3). The drugs targeting multiple targets were paid more attention to. Cyclosporine and valproic acid (VPA) targeted all 10 proteins. In recent years, VPA has been found to be a histone deacetylase inhibitor (HDACi). Many experimental studies have shown that VPA can inhibit the growth and proliferation of tumor cells by inducing cell cycle arrest, apoptosis, and differentiation and by inhibiting tumor angiogenesis and metastasis [11,12]. It is known that the combination of cisplatin (CDDP) and cetuximab (CX) is one of the standard first-line treatments for OSCC. However, this therapeutic regimen is often associated with resistance, suggesting that new combinatorial strategies need to be improved. Federica Iannelli et al. demonstrated that the introduction of VPA to the conventional treatment for recurrent/metastatic HNSCC represents an innovative and feasible antitumor strategy that warrants further clinical evaluation [13]. Another study showed VPA acting as a histone deacetylase inhibitor (HDI) in OSCC cells and normal human keratinocytes (HKs), potentiating the cytotoxic effect of cisplatin in OSCC cell lines and decreasing the viability of OSCC cells as compared to HKs [14]. Taken together, these results provide initial evidence that VPA might be a valuable drug in the development of better therapeutic regimens for HNSCC.

We performed drug sensitivity predictions at single-cell resolution for these drugs, and the drug sensitivity of cell clusters was represented by the mean value of drug sensitivity of the cells in each cluster. According to the pseudo-time trajectory, all cell clusters were divided at the branch point into Paths I and II. Fifty-three drugs were predicted to have higher sensitivity in Path II, suggesting that these drugs are more effective at inhibiting malignant developmental processes (Table S6, Sheet 4). Of these, we found that fulvestrant simultaneously exhibited the highest drug sensitivity in cell clusters 4, 5, and 6, which appeared near the branch point and, thus, likely represented an earlier exacerbation progression (Figure 7A). A study has shown that estrogen can participate in the progression of precancerous lesions of HNSC by inhibiting apoptosis and by promoting the proliferation of advanced HNSC cells [15]. Antiestrogen may be beneficial as a chemopreventive agent for HNSC [15], and fulvestrant is an antiestrogen drug, so our results were consistent with those of the previous study.

For the second respect, marker genes were first calculated using the SC3 [16] method for all cell clusters. With manual examination, a total of 459 genes remained after statistical filtering (Table S7, Sheet 1). These genes showed significant upregulation in specific cell clusters, so they could be used as essential cell-cluster-specific marker genes for drug discovery. As described above, the PPI networks of each cell cluster were constructed (Figure S4), and then, 12 topological methods from cytoHubba were taken into account for identification of the hub genes. Then, 76 hub genes were filtered (Table S7, Sheet 2), and 478 drugs were ultimately discovered (Table S8). Some of these drugs overlap with the blocking drugs found in our study and are all first-line anticancer drugs, such as valproic acid, cisplatin, fluorouracil, methotrexate, temozolomide, etc. Based on CCLE experimental data, 195 drugs were validated as being effective in HNSC cell lines (Table S9, Sheet 1), and 168 of the remaining 283 drugs were validated through the literature (Table S9, Sheets 1 and 2). Many previous studies have shown that the combined use of certain drugs can enhance their effects; for example, the combination of curcumin and copper can enhance the inhibitory effect on the migration and activity of OSCC cells [17]. Our findings show that curcumin and copper can be used for blocking the development of OSCC and targeting cell cluster 1, indicating that the two have the potential for combination, and are consistent with the results of the previous study. Next, we analyzed the sensitivity of drugs and extracted drugs that had higher sensitivity in their targeting of cell clusters. Finally, there were 102 drugs, including many drugs that have been proven to be effective for HNSC treatment (Table S9, Sheet 3). Cell cluster 1 is at the end of the pseudo-time trajectory and, thus, represents highly advanced OSCC cells. Among the selected drugs, there were 71 drugs targeting cell cluster 1, including common anticancer drugs, such as paclitaxel, gemcitabine, carboplatin, decitabine, etc. (Figure 7B). We performed literature validation for all of these drugs, and 91 of the 102 had been reported in previous studies for cancer treatment or combined medication. Therefore, the candidate drugs discovered in our study could be of great significance to changing the current situation of treatment for advanced OSCC.

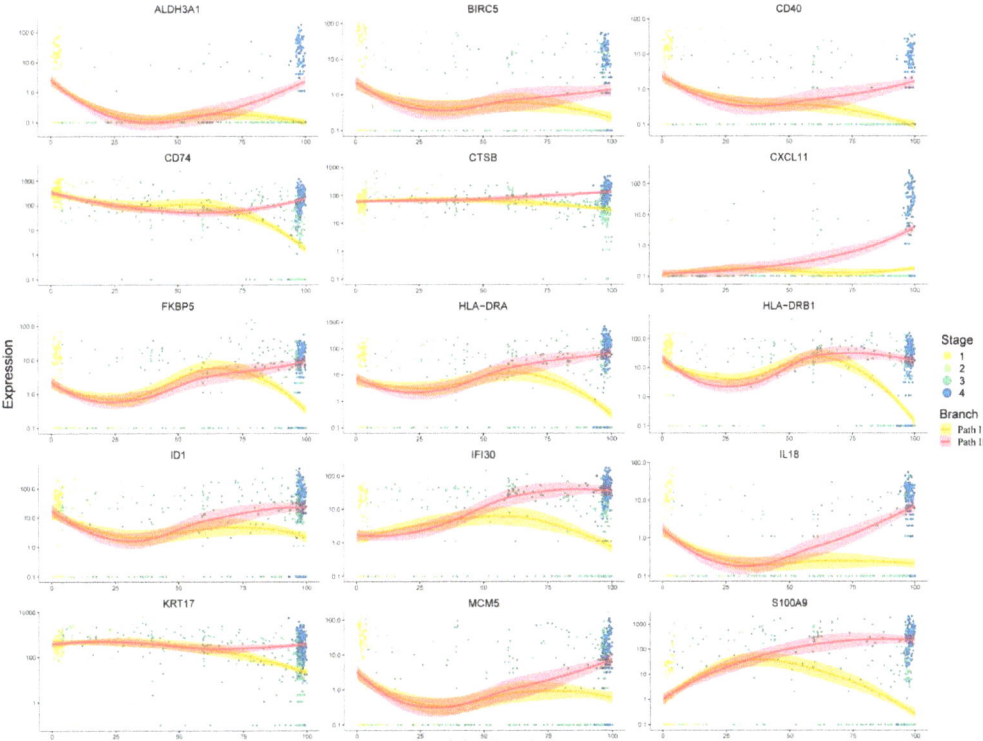

Figure 6. Analysis of 15 target genes' expression trends: This figure shows the expression trends of genes progressing with pseudo-time. The *x*-axis represents pseudo-time, while the *y*-axis represents the gene expression level. Dots represent cells, which are colored according to clinical stages. The curves were fitted by gene expression level, and the colors represent two different development paths in the cell trajectory.

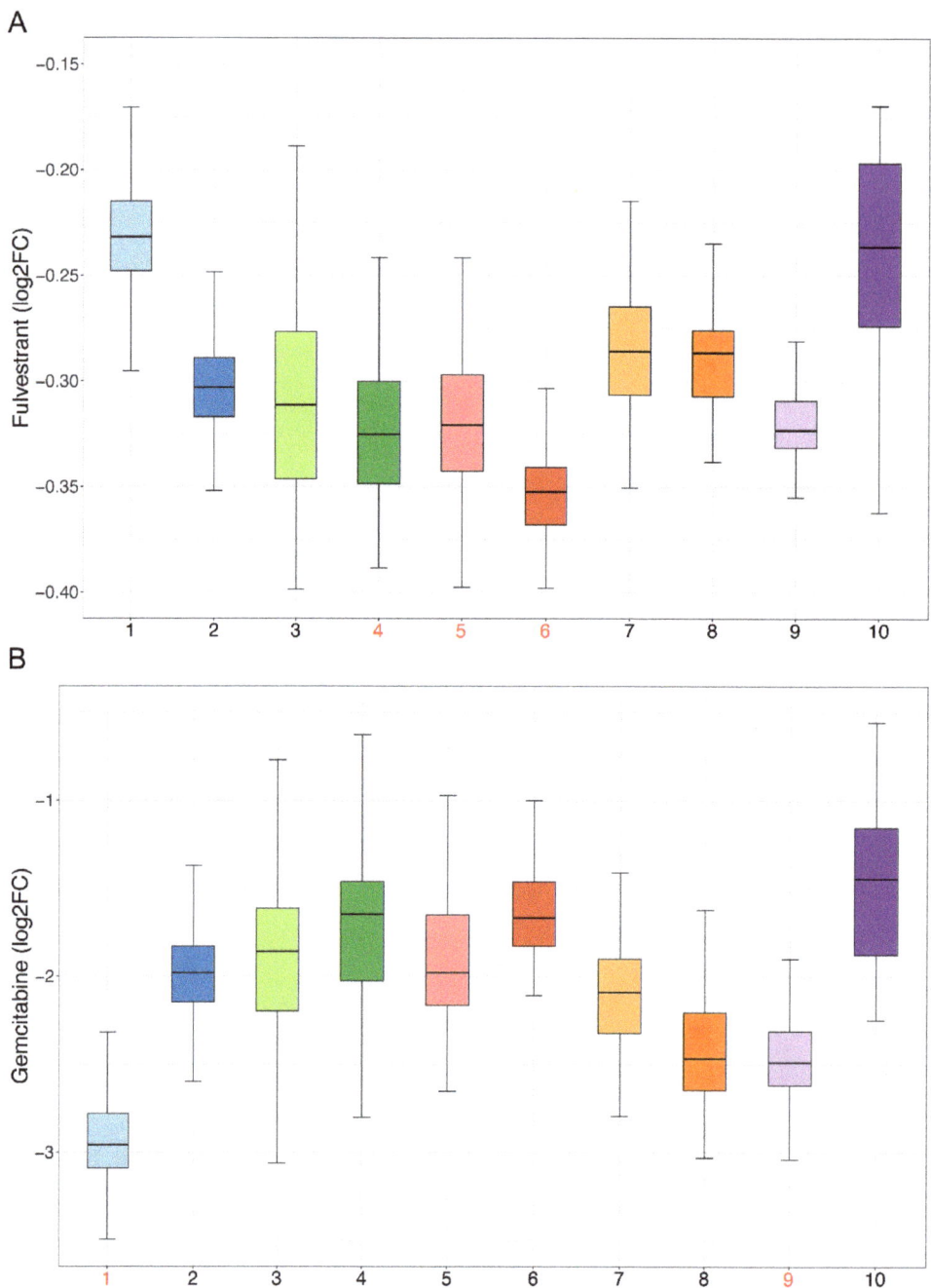

Figure 7. Sensitivity of candidate drugs: The x-axis represents cell clusters, and the y-axis represents the logFC (drug sensitivity data from the CCLE are represented using relative log fold-change values of cell lines' viability to DMSO). Cell clusters with the highest drug sensitivity mentioned in our study are marked in red. (**A**) Sensitivity of fulvestrant. (**B**) Sensitivity of gemcitabine.

3. Methods

3.1. Data and Preprocessing

The single-cell RNA sequencing data of OSCC used in this study were obtained from the GEO database (GSE103322), with a total of 5902 cells from 15 patients [18] including all clinical stages. These data were preprocessed using the method described in the article published by Sidhart V. Puram et al. [18], and all cells were accurately classified into cancer and non-cancer types. The gene expression did not conform to a normal distribution in five patients due to the low number of cells, which may have had a bad impact on the accuracy of the downstream analysis; therefore, these five patients were removed. There were 2200 cancer cells in total. The detailed information of all patients is shown in Table S1. Because our study focused on cancer cells, non-cancer cells were removed.

Bulk sequencing data were obtained from the HNSC cohort of the TCGA database and contained a total of 501 patients.

The dataset used for pseudo-time score validation was obtained from the ICGC database (ORCA-IN, Sequence-Based Gene Expression).

3.2. Unsupervised Clustering of Cells

We used the R package Seurat v4.0 [19]—a toolkit developed specifically for single-cell data. First, the R function "VlnPlot" was used to evaluate the gene expression levels of all cells to ensure that the gene expression level was distributed in an approximately Gaussian manner in each patient, so as to reduce the impact of individual differences on downstream analysis. Then, the expression profiles were log-normalized using the R function "NormalizeData", and 12,000 high variant genes were identified from 23,686 genes using the R function "FindVariableFeatures". Genes with high variation can better reflect the biological similarities and differences between cells, which is conducive to improving the accuracy of downstream unsupervised clustering. Next, we used the R function "ScaleData" to scale the expression of highly variant genes in order to balance the weight of genes in the downstream analysis. Because single-cell data are usually sparser compared with bulk sequencing and their redundancy is higher, principal component analysis (PCA) is an important and essential step in single-cell transcriptome analysis. PCA can effectively remove data noise, extract important information, and improve the accuracy and speed of downstream analysis. PCA was performed using the R function "RunPCA" on the expression profiles of highly variable genes, and then, the R function "ElbowPlot"—which ranks the principal components based on the percentage of variance explained by each component—was used to determine the optimal dimension number of the data. The optimal number of principal components would appear near the "elbow" (i.e., the inflection point). Unsupervised clustering based on the top 20 principal components was implemented for all cells using the R function "FindClusters".

3.3. Trajectory Inference of Cell Development

We used the R package Monocle [20]—a powerful tool for single-cell RNA-Seq data processing and cell trajectory inference—for analysis. Monocle uses algorithms to learn the gene expression changes that each cell experiences during a state transition, to mine the overall trajectory, and then to place each cell at the appropriate location in the trajectory. In addition, Monocle can combine with UMAP (Uniform Manifold Approximation and Projection) [21] so as to make the cell trajectory more intuitive. Therefore, all cells were first embedded by UMAP based on unsupervised clustering results.

The R functions "learn_graph" and "order_cells" were used for the inference of cell trajectory, both of which used default parameter settings. Subsequently, the R function "plot_cells" was used to visualize the results of cell trajectory inference with the pseudo-time.

3.4. Gene Expression Analysis at the Branch Point of the Trajectory

The BEAM (branch expression analysis modeling) [22] algorithm provided by Monocle can analyze the pseudo-time-based gene expression changes at the branch point of the trajectory, revealing the important genes that drive the occurrence of cell trajectory division. The threshold was set as q-value $< 1 \times 10^{-8}$. This stricter threshold was designed to identify essential genes more accurately. In addition, only the genes expressed in more than 20% of cells were retained in order to screen widely expressed genes in cells.

In order to reveal the biological functions of these genes, they were first divided into two gene sets by hierarchical clustering. The genes in the same gene set would have co-expression characteristics and may regulate similar biological processes. Thus, Gene Ontology (GO) [23] enrichment analysis was performed for each gene set separately using the R package clusterProfiler [24] with the threshold p.adjust < 0.05 and q-value < 0.05.

3.5. Cell Communication Analysis

In order to verify the results of cell trajectory inference and to further determine our conclusions, receptor–ligand-based cell communication analysis was performed using the Python package CellPhoneDB [25] for cell clusters adjacent to the branch point. The iteration parameter was set to 2000. The number of receptor–ligand interaction pairs was visualized using a heatmap, and a dot plot was used to show pairs with statistical p-values < 0.05 and mean expression > 0.

3.6. Survival Analysis

In order to reveal the impact of heterogeneity on the survival status of patients, we downloaded the RNA-Seq data from the HNSC cohort with clinical information of patients from the TCGA [26] database. CIBERSORT [27] is a linear support-vector regression-based deconvolution algorithm that enables researchers to perform sample annotation based on a set of background genes. Hence, the selection of the background gene set would have a great impact on the accuracy of the downstream analysis. Since the type of expression profile derived from the TCGA database is at the bulk level, we used the differentially expressed genes that can represent the characteristics of each cluster separately as a background to infer the proportion of cell clusters of each bulk sample using the R package CIBERSORT. For stage III, the threshold for gene background screening was p-value < 0.01 and $\log_2 fc > 1.5$. Since patients in stage IV have greater heterogeneity, the threshold was set as p-value $< 1 \times 10^{-4}$ and $\log_2 fc > 1.5$. This stricter threshold can help identify the genes that represent the characteristics of each cell cluster more effectively and can improve the accuracy of the proportion inference. The results of CIBERSORT were subsequently filtered by setting the threshold as $p < 0.05$ and correlation > 0.3. The Ward.D algorithm [28] was used to perform hierarchical clustering to divide patients in stage III and stage IV into two groups. The survival [29] and survminer [30] R packages were used for survival analysis, plotting of the Kaplan–Meier curve, and the log-rank statistical test.

3.7. Pseudo-Time Score

Here, we hypothesized that patients in the same stage would also have relatively early or advanced cancer cells due to the temporal heterogeneity and that cancer cells in the advanced stage would have more malignant features, leading to a worse prognosis. Therefore, in order to prove our hypothesis, based on the previous trajectory inference results, the pseudo-time score was constructed to quantify the temporal status of each patient. The formula was $S = \sum P_i \times T_i$, where P_i denotes the proportion of cell cluster i of the patient, while T_i denotes the pseudo-time value of cell cluster i. P_i was calculated using CIBERSORT. T_i is the average pseudo-time value of each cell from the cell cluster i, which can be calculated by Monocle. Specifically, for patients in stage III, $S = \sum P_i \times T_i$ (i = 4, 5, 7, or 10), while for patients in stage IV, $S = \sum P_i \times T_i$ (i = 1, 2, 3, 6, 8, or 10). As for the patient groups, the pseudo-time score is the average value of S of each patient from each group.

In order to further reveal the relationship between pseudo-time score and prognosis, all patients were automatically grouped based on their pseudo-time score using survminer to perform survival analysis. Similarly, statistical significance was tested using the log-rank method.

The dataset from the ICGC database was used for further validation. This dataset contains 40 patients, including a stage II patient, 3 stage III patients, and 36 stage IV patients. The cell cluster composition of each patient was inferred using CIBERSORT, based on the same background gene sets as the TCGA data above, and then, the pseudo-time score of each patient was calculated and the patients were grouped for survival analysis as described above.

3.8. Drug Discovery

There may often be many cell clusters in a patient under the single-cell resolution. For such a complex system of multi-cell clusters, we should discover specific drugs for each cell cluster, so as to select multitarget drugs or drug combinations according to the heterogeneity of patients for the elimination of all cell clusters of patients—rather than just the dominant cell cluster, which can often cause drug resistance. Therefore, we first screened specific drugs for each cell cluster. Secondly, discovering drugs to block or delay the development of OSCC would also be an idea to effectively improve the cure rate.

The discovery of drug targets is the first step. The marker genes of each cell cluster were identified using the R package SC3 [16], with the threshold set as p-value < 0.01 and AUROC (the area under the receiver operating characteristic) >0.8. Then, all marker genes were manually checked to ensure that they had significantly high expression characteristics in specific cell clusters. In biomolecular networks, hub nodes often have crucial biological significance, so we used hub genes in the network as targets to find candidate drugs. First, we used STRING [9] and selected the default threshold to construct protein–protein interaction (PPI) networks based on the key genes that drive the occurrence of trajectory branching from BEAM analysis and cell-cluster-specific marker genes from SC3. The visualization of PPI networks and further topological analysis were based on Cytoscape [31] software. To identify hub genes more accurately, we deeply mined the PPI networks based on 12 topological analysis methods built into the cytoHubba [10] plugin. The hub genes were defined as the intersection genes of the top 50% of each of the 12 analysis methods and were used as targets for drug discovery.

Here, we collected 216,428 drug–target relationships including 21,650 human targets and 2470 approved drugs from seven commonly used data sources: the DrugBank database (v5.1.9) [32], the Therapeutic Target Database (TTD) [33], the BindingDB database [34], the PharmGKB database [35], the Drug–Gene Interaction Database (DGIdb, v4.2) [36], the IUPHAR/BPS Guide to PHARMACOLOGY [37], and the Comparative Toxicogenomics Database (CTD) [38]. Finally, using the aforementioned genes as targets, we obtained the preliminary candidate drugs.

3.9. Validation of Candidate Drugs

To validate the candidate drugs identified in our study, we combined experimental data, computational methods, and previous literature to assess the effectiveness of the candidate drugs.

The drug sensitivity experimental data and cell line expression profiles were first obtained from the Cancer Cell Line Encyclopedia (CCLE) [39] database, and all OSCC cell lines were extracted. In order to validate drug effectiveness from experiments indirectly, we computed the mean drug sensitivity of all OSCC cell lines for each drug contained in the CCLE. For drugs that were not included or showed no efficacy in the CCLE, additional literature validation was performed.

In order to reveal the drug specificity during the development of OSCC and of cell clusters, we used the R package oncoPredict [40]—a powerful tool for predicting drug responses based on background data (here, we used drug sensitivity and expression data from the CCLE)—to calculate the drug sensitivity of each cell. Then, the drug sensitivity of each cell cluster was defined as the mean drug sensitivity of cells from this cell cluster. We extracted blocking drugs and cell-specific drugs with high specificity. Drug sensitivity data from the CCLE were represented using the relative log fold-change (logFC) values of cell lines' viability to DMSO. Therefore, for blocking drugs, the following conditions were used for screening: (1) The mean logFC in all cells was lower than 0. (2) The mean logFC of cell clusters located in Path II was lower than that in Path I. For cell-cluster-specific drugs, we screened by the following criteria: (1) The mean logFC in all cells was lower than 0. (2) The mean logFC of targeting cell clusters was lower than that of non-targeting cell clusters.

4. Discussion

The effective curing of advanced OSCC has been a clinical challenge because of its high heterogeneity and metastatic characteristics. Current precision treatment strategies at the single-cell level only focus on static heterogeneity and do not consider dynamic characteristics due to tumor cells' development and evolution. Therefore, our study applied traditional single-cell transcriptome analysis and dynamic cell trajectory inference theory to further explore heterogeneity and precise treatment strategies for OSCC.

During the cell clustering analysis, we found that, with the development of tumor cells, their heterogeneity became greater and greater. This complex heterogeneity reflects the characteristics of multiple evolutionary modes of tumor cells in the same stage that have different sensitivities to chemotherapeutic drugs, which is consistent with the fact that advanced OSCC is difficult to cure. Therefore, we innovatively quantified the drug sensitivity of specific cell clusters and selected drugs with high sensitivities in those specific cell clusters.

The cell trajectory inference with pseudo-time reflects the temporal heterogeneity of OSCC, which forms a complex exacerbation process composed of two paths through a branch point and gives the temporal characteristics of each cell. We integrated this temporal characteristic and cell cluster composition of patients to establish the concept of patients' time score, with significant implications for prognosis—that is, the lower the time score, the better the prognosis. Based on this, it can be seen that even patients in the same clinical stage have different temporal status.

In addition, the patient's response to drug treatment is also dynamic, so RNA-Seq can be performed at different time points during the treatment to focus on the disease progression based on our proposed pipeline. If the time score decreases gradually with the treatment, the prognosis of the patients will be better; otherwise, the medication strategy needs to be adjusted.

Finally, based on the key genes driving the differentiation of cell development trajectory and the cell-cluster-specific marker genes, we used biomolecular network theory and topological analysis to mine hub genes with extremely important biological significance, which were used as targets to find candidate drugs. As a result, there were a total of 167 drugs targeting key genes at the branch point in cell trajectory, which could be used to delay or block the further progression of OSCC. There were a total of 363 cell-cluster-specific drugs, which could be used for targeting medication based on patients' cell composition. These drugs can be combined to treat patients with multiple cell clusters, but some drugs (such as artenimol) can also target multiple cell clusters at the same time. We prefer the latter, so as to maximize the efficiency of the medication while reducing the side effects. Candidate drugs were validated by both literature and computational methods combined with experimental data.

In conclusion, our research provides a new pipeline to dissect the complex heterogeneity of cancer from a dynamic point of view. More importantly, our study proposes the concept of patients' pseudo-time score, which has great clinical value. A series of precision medicine insights for the clinical treatment practice of OSCC were presented—that is, the selection of appropriate drugs for tumor control, which aims to not only block or delay the progression of OSCC but also comprehensively kill various cancer cells. This strategy may also be adapted for other cancers in the future.

However, due to data limitations, no more in-depth research has been carried out. In addition, due to the absence of clinical trials, this study has some limitations. As single-cell spatial sequencing and cell trajectory inference technologies mature, we have reason to believe that the challenges in completely curing OSCC or other cancers will eventually be overcome.

5. Conclusions

Our study confirms the complex heterogeneity of OSCC both statically and dynamically. Advanced-stage patients have greater heterogeneity than early stage patients. The development of OSCC is not a simple pathway, and cell trajectory inference confirms its complex dynamic landscape, which contains multiple developmental pathways. According to this, the proposed pseudo-time score is closely related to the patient's prognosis and has good prognostic prediction potential, as validated by external datasets. We searched for candidate drugs for the treatment and blocking of OSCC, most of which were validated in the literature and via computational methods based on experimental data. In conclusion, our study comprehensively parses the developmental characteristics of OSCC, offering new insights into the basic research and clinical treatment of OSCC.

Supplementary Materials: The following supporting information can be downloaded at: https://www.mdpi.com/article/10.3390/cancers14194801/s1, Figure S1. Principle component selection. The x-axis represents the number of PC and the y-axis represents the standard deviation. The optimal number of principal components appears at the inflection point and was marked by a red arrow. Figure S2: Survival analysis for validation data. The survival curve is shown above, with the x-axis representing the survival time (days), the y-axis representing the survival probability, and the censored values are indicated by "+" in the curve. Below is the risk table showing the number (or percentage) of survivors at each time point. Figure S3. PPI network of key genes of the branch point. The nodes represent genes and the edges represent interaction relationships. Node colors represent gene sets, consistent with Figure 3. Figure S4. PPI networks of cell cluster-specific genes. The nodes represent genes and the edges represent interaction relationships. Node colors represent the auroc of genes generated by SC3 and the legend is shown below. Table S1: The detailed information of patients. Table S2: Key genes which promote the occurrence of the branch in cell trajectory. Table S3: Background genes of stage III for cibersort. Table S4: CIBERSORT result of patients in stage III. Table S5: literature validation for targets. Table S6: In this table, the drug-target relationship is represented as 0-1, and 1 represents that the gene is the target of the drug. Table S7: Marker genes from SC3. Table S8: drug-target-cluster relationships. Table S9: This table shows the literature validation results of CCLE intersection drugs. Only drugs that have not shown efficacy (logFC > 0) on OSCC from the experimental data of CCLE were verified, and drugs that already have been proved effective (logFC < 0) were marked in green color.

Author Contributions: Conceptualization, Q.M. and X.C.; Data curation, Y.L.; Formal analysis, Q.M., F.W., G.L., F.X., Y.L. and H.X.; Funding acquisition, X.C.; Methodology, L.L., G.L., F.X. and D.Z.; Project administration, Q.M. and X.C.; Software, D.Z.; Writing—original draft, Q.M.; Writing—review and editing, L.L., F.W., F.X., D.Z., H.X. and X.C. All authors have read and agreed to the published version of the manuscript.

Funding: This work was supported by the National Natural Science Foundation of China (grant No. 61671191).

Institutional Review Board Statement: Not applicable.

Informed Consent Statement: Not applicable.

Data Availability Statement: The expression data are available through the Gene Expression Omnibus with accession number GSE103322.

Conflicts of Interest: The authors declare no conflict of interest.

References

1. Taghavi, N.; Yazdi, I. Prognostic factors of survival rate in oral squamous cell carcinoma: Clinical, histologic, genetic and molecular concepts. *Arch. Iran. Med.* **2015**, *18*, 314–319. [PubMed]
2. Chow, L.Q.M. Head and Neck Cancer. *N. Engl. J. Med.* **2020**, *382*, 60–72. [CrossRef] [PubMed]

3. Cleary, A.S.; Leonard, T.L.; Gestl, S.A.; Gunther, E.J. Tumour cell heterogeneity maintained by cooperating subclones in Wnt-driven mammary cancers. *Nature* **2014**, *508*, 113–117. [CrossRef] [PubMed]
4. Trapnell, C.; Cacchiarelli, D. Monocle: Differential expression and time-series analysis for single-cell RNA-Seq and qPCR experiments. *Bioconductor. Fmrp. Usp. Br.* **2014**, *2*, 1–13.
5. Stein-O'Brien, G.L.; Ainsile, M.C.; Fertig, E.J. Forecasting cellular states: From descriptive to predictive biology via single cell multi-omics. *Curr. Opin. Syst. Biol.* **2021**, *26*, 24–32. [CrossRef]
6. Zhang, J.; Bajari, R.; Andric, D.; Gerthoffert, F.; Lepsa, A.; Nahal-Bose, H.; Stein, L.D.; Ferretti, V. The International Cancer Genome Consortium Data Portal. *Nat. Biotechnol.* **2019**, *37*, 367–369. [CrossRef]
7. Villarroel-Dorrego, M.; Whawell, S.A.; Speight, P.M.; Barrett, A.W. Transfection of CD40 in a human oral squamous cell carcinoma keratinocyte line upregulates immune potency and costimulatory molecules. *Br. J. Dermatol.* **2006**, *154*, 231–238. [CrossRef]
8. Villarroel-Dorrego, M.; Speight, P.M.; Barrett, A.W. Expression of major histocompatibility complex class II and costimulatory molecules in oral carcinomas in vitro. *Med. Oral Patol. Oral Cir. Bucal* **2005**, *10*, 188–195.
9. Szklarczyk, D.; Gable, A.L.; Lyon, D.; Junge, A.; Wyder, S.; Huerta-Cepas, J.; Simonovic, M.; Doncheva, N.T.; Morris, J.H.; Bork, P.; et al. STRING v11: Protein–protein association networks with increased coverage, supporting functional discovery in genome-wide experimental datasets. *Nucleic Acids Res.* **2019**, *47*, D607–D613. [CrossRef]
10. Chin, C.-H.; Chen, S.-H.; Wu, H.-H.; Ho, C.-W.; Ko, M.-T.; Lin, C.-Y. cytoHubba: Identifying hub objects and sub-networks from complex interactome. *BMC Syst. Biol.* **2014**, *8* (Suppl. S4), S11. [CrossRef]
11. Han, W.; Guan, W. Valproic Acid: A Promising Therapeutic Agent in Glioma Treatment. *Front. Oncol.* **2021**, *11*, 687362. [CrossRef] [PubMed]
12. Blaauboer, A.; van Koetsveld, P.M.; Mustafa, D.A.M.; Dumas, J.; Dogan, F.; van Zwienen, S.; van Eijck, C.H.J.; Hofland, L.J. The Class I HDAC Inhibitor Valproic Acid Strongly Potentiates Gemcitabine Efficacy in Pancreatic Cancer by Immune System Activation. *Biomedicines* **2022**, *10*, 517. [CrossRef] [PubMed]
13. Iannelli, F.; Zotti, A.I.; Roca, M.S.; Grumetti, L.; Lombardi, R.; Moccia, T.; Vitagliano, C.; Milone, M.R.; Ciardiello, C.; Bruzzese, F.; et al. Valproic Acid Synergizes with Cisplatin and Cetuximab in vitro and in vivo in Head and Neck Cancer by Targeting the Mechanisms of Resistance. *Front. Cell Dev. Biol.* **2020**, *8*, 732. [CrossRef] [PubMed]
14. Erlich, R.B.; Rickwood, D.; Coman, W.B.; Saunders, N.A.; Guminski, A. Valproic acid as a therapeutic agent for head and neck squamous cell carcinomas. *Cancer Chemother. Pharmacol.* **2009**, *63*, 381–389. [CrossRef]
15. Shatalova, E.G.; Klein-Szanto, A.J.; Devarajan, K.; Cukierman, E.; Clapper, M.L. Estrogen and Cytochrome P450 1B1 Contribute to Both Early- and Late-Stage Head and Neck Carcinogenesis. *Cancer Prev. Res.* **2011**, *4*, 107–115. [CrossRef]
16. Kiselev, V.Y.; Kirschner, K.; Schaub, M.T.; Andrews, T.; Yiu, A.; Chandra, T.; Natarajan, K.N.; Reik, W.; Barahona, M.; Green, A.R.; et al. SC3: Consensus clustering of single-cell RNA-seq data. *Nat. Methods* **2017**, *14*, 483–486. [CrossRef]
17. Lee, H.-M.; Patel, V.; Shyur, L.-F.; Lee, W.-L. Copper supplementation amplifies the anti-tumor effect of curcumin in oral cancer cells. *Phytomedicine* **2016**, *23*, 1535–1544. [CrossRef]
18. Puram, S.V.; Tirosh, I.; Parikh, A.S.; Patel, A.P.; Yizhak, K.; Gillespie, S.; Rodman, C.; Luo, C.L.; Mroz, E.A.; Emerick, K.S.; et al. Single-Cell Transcriptomic Analysis of Primary and Metastatic Tumor Ecosystems in Head and Neck Cancer. *Cell* **2017**, *171*, 1611–1624.e24. [CrossRef]
19. Hao, Y.; Hao, S.; Andersen-Nissen, E.; Mauck, W.M., 3rd; Zheng, S.; Butler, A.; Lee, M.J.; Wilk, A.J.; Darby, C.; Zager, M.; et al. Integrated analysis of multimodal single-cell data. *Cell* **2021**, *184*, 3573–3587.e29. [CrossRef]
20. Trapnell, C.; Cacchiarelli, D.; Grimsby, J.; Pokharel, P.; Li, S.; Morse, M.A.; Lennon, N.J.; Livak, K.J.; Mikkelsen, T.S.; Rinn, J.L. The dynamics and regulators of cell fate decisions are revealed by pseudotemporal ordering of single cells. *Nat. Biotechnol.* **2014**, *32*, 381–386. [CrossRef]
21. McInnes, L.; Healy, J.; Melville, J. Umap: Uniform manifold approximation and projection for dimension reduction. *arXiv* **2018**, arXiv:1802.03426.
22. Qiu, X.; Hill, A.; Packer, J.; Lin, D.; Ma, Y.-A.; Trapnell, C. Single-cell mRNA quantification and differential analysis with Census. *Nat. Methods* **2017**, *14*, 309–315. [CrossRef] [PubMed]
23. Mi, H.; Muruganujan, A.; Ebert, D.; Huang, X.; Thomas, P.D. PANTHER version 14: More genomes, a new PANTHER GO-slim and improvements in enrichment analysis tools. *Nucleic Acids Res.* **2019**, *47*, D419–D426. [CrossRef]
24. Yu, G.; Wang, L.-G.; Han, Y.; He, Q.-Y. clusterProfiler: An R Package for Comparing Biological Themes Among Gene Clusters. *OMICS J. Integr. Biol.* **2012**, *16*, 284–287. [CrossRef]
25. Efremova, M.; Vento-Tormo, M.; Teichmann, S.A.; Vento-Tormo, R. CellPhoneDB: Inferring cell–cell communication from combined expression of multi-subunit ligand–receptor complexes. *Nat. Protoc.* **2020**, *15*, 1484–1506. [CrossRef] [PubMed]
26. Tomczak, K.; Czerwińska, P.; Wiznerowicz, M. Review The Cancer Genome Atlas (TCGA): An immeasurable source of knowledge. *Contemp. Oncol.* **2015**, *19*, A68–A77. [CrossRef] [PubMed]
27. Newman, A.M.; Steen, C.B.; Liu, C.L.; Gentles, A.J.; Chaudhuri, A.A.; Scherer, F.; Khodadoust, M.S.; Esfahani, M.S.; Luca, B.A.; Steiner, D.; et al. Determining cell type abundance and expression from bulk tissues with digital cytometry. *Nat. Biotechnol.* **2019**, *37*, 773–782. [CrossRef]
28. Murtagh, F.; Legendre, P. Ward's hierarchical clustering method: Clustering criterion and agglomerative algorithm. *arXiv* **2011**, arXiv:1111.6285.
29. Therneau, T.M. *A Package for Survival Analysis in R*; R Package Version 2021; The R Foundation: Great Lakes, MI, USA, 2020.

30. Kassambara, A.; Kosinski, M.; Biecek, P.; Fabian, S. *survminer: Drawing Survival Curves Using 'ggplot2'*; R Package Version 0.3; The R Foundation: Great Lakes, MI, USA, 2017.
31. Shannon, P.; Markiel, A.; Ozier, O.; Baliga, N.S.; Wang, J.T.; Ramage, D.; Amin, N.; Schwikowski, B.; Ideker, T. Cytoscape: A software environment for integrated models of Biomolecular Interaction Networks. *Genome Res.* **2003**, *13*, 2498–2504. [CrossRef]
32. Wishart, D.S.; Feunang, Y.D.; Guo, A.C.; Lo, E.J.; Marcu, A.; Grant, J.R.; Sajed, T.; Johnson, D.; Li, C.; Sayeeda, Z.; et al. DrugBank 5.0: A Major Update to the DrugBank Database for 2018. *Nucleic Acids Res.* **2018**, *46*, D1074–D1082. [CrossRef]
33. Wang, Y.; Zhang, S.; Li, F.; Zhou, Y.; Zhang, Y.; Wang, Z.; Zhang, R.; Zhu, J.; Ren, Y.; Tan, Y.; et al. Therapeutic target database 2020: Enriched resource for facilitating research and early development of targeted therapeutics. *Nucleic Acids Res.* **2020**, *48*, D1031–D1041. [CrossRef] [PubMed]
34. Liu, T.; Lin, Y.; Wen, X.; Jorissen, R.N.; Gilson, M.K. BindingDB: A web-accessible database of experimentally determined protein-ligand binding affinities. *Nucleic Acids Res.* **2007**, *35*, D198–D201. [CrossRef] [PubMed]
35. Barbarino, J.M.; Whirl-Carrillo, M.; Altman, R.B.; Klein, T.E. PharmGKB: A worldwide resource for pharmacogenomic information. *WIREs Syst. Biol. Med.* **2018**, *10*, e1417. [CrossRef] [PubMed]
36. Cotto, K.C.; Wagner, A.H.; Feng, Y.-Y.; Kiwala, S.; Coffman, A.C.; Spies, G.; Wollam, A.; Spies, N.C.; Griffith, O.L.; Griffith, M. DGIdb 3.0: A redesign and expansion of the drug–gene interaction database. *Nucleic Acids Res.* **2018**, *46*, D1068–D1073. [CrossRef]
37. Armstrong, J.F.; Faccenda, E.; Harding, S.D.; Pawson, A.J.; Southan, C.; Sharman, J.L.; Campo, B.; Cavanagh, D.R.; Alexander, S.; Davenport, A.P.; et al. The IUPHAR/BPS Guide to PHARMACOLOGY in 2020: Extending immunopharmacology content and introducing the IUPHAR/MMV Guide to MALARIA PHARMACOLOGY. *Nucleic Acids Res.* **2020**, *48*, D1006–D1021. [CrossRef]
38. Davis, A.P.; Grondin, C.J.; Johnson, R.J.; Sciaky, D.; McMorran, R.; Wiegers, J.; Wiegers, T.C.; Mattingly, C. The Comparative Toxicogenomics Database: Update 2019. *Nucleic Acids Res.* **2019**, *47*, D948–D954. [CrossRef]
39. Barretina, J.; Caponigro, G.; Stransky, N.; Venkatesan, K.; Margolin, A.A.; Kim, S.; Wilson, C.J.; Lehár, J.; Kryukov, G.V.; Sonkin, D.; et al. The Cancer Cell Line Encyclopedia enables predictive modelling of anticancer drug sensitivity. *Nature* **2012**, *483*, 603–607. [CrossRef]
40. Maeser, D.; Gruener, R.F.; Huang, R.S. oncoPredict: An R package for predicting in vivo or cancer patient drug response and biomarkers from cell line screening data. *Brief. Bioinform.* **2021**, *22*, bbab260. [CrossRef]

Article

Oral *Candida* spp. Colonisation Is a Risk Factor for Severe Oral Mucositis in Patients Undergoing Radiotherapy for Head & Neck Cancer: Results from a Multidisciplinary Mono-Institutional Prospective Observational Study

Cosimo Rupe [1,*], Gioele Gioco [1], Giovanni Almadori [2], Jacopo Galli [2], Francesco Micciché [3], Michela Olivieri [3], Massimo Cordaro [1] and Carlo Lajolo [1]

[1] Head and Neck Department, Fondazione Policlinico Universitario A. Gemelli—IRCCS, School of Dentistry, Università Cattolica del Sacro Cuore, Largo A. Gemelli, 8, 00168 Rome, Italy
[2] Head and Neck Department, Fondazione Policlinico Universitario A. Gemelli—IRCCS, Institute of Otolaryngology, Università Cattolica del Sacro Cuore, Largo A. Gemelli, 8, 00168 Rome, Italy
[3] Department of Radiation Oncology, Fondazione Policlinico Universitario A. Gemelli—IRCCS, Institute of Radiology, Università Cattolica del Sacro Cuore, Largo A. Gemelli, 8, 00168 Rome, Italy
* Correspondence: cosimorupe@gmail.com

Simple Summary: This study aims to find a correlation between *Candida* spp. oral colonisation prior to radiotherapy and (i) the development of severe oral mucositis (OM) (grade 3/4) and (ii) early development of severe OM (EOM). *Candida* spp. in the oral cavity appears to be a predictive factor of EOM. Preventive treatment could aid in reducing incidence of EOM. Further clinical trials are required to confirm our findings.

Abstract: Background: This study aims to find a correlation between *Candida* spp. oral colonisation prior to radiotherapy (RT) and (i) the development of severe oral mucositis (OM) (grade 3/4) and (ii) early development of severe OM (EOM). Methods: The protocol was registered on ClinicalTrials.gov (ID: NCT04009161) and approved by the ethical committee of the 'Fondazione Policlinico Universitario Gemelli IRCCS' (22858/18). An oral swab was obtained before RT to assess the presence of *Candida* spp. Severe OM occurring before a dose of 40 Gy was defined as EOM. Results: No patient developed G4 OM, and only 36/152 patients (23.7%) developed G3 OM. Tumour site and lymphocytopenia were risk factors for severe OM (OR for tumour site: 1.29, 95% CI: 1–1.67, $p = 0.05$; OR for lymphocytopenia: 8.2, 95% CI: 1.2–55.8, $p = 0.03$). We found a correlation between *Candida* spp. and EOM (OR: 5.13; 95% CI: 1.23–21.4 $p = 0.04$). Patients with oral colonisation of *Candida* spp. developed severe OM at a mean dose of 38.3 Gy (range: 28–58; SD: 7.6), while negative patients did so at a mean dose of 45.6 Gy (range: 30–66; SD: 11.1). Conclusions: *Candida* spp. in the oral cavity appears to be a predictive factor of EOM.

Keywords: oral mucositis; radiotherapy; head and neck cancer; oral *Candida* spp.; oral candidiasis; chemotherapy; radiochemotherapy

1. Introduction

More than 900,000 new cases of head–neck cancer (HNC) are diagnosed worldwide, with 40,000 new cases and 7890 deaths reported annually in the United States. HNC can arise in multiple anatomic subsites (i.e., the oral cavity, oropharynx, hypopharynx, nasopharynx, larynx, and salivary glands) [1].

HNC treatment is challenging and requires a multidisciplinary approach with a team of specialists, including head and neck surgeons, radiation oncologists, medical oncologists, nutritionists, nuclear physicians, and oral oncologists [2,3].

Approximately 60% of patients with HNC require radiotherapy (RT), with or without induction chemotherapy [4], and a substantial proportion of patients suffer significant treatment-related adverse effects [5], including acute adverse effects (i.e., mucositis and dermatitis) that occur during treatment and late adverse effects (i.e., dysgeusia, osteoradionecrosis, and trismus) that occur in the weeks following the end of therapy [6–8].

Oral and oropharyngeal mucositis (OM) caused by RT and combined systemic therapies appears to be a significant side effect that presents numerous clinical signs and symptoms [9]. It affects the patient's quality of life (QoL) and is associated with symptoms such as pain, bleeding, dysphagia, local infections, increased susceptibility to secondary and systemic infections, impaired food intake, and weight loss [10,11]. The incidence of OM in patients treated with RT is estimated to be approximately 80%, becoming nearly ubiquitous in patients undergoing radiochemotherapy (RTCT) [12].

Severe OM (grade 3/4), according to the Radiation Therapy Oncology Group (RTOG), appears in approximately 43% of patients undergoing combination treatment [13]. It may cause inadequate food intake; this further results in the development of severe nutritional deficiencies and a need for parenteral nutrition. In addition, approximately 15% of patients require an interruption of RT or dose reshaping of concomitant systemic therapy, thus influencing the effectiveness of the treatment [14]. However, the incidence and severity of this condition varies depending on several factors (i.e., cancer subsite, radiation dose, volume of the irradiated mucosa, daily fractionation, association with CT, habit history, oral health prior to initiation of treatment, and neutrophil recovery period) [15].

Nevertheless, while dosimetric parameters are best known to correlate with the time of onset and severity of side effects, the available literature does not provide clear evidence about the clinical parameters that can predict OM development or may indicate worsening of OM [16].

Oral candidiasis is a common fungal disease caused by overgrowth of *Candida* spp. in the mouth. Acute pseudomembranous candidiasis and acute erythematous candidiasis are the most frequent clinical patterns of oral candidiasis, requiring complex treatments (i.e., adequate oral hygiene, topical agents, and systemic medications) that often lead to chronic candidiasis in patients with HNC [17,18]. Oral candidiasis, especially in its acute-erythematous manifestation, may enhance OM-related symptoms and result in worsening of the clinical condition of patients. Thus, treatment of oral candidiasis is recommended when RT in the head and neck region is scheduled. Nevertheless, *Candida* spp. can be found in 50% of the population as a component of the oral microbiota, and it can become a pathogen even after the initiation of RT [19]. Furthermore, alterations in the mucosal layer structure caused by OM often allow bacteria and fungi to penetrate damaged tissue and cause infections, increasing the risk of oral candidiasis development [20].

The primary objective of this observational prospective cohort study was to understand whether the presence of *Candida* spp. in the oral cavity, evaluated using an oral swab taken prior to initiation of RT, is a risk factor for the development of severe OM during RT. The secondary objectives were (i) to understand whether oral colonisation of *Candida* spp. is a risk factor for the early development of severe OM (EOM), defined as an OM developed at 40 Gy of the cumulative radiation dose, (ii) to understand whether other clinical parameters (radiation dose, dose received by the oral cavity and oropharynx, smoking history, white blood cell count (WBC), chemotherapy (CT), and cancer subsite) are risk factors for the development of severe OM or (iii) EOM, and (iv) to evaluate the overall incidence of OM in the studied cohort.

2. Materials and Methods

2.1. Setting

The protocol was registered on ClinicalTrials.gov (ID: NCT04009161) and was approved by the ethical committee of the 'Fondazione Policlinico Universitario A. Gemelli IRCCS in Rome' (22858/18). The study was conducted in accordance with the Declaration of Helsinki, and all patients signed an informed consent form. Patients with HNC seeking treatment at the Oral Medicine, Head and Neck Department, with a scheduled external beam RT at Gemelli Advanced Radiation Therapy (ART), Fondazione Policlinico Universitario A. Gemelli-IRCSS, between March 2017 and August 2021, were consecutively recruited for this study. All included patients visited the hospital prior to initiation of RT. This paper was written in accordance with the STROBE guidelines (Table S1).

2.2. Participants

The inclusion criteria were HNC diagnosis, indication for RT (either adjuvant or neoadjuvant), and treatment with a curative intent. The exclusion criteria were as follows: indication for palliative treatment, presence of clinically detectable signs of oral candidiasis, patients who received neoadjuvant CT before RT, and metastatic disease.

2.3. Variables—Anamnesis

Before the clinical examination, anagraphic and anamnestic data (age, sex, and co-morbidities) were recorded, particularly focusing on the oncologic history of the patient (tumour site, histological type of cancer, stage of the tumour, and previous oncologic treatments) and on the exposure to risk factors for the oncologic disease (i.e., smoking).

2.4. Variables—Oral Examination

Subsequently, clinical evaluation of the oral mucosal conditions was performed, focusing on the presence of signs of oral candidiasis.

Furthermore, oral colonisation by *Candida* spp. was recorded using a sterile swab (eSwab®®, Copan's Liquid Amies Elution Swab, Copan Italia SPA, Brescia, Italy); it was rubbed on the following mucosal surfaces of the oral cavity: hard palate, tongue, upper and lower vestibule, and ending at the commissures of the mouth. Post sample collection, sterile swabs were placed in tubes containing 1 mL of transport medium. The tubes were then stored at 4 °C until further processing. Processing involved streak inoculation of the swab onto Sabouraud dextrose agar (SDA) plates, followed by incubation at 37 °C for 48 h, according to the manufacturer's instructions.

The unstimulated salivary flow rate was assessed using the spitting method. Patients were instructed to collect saliva for 5 min in a graded tube. The stimulated salivary flow was determined in a similar manner. Saliva secretion was stimulated by applying a solution of 2% citric acid to the sides of the tongue at intervals of 30 s. An unstimulated salivary flow (USF) of over 0.4 mL/min was considered normal [21]. Furthermore, a blood count was performed before the beginning of RT, and the following variables were recorded: number of leukocytes, neutrophils, and lymphocytes. Leukopenia was defined as a leukocyte count $< 4 \times 10^9$/L, neutropenia as $<1.5 \times 10^9$/L neutrophils, and lymphocytopenia as $<1 \times 10^9$/L lymphocytes.

2.5. Variables—RT and OM

RT was delivered using the volumetric-modulated arc radiotherapy (VMAT) technique with a linear accelerator, and treatment was administered in five daily fractions per week for 6–7 weeks. The definition of volume is in accordance with international RT guidelines [22,23].

The treatment plan was optimised to ensure adequate coverage of the target (D95% of the treatment volume received > 95% of the prescribed dose) and to respect the constraints of the various organs at risk, identified during contouring.

Treatment included a daily image-guided radiation therapy (IGRT) check with Cone-Beam CT and, if necessary, the radiation dose was re-planned between 30 Gy and 40 Gy, in case of tumour shrinkage or anatomical changes. Patients were instructed to receive supportive therapy according to the centre's procedures and international guidelines [24]. Each patient underwent at least one weekly examination during RT, in which the diagnosis of OM took place: if present, OM was recorded according to the National Cancer Institute Common Toxicity Criteria for Adverse Events (CTCae, version 4.0) [25]. Each patient was assigned a single OM grade, corresponding to the most severe OM grade recorded during

RT and during the immediate RT follow-up. When OM signs disappeared, the patients terminated their study involvement. For patients who developed severe OM, the dose at which OM developed was also recorded.

According to Mallick et al., since the onset of G3-G4 OM occurs between 50 Gy and 60 Gy [26], we assumed that the onset of severe toxicity at 40 Gy should be considered as early acute toxicity. Onset of OM at a dose of 40 Gy or less was defined as an 'early onset mucositis (EOM)'.

Severe OM was managed according to the centre's procedures and international guidelines: in case of G3 OM, the patients were treated by analgesic drugs to reduce the pain [24].

2.6. Statistical Analysis

The sample size was calculated, with a 90% confidence level and 80% power, by comparing two proportions: considering 45% as the expected incidence of severe OM in the presence of *Candida* spp. in the oral cavity and 25% as the expected incidence in the absence of oral colonisation of *Candida* spp. The required sample size was 136 patients, with 68 in each group (positive or negative for oral cavity swabs). Considering a dropout rate of 10%, the final sample size was 150 patients.

The following variables were recorded as baseline patient characteristics (sex, age, histological type and stage of the tumour, site of the tumour, risk factors such as smoking history, previous oncological surgery, salivary flow, presence of *Candida* spp. oral colonisation), basal treatment characteristics (scheduled CT, Total Radiation Dose, daily fraction, dose received by the oral cavity and oropharynx), and treatment-related toxicity parameters (presence and grade of OM).

Qualitative variables were described using absolute and percentage frequencies, while the Kolmogorov–Smirnov test was performed to evaluate the normal distribution of quantitative variables. Quantitative variables were summarised either as mean and standard deviation (SD) if normally distributed, or as median and percentiles otherwise.

OM was reclassified into three categories: absence of OM, grade I or II OM, and grade 3 or 4 OM.

Correlation analysis between OM onset and clinical characteristics of the patients was performed. The Mann–Whitney U test and Kruskall–Wallis test were performed to compare the continuous variables with non-parametric distribution, while the parametric variables were analysed through an ANOVA test; Pearson's χ^2 test and Fisher's exact test were used to compare the discontinuous variables. Statistical analysis was stratified according to the following variables: development of severe OM and early onset of severe OM.

Univariate analysis was performed to determine the risk factors associated with the onset of OM, and risk factors were introduced in a stepwise logistic regression analysis to identify independent predictors of OM. The same statistical analysis was used to determine risk factors for EOM. All statistical analyses were performed using IBM SPSS Statistics software (IBM Corp. Released 2017. IBM SPSS Statistics for Apple, Version 25.0 (IBM Corp., Armonk, NY, USA).

3. Results

One hundred and sixty-three patients were enrolled in the study; 11 patients were excluded per the inclusion criteria: 5 patients suffered from oral candidiasis at baseline, so they were treated but excluded from the final sample, whereas 6 patients had received a planning for a palliative treatment. The final sample included 152 patients (49 female and 103 male), with a mean age of 60.3 years (range: 22–86). One hundred and fifteen (75.7%) patients had locally advanced oncologic disease (stage III–IV), 93 patients (61.2%) received treatment with curative intent, and 59 patients (38.8%) received adjuvant treatment. Oral cavity swabs were positive in 68 of the 152 patients (44.7%), and the remaining (84/152, 55.3%) swabs showed negative results prior to the initiation of RT. The mean total RT dose was 67.6 Gy (50–72), and the dose was fractionated in 2 Gy/die in majority of the patients (136/152, 89.5%). One hundred and twenty patients out of 152 (78.9% of the total sample) developed OM. Severe OM occurred in 36 patients (23.7% of the total sample). None of the patients developed G4 OM. Termination of RT before reaching the target dose was not required in any patient, and all patients completed their scheduled treatment; three patients had to discontinue RT for a few days. However, they still finished their RT course. Patient and treatment characteristics and related toxicity parameters are shown in Table 1.

Table 1. Basal patients' characteristics, basal treatment characteristics of the studied population and treatment related toxicity parameters. SD: standard deviation; SCC: squamous cell carcinoma, RT: radiotherapy.

Variable	Group	N (%)
Gender	Men	103 (67.8%)
	Women	49 (32.2%)
	Total	152 (100%)
Age	Mean	60.3 (22–86; SD: 11.5)
Comorbidities	Yes	75 (49.3%)
	No	77 (50.7%)
	Total	152 (100%)
Tumour Type	SCC	130 (85.5%)
	Other types	22 (14.5%)
	Total	152 (100%)
Tumour Stage	Stage 1	10 (6.5%)
	Stage 2	27 (17.8%)
	Stage 3	38 (25%)
	Stage 4	77 (50.7%)
	Total	152 (100%)
Tumour Site	Hipopharynx	9 (5.9%)
	Larynx	28 (18.4%)
	Oral cavity	28 (18.4%)
	Oropharynx	38 (25%)
	Rhinopharynx	19 (12.6%)
	Salivary Glands	14 (9.2%)
	Other sites	16 (10.5%)
	Total	152 (100%)
Smoking	Smokers	87 (57.2%)
	Non smokers	65 (42.8%)
	Total	152 (100%)
Surgery	Performed	59 (38.8%)
	Not performed	93 (61.2%)
	Total	152 (100%)

Table 1. Cont.

Variable	Group	N (%)
Chemotherapy	Performed	86 (56.6%)
	Not Performed	66 (43.4%)
	Total	152 (100%)
White Blood Cell Count	Leucocytes (10^9/L, Mean)	6.7 (1.6–15.1; SD: 2.5)
	Neutrophils (10^9/L, Mean)	4.6 (0.7–11.8; SD: 2.1)
	Lymphocytes (10^9/L, Mean)	2.2 (0.6–11.4; SD: 1.2)
Leukopenia	Yes	19
	No	133
	Total	152 (100%)
Neutropenia	Yes	4
	No	148
	Total	152 (100%)
Lymphocytopenia	Yes	15
	No	137
	Total	152 (100%)
Salivary Flow	mL (Mean)	2.6 (0–15; SD: 2.2)
Hyposalivation (<2 mL)	Yes (n. of Patients)	79 (51.9%)
	No (n. of Patients)	73 (48.1%)
	Total	152 (100%)
Oral Candida	Positive Oral Cavity Swab	68 (44.7%)
	Negative Oral Cavity Swab	84 (55.3%)
	Total	152 (100%)
Total RT Dose	Gy (Mean)	67.6 (50–72; SD: 3.9)
Fractioning Schedule	1.8 Gy/die	1 (0.7%)
	2 Gy/die	136 (89.5%)
	2.2 Gy/die	14 (9.2%)
	2.4 Gy/die	1 (0.7%)
	Total	152 (100%)
Oral RT Dose	Gy (Mean)	36.8 (0–75.2; SD: 16.9)
Oropharynx RT Dose	Gy (Mean)	50.3 (0–71.3; SD: 18.9)
Oral Mucositis	Absence	32 (21.1%)
	Grade 1	40 (26.3%)
	Grade 2	44 (28.9%)
	Grade 3	36 (23.7%)
	Grade 4	0 (0%)
	Total	152 (100%)

The study flow chart is presented in Figure 1.

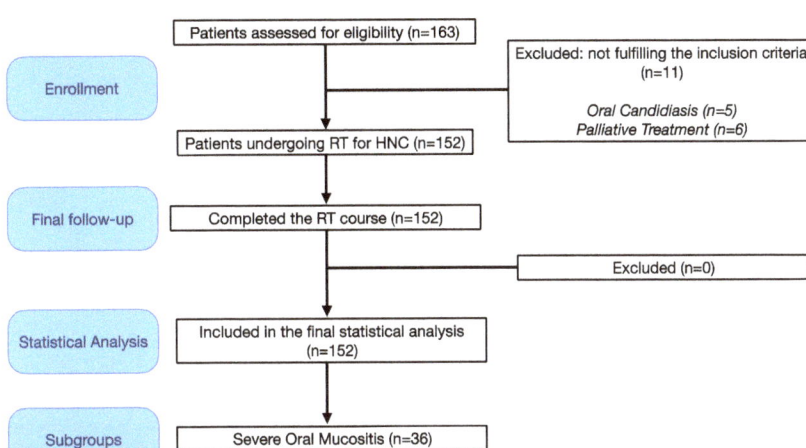

Figure 1. Strobe flow chart of the study.

Results of the statistical analysis stratified according to the development of severe OM are shown in Table 2.

In the univariate analysis, the clinical parameters associated with severe OM onset were the tumour site and RT-CT treatment. Patients with different tumour sites showed a different incidence of severe OM (χ^2 test, $p < 0.05$), and nasopharyngeal cancers were associated with the highest incidence of OM (9/19 patients, 47.4%), while laryngeal cancers had the lowest incidence of OM (1/28, 3.6%). Patients who developed severe OM (25/36 patients; 69.4%) were more frequently treated with combined RT-CT (χ^2 test, $p = 0.05$), while patients who did not develop severe OM often did not receive combined treatment (61/116; 52.6%). The prevalence of oral colonisation of *Candida* spp. was higher in patients with severe OM (20/36; 55.6%) than in other patients in the cohort (48/116; 41.4%), but the correlation was not statistically significant. Furthermore, severe OM correlated with leukopenia, neutropenia, and lymphocytopenia (χ^2 test, $p < 0.05$). However, when inserted in a multiple logistic regression model, only tumour site and lymphocytopenia were statistically significant risk factors for severe OM development (OR for tumour site: 1.29, 95% CI: 1–1.67, $p = 0.05$; OR for lymphocytopenia: 8.2, 95% CI: 1.2–55.8, $p = 0.03$).

Table 3 summarises the characteristics of patients who developed EOM. Oral colonisation by *Candida* spp. was correlated with an early onset of severe OM in the univariate analysis (χ^2 test, $p < 0.05$), showing that the presence of *Candida* spp. in the oral cavity is a risk factor for the development of EOM (OR: 5.13, 95% CI: 1.23–21.4 $p = 0.04$). Patients with oral colonisation by *Candida* spp. developed severe OM at a mean dose of 38.3 Gy (range: 28–58), while patients with negative oral swabs developed severe OM at a mean dose of 45.6 Gy (range: 30–66). From a clinical point of view, these patients experienced severe OM approximately four days before those with a negative swab.

Table 2. Clinical variables of the studied population, according to the development of severe mucositis.

		Total Sample	Severe Mucositis		Statistical Significance
		152 (100%)	Yes 36 (23.7%)	No 116 (76.3%)	
Gender	Male	103 (67.8%)	28 (27.2%)	75 (72.8%)	χ^2 Test—$p = 0.64$
	Female	49 (32.2%)	8 (16.3%)	41 (83.7%)	
Age	Mean (Range; SD)	60.3 (22–86; 11.5)	58.7 (22–75; 10.5)	60.8 (29–86, 11.8)	ANOVA—$p = 0.83$
Total RT dose (Gy)	Mean (Range; SD)	67.6 (50–72; 3.9)	68.2 (60–70; 2.7)	67.4 (50–72; 4.2)	Mann–Whitney—$p = 0.56$
Mean oral cavity dose (Gy)	Mean (Range; SD)	36.8 (0–70; 16.9)	38.8 (0.8–65.9; 17.1)	36.2 (0–70; 16.9)	ANOVA—$p = 0.427$
Mean oropharynx dose (Gy)	Mean (Range; SD)	50.3 (0–71.3; 18.9)	50.7 (2.5–70.4; 22.3)	50.2 (0–71.3; 17.8)	Mann–Whitney—$p = 0.22$
Leucocytes ($10^9/l$) [a,e]	Mean (Range; SD)	6.7 (1.6–15.1; 2.5)	4.9 (1.6–13.5; 2.4)	7.2 (3.0–15.1; 2.4)	Mann–Whitney—$p = 0.001$
Neutrophils ($10^9/l$) [b]	Mean (Range; SD)	4.6 (0.7–11.8; 2.1)	3.7 (0.7–11.8; 2.1)	4.8 (1.5–10.9; 2.0)	Mann–Whitney—$p = 0.01$
Lymphocytes ($10^9/l$) [c]	Mean (Range; SD)	2.2 (0.6–11.4; 1.2)	1.3 (0.7–5.8; 0.8)	2.5 (0.6–11.4; 1.1)	Mann–Whitney—$p = 0.001$
Leukopenia [d]	Yes	19 (12.5%)	15 (41.7%)	4 (3.5%)	χ^2 Test—$p = 0.001$
	No	133 (87.5%)	21 (58.3%)	112 (96.5%)	
Neutropenia [e]	Yes	4 (2.6%)	3 (8.4%)	1 (0.9%)	χ^2 Test—$p = 0.04$
	No	148 (97.4%)	33 (91.6%)	115 (99.1%)	
Lymphocytopenia [f,i]	Yes	15 (9.9%)	13 (36.1%)	2 (1.8%)	χ^2 Test—$p = 0.001$
	No	137 (90.1%)	23 (63.9%)	114 (98.2%)	
Comorbidities	Yes	75 (49.3%)	15 (20%)	60 (80%)	χ^2 Test—$p = 0.34$
	No	77 (50.7%)	21 (27.3%)	56 (72.7%)	
Tumour type	SCC	130 (85.5%)	32 (24.6%)	98 (75.4%)	χ^2 Test—$p = 0.13$
	Other types	22 (14.5%)	3 (13.6%)	19 (86.4%)	
Tumour site [g,i]	Larynx	28 (18.4%)	1 (3.6%)	27 (96.4%)	
	Oral cavity	28 (18.4%)	9 (32.1%)	19 (67.9%)	
	Oropharynx	38 (25%)	12 (31.6%)	26 (68.4%)	
	Rhinopharynx	19 (12.5%)	9 (47.4%)	10 (52.6%)	χ^2 Test—$p = 0.006$
	Salivary Glands	14 (9.2%)	1 (7.1%)	13 (92.9%)	
	Hypoparynx	9 (5.9%)	1 (11.1%)	8 (88.9%)	
	Other sites	16 (10.5%)	3 (18.7%)	13 (81.3%)	
	Stage I	10 (6.6%)	2 (20%)	8 (80%)	
	Stage II	27 (17.8%)	4 (14.8%)	23 (85.2%)	
	Stage III	38 (25%)	10 (26.3%)	28 (73.7%)	
	Stage IV	77 (50.6%)	20 (25.9%)	57 (74.1%)	
Chemotherapy [h]	Yes	86 (56.6%)	25 (29.1%)	61 (70.9%)	χ^2 Test—$p = 0.05$
	No	66 (43.4%)	11 (16.7%)	55 (83.3%)	
Surgery	Performed	59 (38.8%)	11 (18.6%)	48 (81.4%)	χ^2 Test—$p = 0.32$
	Non performed	93 (61.2%)	25 (26.9%)	68 (73.1%)	
Smoking	Yes	87 (57.2%)	21 (24.1%)	66 (75.9%)	χ^2 Test—$p = 0.52$
	No	65 (42.8%)	15 (23.1%)	50 (76.9%)	
Oral candida swab	Positive	68 (44.7%)	20 (29.4%)	48 (70.6%)	χ^2 Test—$p = 0.097$
	Negative	84 (55.3%)	16 (19%)	68 (81%)	
Hyposalivation (<2 mL)	Yes	79 (51.9%)	60 (75.9%)	19 (24.1%)	χ^2 Test—$p = 0.53$
	No	73 (48.1%)	56 (76.7%)	17 (23.3%)	

[a] Correlation between leucocytes and severe OM—Mann–Whitney test—$p < 0.05$. [b] Correlation between neutrophils and severe OM—Mann–Whitney test—$p < 0.05$. [c] Correlation between lymphocytes and severe OM—Mann–Whitney test—$p < 0.05$. [d] Correlation between Leukopenia and severe OM—χ^2 Test—$p < 0.05$. [e] Correlation between neutropenia and severe OM—χ^2 Test—$p < 0.05$. [f] Correlation between lymphocytopenia and severe OM—χ^2 Test—$p < 0.05$. [g] Correlation between tumour site and severe OM—χ^2 Test—$p < 0.05$. [h] Correlation between chemotherapy and severe OM—χ^2 Test—$p = 0.05$. [i] Multiple Logistic Regression showed how tumour site and lymphocytopenia are risk factors for severe OM: tumour site—OR: 1.29, 95% CI: 1–1.67, $p = 0.05$. Lymphocytopenia-OR: 8.2, 95% CI: 1.2–55.8, $p = 0.03$.

Table 3. Clinical variables of the studied population, according to the development of severe mucositis. WBC: white blood cell count.

		Total Sample	Early Onset Severe OM		Statistical Significance
		36 (100%)	Yes 19 (52.8%)	No 17 (47.2%)	
Gender	Male	28 (77.8%)	13 (46.4%)	15 (53.6%)	χ^2 Test—$p = 0.24$
	Female	8 (22.2%)	6 (75%)	2 (25%)	
Comorbidities	Yes	15 (43.1%)	8 (53.3%)	7 (46.7%)	χ^2 Test—$p = 0.9$
	No	21 (56.9%)	11 (52.4%)	10 (47.5%)	
Age	Mean (Range; SD)	58.7 (22–75; 10.5)	59.1 (22–70; 11.7)	58.3 (43–75; 9.2)	ANOVA—$p = 0.19$
Total rt dose (Gy)	Mean (Range; SD)	68.2 (60–70; 2.7)	68.4 (60–70; 2.7)	68 (60–70; 2.8)	Mann-Whitney—$p = 0.69$
Mean oral cavity dose (Gy)	Mean (Range; SD)	38.8 (0.8–65.9; 17.1)	37.9 (3.4–65.9; 17.1)	39.7 (0.8–63.7; 17.6)	ANOVA—$p = 0.75$
Mean oropharynx dose (Gy)	Mean (Range; SD)	50.7 (2.5–70.4; 22.3)	49.4 (2.7–70.4; 24.6)	52 (2.5–69.2; 19.9)	Mann-Whitney—$p = 0.75$
WBC (10^9/l)	Leucocytes (Range; SD)	4.9 (1.6–13.5; 2.4)	5.1 (2.5–8.9; 1.9)	4.6 (1.6–13.5; 2.9)	Mann-Whitney—0.45
	Neutrophils (Range; SD)	3.7 (0.7–11.8; 2.1)	3.7 (1.7–7.1; 1.5)	3.5 (0.7–11.7; 2.4)	Mann-Whitney—0.21
	Lymphocytes (Range; SD)	1.3 (0.7–5.8; 0.8)	1.4 (0.7–5.7; 1.1)	1.1 (0.6–1.7; 0.3)	Mann-Whitney—0.18
Leukopenia	Yes	15 (41.7%)	7 (46.7%)	8 (53.3%)	χ^2 Test—$p = 0.73$
	No	21 (58.3%)	12 (57.1%)	9 (42.9%)	
Neutropenia	Yes	3 (8.4%)	0 (-)	3 (100%)	χ^2 Test—$p = 0.09$
	No	33 (91.6%)	19 (57.6%)	14 (42.4%)	
Lymphocytopenia	Yes	13 (36.1%)	5 (38.4%)	8 (61.6%)	χ^2 Test—$p = 0.3$
	No	23 (63.9%)	14 (60.9%)	9 (39.1%)	
Tumour type	SCC	32 (88.9%)	17 (53.1%)	15 (46.9%)	χ^2 Test—$p = 0.79$
	Other types	4 (11.1%)	2 (50%)	2 (50%)	
Tumour site	Larynx	1 (2.8%)	1 (100%)	0 (-)	
	Oral cavity	9 (25%)	5 (55.6%)	4 (44.4%)	
	Oropharynx	12 (66.7%)	4 (33.3%)	8 (66.7%)	
	Rhinopharynx	9 (25%)	6 (66.7%)	3 (33.3%)	χ^2 Test—$p = 0.17$
	Salivary Glands	1 (2.8%)	0 (-)	1 (100%)	
	Hypoparynx	1 (2.8%)	0 (-)	1 (100%)	
	Other sites	3 (2.8%)	3 (100%)	0 (-)	
	Stage I	2 (5.6%)	2 (100%)	0 (-)	
	Stage II	4 (11.2%)	1 (25%)	3 (75%)	
	Stage III	10 (27.8%)	6 (60%)	4 (40%)	
	Stage IV	20 (55.6%)	10 (50%)	10 (50%)	
Chemotherapy	Yes	25 (69.4%)	14 (56%)	11 (44%)	χ^2 Test—$p = 0.72$
	No	11 (30.6%)	5 (45.5%)	6 (54.5%)	
Surgery	Performed	11 (30.6%)	5 (45.5%)	6 (54.5%)	χ^2 Test—$p = 0.72$
	Non performed	25 (69.4%)	14 (56%)	11 (44%)	
Smoking	Yes	21 (58.3%)	11 (52.4%)	10 (47.6%)	χ^2 Test—$p = 0.61$
	No	15 (41.7%)	8 (53.3%)	7 (46.7%)	
Oral candida swab [a]	Positive	20 (55.6%)	14 (70%)	6 (30%)	χ^2 Test—$p = 0.04$
	Negative	16 (44.4%)	5 (31.3%)	11 (68.7%)	
Hyposalivation (<2 mL)	Yes	17 (47.2%)	5 (29.4%)	12 (70.6%)	χ^2 Test—$p = 0.06$
	No	19 (52.8%)	12 (63.2%)	7 (36.8%)	

[a] Correlation between oral candida and early onset severe OM—χ^2 Test—$p < 0.05$; (OR: 5.13, 95% CI: 1.23–21.4 $p = 0.04$).

4. Discussion

RT has played a fundamental role in the multidisciplinary management of patients with HNC over the last few decades. Nevertheless, some adverse events such as OM are a major concern for clinicians. OM is an acute inflammation that may initially manifest as redness of the mucous membrane, which eventually evolves into ulceration and formation of a pseudomembrane, leading to a temporary disruption of mucosal integrity [27]. OM pathogenesis, according to the most widely accepted biological model, appears to be a complex multistep process. This theory, proposed by Sonis et al. [28], describes an initiation phase, followed by upregulation and activation, signal amplification, ulceration, and ultimately a healing phase. It is crucial to understand that OM does not simply result from the epithelial injury caused during RT or CT; the epithelium, the underlying connective tissue, and the type of injury are the main characteristics of this mechanism, although other factors (the oral environment, immunological conditions, and performance status) also play a role in OM pathogenesis. Despite the wide interest in this topic, evidence regarding the risk factors for OM is limited, representing a challenge for healthcare professionals involved in the supportive care field [29]; in particular, mycetes harbouring in the oral cavity could play a pathogenic role in the onset and perpetuation of OM. Few studies have investigated the possible role of *Candida* spp. in the onset of OM.

The main objective of this study was to identify the clinical impact of oral *Candida* spp. colonisation on OM onset and its possible effects on OM severity. Although the prevalence of *Candida* spp. in the oral cavity was higher in patients with severe OM (20/36; 55.6%) than in other patients of the cohort (48/116; 41.4%), this correlation was not statistically significant (χ^2 test, $p = 0.097$). Nevertheless, in our population, *Candida* spp. was identified as the only risk factor for EOM (OR: 5.13, 95% CI: 1.23–21.4 $p = 0.04$; Table 3).

The early onset of severe OM is a critical issue in the HNC patients' management, since it may further reduce the QoL of patients [30] and may increase the need for intensive supportive care and hospitalisation [31] and the need for treatment interruption, impairing the control of the disease [32]. Several studies have demonstrated a correlation between EOM and different CT regimens, RT dose per fraction, and treatment timing; however, [33] no studies have demonstrated a correlation between EOM and *Candida* spp. colonisation. Although the reason why *Candida* spp. colonisation resulted as the only risk factor for EOM is unclear, several hypotheses can be put forward. First, *Candida* spp. may accelerate the cascade of events leading to OM through their virulence factors, which can directly damage the epithelial layer by the production of cytolytic enzymes (proteinases, hemolysins, siderophores, and phospholipases) [34]. In addition, as highlighted by in vitro studies [35], *Candida* spp. blastospores may stimulate peripheral blood mononuclear cells to secrete tumour necrosis α (TNF-α) and the type 1 cytokine interferon-γ (IFN-γ), which contribute to OM pathogenesis [28]. However, it has been demonstrated that *Candida* spp. may influence bacterial growth, especially in the oral cavity, through different interaction mechanisms (adhesion and quorum sensing) [36]. This condition may cause a worsening of OM; in fact, it has been hypothesized that dynamic changes in the oral microbial community composition may be involved in OM pathogenesis [37]. HNC patients, often dentally compromised even before the initiation of RT [38], show microbial and inflammatory profiles different from healthy individuals [39], which probably contributes to the high incidence of OM in this group of patients.

Furthermore, an irradiated oral and oropharyngeal mucosa presents an ideal environment that favours opportunistic oral candidiasis; and ulcerations in the mucosal layer structure caused by OM may allow fungal penetration into the damaged tissue [20], enhancing the interactions between *Candida* spp. and the connective tissues. The ongoing inflammatory process, resulting in an anaerobic condition, could promote interactions between *Candida* spp. and pathogenic bacteria of the oral cavity [36]. Although not definitively proven, it is likely that RT may slightly change the oral microbiota composition, favouring the onset of oral candidiasis [40]. Another issue is that irradiated patients may often experience an impairment of the local and systemic immune systems, as highlighted by our findings (leukopenia was present in 12.5% of our samples) and previously published papers [41]. Furthermore, *Candida* spp. hyphae induce a higher production of IL-10, an immunosuppressive cytokine, indirectly worsening the local immune response [35]. Another factor that can be involved in this process is the reduction in salivary flow in irradiated patients. Although hyposalivation is considered a late-onset RT adverse event, it has been demonstrated that salivary flow may be reduced to 50–70% of the baseline after 10–16 Gy of RT [20,42]. Radiation induces a decrease in amylase activity, bicarbonate levels, and pH and a significant increase in the viscosity [43] of saliva, mainly due to the disruption of the mucin network [44], which could promote the transformation of Candida spp. into a pathogen. A recent observational study demonstrated that Candida spp. had higher biofilm formation capability in a population of irradiated patients than in healthy individuals [45]. Nevertheless, our findings do not demonstrate a direct correlation between hyposalivation and EOM; thus, further studies are required to evaluate this hypothesis.

Previous studies have investigated the role of Candida spp. in irradiated HNC patients, with contradictory results. Singh et al. [19] argued that OM is a risk factor for oral candidiasis, suggesting that Candida spp. may overinfect pre-existing lesions. Suryawanshi et al. [46] concluded that Candida spp. colonisation does not influence the severity of OM, whereas oropharyngeal candidiasis may play a role in increasing the duration and discomfort of OM. In contrast, Rao et al. [47] found that biweekly prophylactic administration of fluconazole, an antimycotic, during RT-CT for HNC reduced the incidence of OM. Although their study was retrospective and lacked a control group or a pre-RT Candida spp. colonisation assessment, our findings may confirm their interesting results. Further clinical trials, designed to investigate this specific outcome, are needed to confirm this hypothesis; performing an oral swab before starting RT should be considered a routine procedure during pre-RT dental evaluation, given its low cost and the potential impact of Candida spp. on OM. Future studies should evaluate the preventive eradication of Candida spp. and assess whether this therapy has a positive effect in reducing the incidence of EOM.

Other important results retrieved by this study include the incidence of OM in a cohort of patients with HNC and the role of other possible risk factors for OM. Among the studied population, while the overall incidence of OM was 78.9%, in accordance with the 80% estimate reported by Trotti et al. [13], only 36 of 152 (23.7%) patients developed severe OM, which is a lower rate than that reported in previous studies [30]. While severe OM occurred in 36 out of the 152 patents, no patient developed G4 or G5 OM. The low incidence of severe OM might have been due to the use of the VMAT technique, which helps reduce the duration of RT sessions and spares healthy tissues [48].

Based on the results of the multiple logistic regression, two main clinical parameters were significantly associated with a higher incidence of severe OM: the site of the tumour (OR: 1.29, 95% CI: 1–1.67, $p = 0.05$) and lymphocytopenia (OR: 8.2, 95% CI: 1.2–55.8, $p = 0.03$).

As expected, the larynx had the lowest incidence of severe OM (1/28 patients, 3.6%), followed by the hypopharynx (1/9 patients, 11%). In contrast, the nasopharynx was the site that showed the highest incidence (9/19 patients, 47.7%). This finding confirms the results of the vast majority of the literature [41,49], and can be due to the introduction of more targeted radiation therapy techniques and the use of increasingly smaller treatment volumes (PTV) in clinical practice, which helped to spare the oral and oropharyngeal mucosa, maintaining clinical efficacy on the tumoural tissues.

Although a few studies have investigated the role of lymphocytopenia in the onset of OM [41] and found a correlation, the evidence is still limited [29]. It is reasonable to think that lymphocytopenia may have a direct or indirect role in modulating the inflammatory process leading to OM (i.e., dysregulation of the inflammatory processes and enhancement of the risk of bacterial colonisation of the epithelium, which stimulates cytokine production); however, the effective role of lymphocytes in the pathogenesis of OM needs to be clarified by other studies. Notably, Munneke et al., in a randomised clinical trial, highlighted how activated innate lymphoid cells are associated with reduced susceptibility to OM in a cohort of patients undergoing allogeneic haematopoietic stem cell transplantation (HSCT) [50], thus indirectly confirming our findings.

Previous studies have revealed how concomitant CT can predict OM in patients with HNC [10,16,51]. Our results, in accordance with the previous results, showed a higher incidence (χ^2 test, $p < 0.05$) of severe OM (29.1%) in RT-CT-treated patients than in patients treated with RT alone (16.7%). However, when included in a logistic regression model, this correlation was not statistically significant. Similarly, CT was not a statistically significant risk factor for EOM. It is likely that the number of patients treated with concomitant CT (86 patients) within our sample was not sufficient to draw statistically significant results.

This study has several strengths. Our results revealed how severe OM developed significantly earlier in patients with HNC with oral *Candida* spp. colonisation prior to initiation of RT. To our knowledge, this is the first study to prospectively investigate this relationship in patients with HNC undergoing RT, and its novelty lies in the fact that it highlights how oral *Candida* spp. can also play a crucial role in the onset of severe OM, apart from the simple overinfection of already existing lesions.

Furthermore, since this was a monocentric study, the RT treatment plan was always decided by the same radiotherapist (F.M.) with the same device, and the whole sample was homogeneous by mean total dose of radiation, which allowed the identification of risk factors different from the RT dose or RT technique.

This study also had some limitations. Its monocentric nature may have limited the reliability of our results on a larger scale, especially regarding the effects of different types of RT and other devices. Furthermore, because this study aimed to evaluate the onset of OM as a primary outcome, the duration of severe OM was not recorded. These data, however, need to be recorded in future studies and will contribute to a deeper description and understanding of the clinical impact of OM in terms of the number of visits during therapy, supportive therapy, economic burden, and perceived QoL changes. Another possible limitation of this study may be the lack of evaluation of the oral microbiota of included patients; it was not possible to carry out this analysis given its high economic impact. Nevertheless, given its significance in promoting the occurrence of oral candidiasis, further studies should evaluate its impact on opportunistic infection-related diseases.

5. Conclusions

In conclusion, our findings show that oral colonisation by *Candida* spp. is a predictive factor for EOM. Performing an oral swab test before initiation of RT should be considered as a routine procedure during pre-RT dental evaluation, given its low cost and the impact of *Candida* spp. on OM. Therefore, physicians, dentists, and otolaryngologists should be aware that OM prevention strategies should be implemented before the initiation of RT in patients with positive oral cavity swabs. Future studies should evaluate the preventive eradication of *Candida* spp. and assess whether this therapy has a positive effect in reducing the incidence of EOM.

Supplementary Materials: The following supporting information can be downloaded at https://www.mdpi.com/article/10.3390/cancers14194746/s1: Table S1: STROBE Guidelines.

Author Contributions: Conceptualization, C.R., C.L. and F.M.; methodology, C.R. and C.L; software, C.R. and C.L.; validation, M.C., J.G. and G.A.; formal analysis, C.R. and C.L.; investigation, M.O. and G.G.; data curation, C.R. and C.L.; writing—original draft preparation, C.R.; writing—review and editing, C.L. and F.M.; visualization, G.G.; supervision, M.C., J.G. and G.A.; project administration, C.L. All authors have read and agreed to the published version of the manuscript.

Funding: This research received no external funding.

Institutional Review Board Statement: This study was conducted in accordance with the Declaration of Helsinki, approved by the Ethics Committee of the Università Cattolica del Sacro Cuore (Ref. 22858/18) and registered at ClinicalTrials.gov (ID: NCT04009161).

Informed Consent Statement: Informed consent was obtained from all subjects involved in the study.

Data Availability Statement: The data presented in this study are available on request from the corresponding authors. The data are not publicly available because of privacy concerns.

Acknowledgments: The authors would like to acknowledge the help received from Sunstar Europe S.A., Route de Pallatex 11, P.O. Box 32, 1163 Etoy, Switzerland. (prot. CA-19–0888).

Conflicts of Interest: The authors declare no conflict of interest.

References

1. Sung, H.; Ferlay, J.; Siegel, R.; Laversanne, M.; Soerjomataram, I.; Jemal, A.; Bray, F. Global Cancer Statistics 2020: GLOBOCAN Estimates of Incidence and Mortality Worldwide for 36 Cancers in 185 Countries. *CA Cancer J. Clin.* **2021**, *71*, 209–249. [CrossRef] [PubMed]
2. Berrone, M.; Lajolo, C.; De Corso, E.; Settimi, S.; Rupe, C.; Crosetti, E.; Succo, G. Cooperation between ENT surgeon and dentist in head and neck oncology. *Acta Otorhinolaryngol. Ital.* **2021**, *41*, S124–S137. [CrossRef] [PubMed]
3. Liu, J.; Kaplon, A.; Mph, M.; Miyamoto, C.; Savior, D.; Ragin, C. The impact of the multidisciplinary tumor board on head and neck cancer outcomes. *Laryngoscope* **2019**, *130*, 946–950. [CrossRef] [PubMed]
4. Marur, S.; Forastiere, A.A. Head and Neck Squamous Cell Carcinoma: Update on Epidemiology, Diagnosis, and Treatment. *Mayo Clin. Proc.* **2016**, *91*, 386–396. [CrossRef]
5. Langendijk, J.A.; Doornaert, P.; Leeuw, I.V.-D.; Leemans, C.R.; Aaronson, N.K.; Slotman, B. Impact of Late Treatment-Related Toxicity on Quality of Life Among Patients with Head and Neck Cancer Treated with Radiotherapy. *J. Clin. Oncol.* **2008**, *26*, 3770–3776. [CrossRef]
6. Lajolo, C.; Gioco, G.; Rupe, C.; Troiano, G.; Cordaro, M.; Lucchese, A.; Paludetti, G.; Giuliani, M. Tooth extraction before radiotherapy is a risk factor for developing osteoradionecrosis of the jaws: A systematic review. *Oral Dis.* **2020**, *27*, 1595–1605. [CrossRef]
7. Lajolo, C.; Rupe, C.; Gioco, G.; Troiano, G.; Patini, R.; Petruzzi, M.; Micciche', F.; Giuliani, M. Osteoradionecrosis of the Jaws Due to Teeth Extractions during and after Radiotherapy: A Systematic Review. *Cancers* **2021**, *13*, 5798. [CrossRef]
8. Massaccesi, M.; Dinapoli, N.; Fuga, V.; Rupe, C.; Panfili, M.; Calandrelli, R.; Settimi, S.; Olivieri, M.; Bartoli, F.B.; Mazzarella, C.; et al. A predictive nomogram for trismus after radiotherapy for head and neck cancer. *Radiother. Oncol.* **2022**, *173*, 231–239. [CrossRef]
9. De Sanctis, V.; Bossi, P.; Sanguineti, G.; Trippa, F.; Ferrari, D.; Bacigalupo, A.; Ripamonti, C.I.; Buglione, M.; Pergolizzi, S.; Langendijk, J.A.; et al. Mucositis in head and neck cancer patients treated with radiotherapy and systemic therapies: Literature review and consensus statements. *Crit. Rev. Oncol. Hematol.* **2016**, *100*, 147–166. [CrossRef]
10. Elting, L.S.; Cooksley, C.D.; Chambers, M.S.; Garden, A.S. Risk, Outcomes, and Costs of Radiation-Induced Oral Mucositis Among Patients with Head-and-Neck Malignancies. *Int. J. Radiat. Oncol. Biol. Phys.* **2007**, *68*, 1110–1120. [CrossRef]
11. Elting, L.; Keefe, D.M.; Sonis, S.T.; Garden, A.S.; Spijkervet, F.K.; Barasch, A.; Tishler, R.B.; Canty, T.P.; Kudrimoti, M.K.; Vera-Llonch, M. Patient-reported measurements of oral mucositis in head and neck cancer patients treated with radiotherapy with or without chemotherapy: Demonstration of increased frequency, severity, resistance to palliation, and impact on quality of life. *Cancer* **2008**, *13*, 2704–2713. [CrossRef] [PubMed]
12. Sonis, S.T. Oral Mucositis in Head and Neck Cancer: Risk, Biology, and Management. *Am. Soc. Clin. Oncol. Educ. Book* **2013**, *33*, e236–e240. [CrossRef]
13. Trotti, A.; Bellm, L.A.; Epstein, J.B.; Frame, D.; Fuchs, H.J.; Gwede, C.K.; Komaroff, E.; Nalysnyk, L.; Zilberberg, M.D. Mucositis incidence, severity and associated outcomes in patients with head and neck cancer receiving radiotherapy with or without chemotherapy: A systematic literature review. *Radiother. Oncol.* **2003**, *66*, 253–262. [CrossRef]
14. Bese, N.; Hendry, J.; Jeremic, B. Effects of Prolongation of Overall Treatment Time Due to Unplanned Interruptions During Radiotherapy of Different Tumor Sites and Practical Methods for Compensation. *Int. J. Radiat. Oncol.* **2007**, *68*, 654–656. [CrossRef]
15. Mazzola, R.; Ricchetti, F.; Fersino, S.; Fiorentino, A.; Levra, N.G.; Ms, G.D.P.; Ruggieri, R.; Alongi, F. Predictors of mucositis in oropharyngeal and oral cavity cancer in patients treated with volumetric modulated radiation treatment: A dose-volume analysis. *Head Neck* **2015**, *38*, E815–E819. [CrossRef]
16. Sunaga, T.; Nagatani, A.; Fujii, N.; Hashimoto, T.; Watanabe, T.; Sasaki, T. The association between cumulative radiation dose and the incidence of severe oral mucositis in head and neck cancers during radiotherapy. *Cancer Rep.* **2020**, *4*, e1317. [CrossRef]
17. Millsop, J.; Fazel, N. Oral Candidiasis. *Clin. Dermatol.* **2016**, *34*, 487–494. [CrossRef]
18. Contaldo, M.; Di Stasio, D.; Romano, A.; Fiori, F.; Vella, F.D.; Rupe, C.; Lajolo, C.; Petruzzi, M.; Serpico, R.; Lucchese, A. Oral candidiasis and novel therapeutic strategies: Antifungals, phytotherapy, probiotics, and photodynamic therapy. *Curr. Drug Deliv.* **2022**, *18*, 780. [CrossRef]
19. Singh, G.; Capoor, M.; Nair, D.; Bhowmik, K. Spectrum of fungal infection in head and neck cancer patients on chemoradiotherapy. *J. Egypt. Natl. Cancer Inst.* **2017**, *29*, 33–37. [CrossRef]
20. Aghamohamamdi, A.; Hosseinimehr, S. Natural Products for Management of Oral Mucositis Induced by Radiotherapy and Chemotherapy. *Integr. Cancer Ther.* **2016**, *15*, 60–68. [CrossRef]
21. Villa, A.; Connell, C.L.; Abati, S. Diagnosis and management of xerostomia and hyposalivation. *Ther. Clin. Risk Manag.* **2014**, *11*, 45–51. [CrossRef] [PubMed]
22. Brouwer, C.L.; Steenbakkers, R.J.; Bourhis, J.; Budach, W.; Grau, C.; Grégoire, V.; van Herk, M.; Lee, A.; Maingon, P.; Nutting, C.; et al. CT-based delineation of organs at risk in the head and neck region: DAHANCA, EORTC, GORTEC, HKNPCSG, NCIC CTG, NCRI, NRG Oncology and TROG consensus guidelines. *Radiother. Oncol.* **2015**, *117*, 83–90. [CrossRef]
23. Grégoire, V.; Evans, M.; Le, Q.-T.; Bourhis, J.; Budach, V.; Chen, A.; Eisbruch, A.; Feng, M.; Giralt, J.; Gupta, T.; et al. Delineation of the primary tumour Clinical Target Volumes (CTV-P) in laryngeal, hypopharyngeal, oropharyngeal and oral cavity squamous cell carcinoma: Consensus guidelines. *Radiother. Oncol.* **2018**, *126*, 3–24. [CrossRef] [PubMed]

24. Lalla, R.V.; Bowen, J.; Barasch, A.; Elting, L.; Epstein, J.; Keefe, D.M.; McGuire, D.B.; Migliorati, C.; Nicolatou-Galitis, O.; Dmd, D.E.P.; et al. MASCC/ISOO clinical practice guidelines for the management of mucositis secondary to cancer therapy. *Cancer* **2014**, *120*, 1453–1461. [CrossRef] [PubMed]
25. National Cancer Institute. *Common Terminology Criteria for Adverse Events (CTCAE)*; National Cancer Institute: Bethesda, MD, USA, 2018; pp. 1–147.
26. Mallick, S.; Benson, R.; Rath, G.K. Radiation induced oral mucositis: A review of current literature on prevention and management. *Eur. Arch. Otorhinolaryngol.* **2016**, *273*, 2285–2293. [CrossRef]
27. Sroussi, H.; Epstein, J.B.; Bensadoun, R.J.; Saunders, D.P.; Lalla, R.V.; Migliorati, C.A.; Heaivilin, N.; Zumsteg, Z.S. Common oral complications of head and neck cancer radiation therapy: Mucositis, infections, saliva change, fibrosis, sensory dysfunctions, dental caries, periodontal disease, and osteoradionecrosis. *Cancer Med.* **2017**, *6*, 2918–2931. [CrossRef] [PubMed]
28. Sonis, S. The pathobiology of mucositis. *Nat. Rev. Cancer* **2004**, *4*, 277–284. [CrossRef]
29. Wardill, H.; Sonis, S.T.; Blijlevens, N.M.A.; Van Sebille, Y.Z.A.; Ciorba, M.A.; Loeffen, E.A.H.; Cheng, K.K.F.; Bossi, P.; Porcello, L.; Castillo, D.A.; et al. Mucositis Study Group of the Multinational Association of Supportive Care in Cancer/International Society of Oral Oncology (MASCC/ISOO). Prediction of mucositis risk secondary to cancer therapy: A systematic review of current evidence and call to action. *Support Care Cancer* **2020**, *28*, 5059–5073. [CrossRef]
30. Oba, M.; Innocentini, L.M.A.R.; Viani, G.; Ricz, H.M.A.; Reis, T.D.C.; Ferrari, T.C.; de Macedo, L.D. Evaluation of the correlation between side effects to oral mucosa, salivary glands, and general health status with quality of life during intensity-modulated radiotherapy for head and neck cancer. *Support Care Cancer* **2021**, *29*, 127–134. [CrossRef]
31. McCullough, R.W. US oncology-wide incidence, duration, costs and deaths from chemoradiation mucositis and antimucositis therapy benefits. *Future Oncol.* **2017**, *13*, 2823–2852. [CrossRef]
32. Barik, S.; Singh, A.K.; Mishra, M.; Amritt, A.; Sahu, D.P.; Das Majumdar, S.K.; Parida, D.K. Effect of treatment interruptions and outcomes in cancer patients undergoing radiotherapy during the first wave of COVID-19 pandemic in a tertiary care institute. *J. Egypt Natl. Cancer Inst.* **2022**, *4*, 28. [CrossRef] [PubMed]
33. Pulito, C.; Cristaudo, A.; La Porta, C.; Zapperi, S.; Blandino, G.; Morrone, A.; Strano, S. Oral mucositis: The hidden side of cancer therapy. *J. Exp. Clin. Cancer Res.* **2020**, *39*, 210. [CrossRef] [PubMed]
34. Mba, I.E.; Nweze, E. Mechanism of Candida pathogenesis: Revisiting the vital drivers. *Eur. J. Clin. Microbiol. Infect. Dis.* **2020**, *39*, 1797–1819. [CrossRef]
35. Filler, S. Candida-host cell receptor-ligand interactions. *Curr. Opin. Microbiol.* **2006**, *9*, 333–339. [CrossRef] [PubMed]
36. Bernard, C.; Girardot, M.; Imbert, C. Candida albicans interaction with Gram-positive bacteria within interkingdom biofilms. *J. Mycol. Med.* **2019**, *30*, 100909. [CrossRef]
37. Vanhoecke, B.; De Ryck, T.; Stringer, A.; Van De Wiele, T.; Keefe, D. Microbiota and their role in the pathogenesis of oral mucositis. *Oral Dis.* **2014**, *21*, 17–30. [CrossRef] [PubMed]
38. Rupe, C.; Basco, A.; Schiavelli, A.; Cassano, A.; Micciche', F.; Galli, J.; Cordaro, M.; Lajolo, C. Oral Health Status in Patients with Head and Neck Cancer before Radiotherapy: Baseline Description of an Observational Prospective Study. *Cancers* **2022**, *14*, 1411. [CrossRef] [PubMed]
39. Vesty, A.; Gear, K.; Biswas, K.; Mackenzie, B.W.; Taylor, M.W.; Douglas, R.G. Oral microbial influences on oral mucositis during radiotherapy treatment of head and neck cancer. *Support Care Cancer* **2020**, *28*, 2683–2691. [CrossRef]
40. Musha, A.; Hirai, C.; Kitada, Y.; Tsunoda, A.; Shimada, H.; Kubo, N.; Kawamura, H.; Okano, N.; Sato, H.; Okada, K.; et al. Relationship between oral mucositis and the oral bacterial count in patients with head and neck cancer undergoing carbon ion radiotherapy: A prospective study. *Radiother. Oncol.* **2021**, *167*, 65–71. [CrossRef]
41. Nishii, M.; Soutome, S.; Kawakita, A.; Yutori, H.; Iwata, E.; Akashi, M.; Hasegawa, T.; Kojima, Y.; Funahara, M.; Umeda, M.; et al. Factors associated with severe oral mucositis and candidiasis in patients undergoing radiotherapy for oral and oropharyngeal carcinomas: A rundergoing radiotherapy for oral and oropharyngeal carcinomas: A retrospective multicenter study of 326 patients. *Support Care Cancer* **2020**, *28*, 1069–1075. [CrossRef]
42. Radfar, L.; Sirois, D. Structural and functional injury in minipig salivary glands following fractionated exposure to 70 Gy of ionizing radiation: An animal model for human radiation-induced salivary gland injury. *Oral Surg. Oral Med. Oral Pathol. Oral Radiol. Endod.* **2003**, *96*, 267–274. [CrossRef]
43. Kałużny, J.; Wierzbicka, M.; Nogala, H.; Milecki, P.; Kopeć, T. Radiotherapy induced xerostomia: Mechanisms, diagnostics, prevention and treatment-evidence based up to 2013. *Otolaryngol. Pol.* **2014**, *68*, 1–14. [CrossRef] [PubMed]
44. Winter, C.; Keimel, R.; Gugatschka, M.; Kolb, D.; Leitinger, G.; Roblegg, E. Investigation of Changes in Saliva in Radiotherapy-Induced Head Neck Cancer Patients. *Int. J. Environ. Res. Public Health* **2021**, *18*, 1629. [CrossRef]
45. Leerahakan, P.; Matangkasombut, O.; Tarapan, S.; Lam-Ubol, A. Biofilm formation of Candida isolates from xerostomic post-radiotherapy head and neck cancer patients. *Arch. Oral Biol.* **2022**, *142*, 105495. [CrossRef] [PubMed]
46. Suryawanshi, H.; Ganvir, S.M.; Hazarey, V.K.; Wanjare, V.S. Oropharyngeal candidosis relative frequency in radiotherapy patient for head and neck cancer. *J. Oral Maxillofac. Pathol.* **2012**, *16*, 31–37. [CrossRef]
47. Rao, N.G.; Han, G.; Greene, J.N.; Tanvetyanon, T.; Kish, J.A.; De Conti, R.C.; Chuong, M.D.; Shridhar, R.; Biagioli, M.C.; Caudell, J.J.; et al. Effect of prophylactic fluconazole on oral mucositis and candidiasis during radiation therapy for head-and-neck cancer. *Pr. Radiat. Oncol.* **2013**, *3*, 229–233. [CrossRef] [PubMed]
48. Osborn, J. Is VMAT beneficial for patients undergoing radiotherapy to the head and neck? *Radiography* **2017**, *23*, 73–76. [CrossRef]

49. Vera-Llonch, M.; Oster, G.; Hagiwara, M.; Sonis, S. Oral mucositis in patients undergoing radiation treatment for head and neck carcinoma. *Cancer* **2005**, *106*, 329–336. [CrossRef]
50. Munneke, J.M.; Björklund, A.T.; Mjösberg, J.M.; Garming-Legert, K.; Bernink, J.H.; Blom, B.; Huisman, C.; Van Oers, M.H.J.; Spits, H.; Malmberg, K.-J.; et al. Activated innate lymphoid cells are associated with a reduced susceptibility to graft-versus-host disease. *Blood* **2014**, *124*, 812–821. [CrossRef] [PubMed]
51. Nagarajan, K. Chemo-radiotherapy induced oral mucositis during IMRT for head and neck cancer—An assessment. *Med. Oral Patol. Oral Cir. Bucal.* **2015**, *20*, e273–e277. [CrossRef]

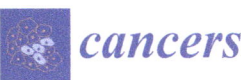

Article

Trimodal Therapy in Esophageal Squamous Cell Carcinoma: Role of Adjuvant Therapy Following Neoadjuvant Chemoradiation and Surgery

Xiaokun Li [†], Siyuan Luan [†], Yushang Yang [†], Jianfeng Zhou, Qixin Shang, Pinhao Fang, Xin Xiao, Hanlu Zhang and Yong Yuan *

Department of Thoracic Surgery, West China Hospital, Sichuan University, Chengdu 610000, China; drlixiaokun@163.com (X.L.); luansiyuan30@163.com (S.L.); yangysh07@163.com (Y.Y.); 2020224020107@stu.scu.edu.cn (J.Z.); qixinshang0405@gmail.com (Q.S.); 15877929137@163.com (P.F.); drxiaoxin@foxmail.com (X.X.); drzhanghanlu@wchscu.cn (H.Z.)
* Correspondence: yongyuan@scu.edu.cn
† These authors contributed equally to this work.

Simple Summary: In this work, we aimed to explore the effectiveness of adjuvant therapy after trimodal therapy (neoadjuvant chemoradiotherapy and esophagectomy) in patients with thoracic esophageal squamous cell carcinoma (ESCC). Overall survival (OS) and disease-free survival (DFS) were both compared for adjuvant and non-adjuvant groups. Propensity score matching was used to eliminate the confounding factors between the two groups. Meanwhile, subgroup analysis based on a neoadjuvant-treated node stage (ypN) was performed to precisely stratify the patients and to guide the clinical decision-making at the point of care. As of now, there is no guideline or recommendation on the treatment of ESCC patients with adjuvant therapy after neoadjuvant chemoradiotherapy followed by surgery. The results of our study indicate that adjuvant therapy after trimodal therapy could shorten OS and DFS in patients with ESCC. Meanwhile, adjuvant therapy is an independently unfavorably prognostic factor for DFS. Therefore, adjuvant therapy is not recommended for ESCC patients after trimodal therapy, especially patients without nodal metastases after neoadjuvant therapy. To our knowledge, this is the first retrospective study using subgroup analysis to examine the effect of adjuvant therapy in ESCC patients after trimodal therapy by comparing overall survival and disease-free survival. The results of our study add useful evidence to recent guidelines.

Abstract: Background: The aim of this study was to determine the role of adjuvant therapy after neoadjuvant chemoradiotherapy and esophagectomy for esophageal squamous cell carcinoma (ESCC). **Methods:** The study retrospectively reviewed 447 ESCC patients who underwent neoadjuvant chemoradiotherapy and esophagectomy. Patients were divided into an adjuvant therapy group and no adjuvant therapy group. Propensity score matching was used to adjust the confounding factors. **Results:** 447 patients with clinical positive lymph nodes and no distant metastasis treated with neoadjuvant chemoradiotherapy and esophagectomy were eligible for analysis. After propensity score matching, there were 120 patients remaining in each group. Patients receiving adjuvant therapy had a significantly shorter post-resection overall survival (OS) and disease-free survival (DFS) when compared to patients not receiving adjuvant therapy (log-rank, OS: $p = 0.046$, DFS: $p < 0.001$). Receiving adjuvant therapy is not an independently prognostic factor for OS (hazard ratio (HR): 1.270, HR: 0.846–1.906, $p = 0.249$) but a significantly unfavorable independent prognostic factor for DFS (HR: 2.061, HR: 1.436–2.958, $p < 0.001$). **Conclusions:** The results of our study indicate that adjuvant therapy after neoadjuvant chemoradiotherapy and surgery could reduce the OS and DFS in patients with ESCC. Therefore, adjuvant therapy is not recommended for ESCC patients after neoadjuvant chemoradiotherapy and esophagectomy, especially patients without nodal metastases after neoadjuvant therapy.

Keywords: esophageal cancer; neoadjuvant chemoradiotherapy; esophagectomy; adjuvant therapy

Citation: Li, X.; Luan, S.; Yang, Y.; Zhou, J.; Shang, Q.; Fang, P.; Xiao, X.; Zhang, H.; Yuan, Y. Trimodal Therapy in Esophageal Squamous Cell Carcinoma: Role of Adjuvant Therapy Following Neoadjuvant Chemoradiation and Surgery. *Cancers* **2022**, *14*, 3721. https://doi.org/10.3390/cancers14153721

Academic Editor: David Wong

Received: 16 June 2022
Accepted: 27 July 2022
Published: 30 July 2022

Publisher's Note: MDPI stays neutral with regard to jurisdictional claims in published maps and institutional affiliations.

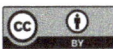

Copyright: © 2022 by the authors. Licensee MDPI, Basel, Switzerland. This article is an open access article distributed under the terms and conditions of the Creative Commons Attribution (CC BY) license (https://creativecommons.org/licenses/by/4.0/).

1. Introduction

Esophageal cancer (EC) is the sixth leading cause of cancer deaths worldwide and the second deadliest gastrointestinal cancer after gastric carcinoma [1]. The literature reports that approximately 200,000 people die of EC annually worldwide, and most cases of EC are diagnosed at advanced stages [1]. Esophageal squamous cell carcinoma (ESCC) represents the predominant subtype of EC, with most cases occurring in eastern Asia. The morbidity rate varies extremely across areas and countries [2,3].

Although a tremendous improvement of therapeutic modalities has been recently observed, patients' quality of life remains poor, and the five-year survival rate rarely exceeds 40% [3]. Currently, surgery remains the major treatment for patients with early stage resectable ESCC, whereas neoadjuvant therapy (chemotherapy, radiotherapy, or their combination prior to surgery) followed by esophagectomy is the standard of care for those with locally advanced disease (cT1-2N+ or cT3-4aN1-3). It has been proven that patients with locally advanced esophageal cancer can benefit from trimodal therapy (neoadjuvant concurrent chemoradiation followed by surgery), when compared to surgery alone [2]. However, additional adjuvant therapy (chemotherapy and/or radiotherapy after surgery) may be necessary for patients that do not fully respond to neoadjuvant therapy, characterized by pathologically confirmed residual disease and lymph node metastasis. Nevertheless, the use of adjuvant therapy remains controversial for these patients because the therapeutic efficacy may be insufficient to control the residual disease. In addition, patients are at an additional risk of adverse events. Currently, there is no guideline recommendation to treat ESCC patients with adjuvant therapy after they receive neoadjuvant chemoradiotherapy and esophagectomy [2]. Due to a restricted number of clinical studies concerning this topic, the indication for adjuvant therapy after trimodal therapy is highly dependent on the patient and the institution [4]. Although there are several large-scale studies investigating the utility of adjuvant therapy after neoadjuvant therapy and surgery in western populations, the majority of the cases included in these cohorts are esophageal adenocarcinoma and the information regarding treatment regimens is missing [5–7]. Therefore, no clear evidence could guide the utilization of adjuvant therapy after trimodal therapy in patients with ESCC, especially in the east Asian region.

To add evidence to this important clinical question, we conducted a single-center and retrospective cohort study to investigate the role of adjuvant therapy following neoadjuvant chemoradiotherapy and surgery in patients with thoracic ESCC. Meanwhile, subgroup analysis based on neoadjuvant treated node stage (ypN) was performed to further explore the impact of adjuvant therapy on ESCC patients.

2. Materials and Methods

2.1. Patients

There were 447 ESCC patients undergoing neoadjuvant chemoradiotherapy and esophagectomy retrospectively reviewed at the West China Hospital from January 2014 to July 2020. The study was approved by the human participants' committee of the West China Hospital of Sichuan University. Surgeons informed the patients concerning the risks of the neoadjuvant/adjuvant therapy and esophagectomy. The written consent of the study's participants and permission to use resected specimens were obtained preoperatively. This study was approved by the Institutional Review Board of West China Hospital, Sichuan University in April 2021 (2022-636).

The inclusion criteria are listed as follows: (1) patients were pathologically diagnosed with ESCC before treatment, (2) patients received neoadjuvant chemoradiotherapy and esophagectomy, (3) patients were staged according to the American Joint Committee on Cancer (AJCC) 8th edition (the patients from 2014 to 2016 were staged according to AJCC 7th edition and then re-staged for the purpose of the study) [8], (4) patients were diagnosed as clinical lymph node metastasis positive (cN+) based on imaging evidence and no distant metastasis (cM0) before any treatments, (5) detailed data of the pathological information and adjuvant therapy were collected, and (6) patients were assessed as negative surgical margin pathologically after radical esophagectomy with complete tumor resection (R0 resection).

Patients were excluded if they had missing pathological information data, had unknown adjuvant treatment status, died prior to eligibility (≤60 days) for adjuvant therapy, had pathologic M1 disease, or had a documented recurrence of cancer prior to administration of adjuvant therapy. Only patients with ESCC were included. The CONSORT diagram (Figure 1) shows the inclusion and exclusion criteria of our study.

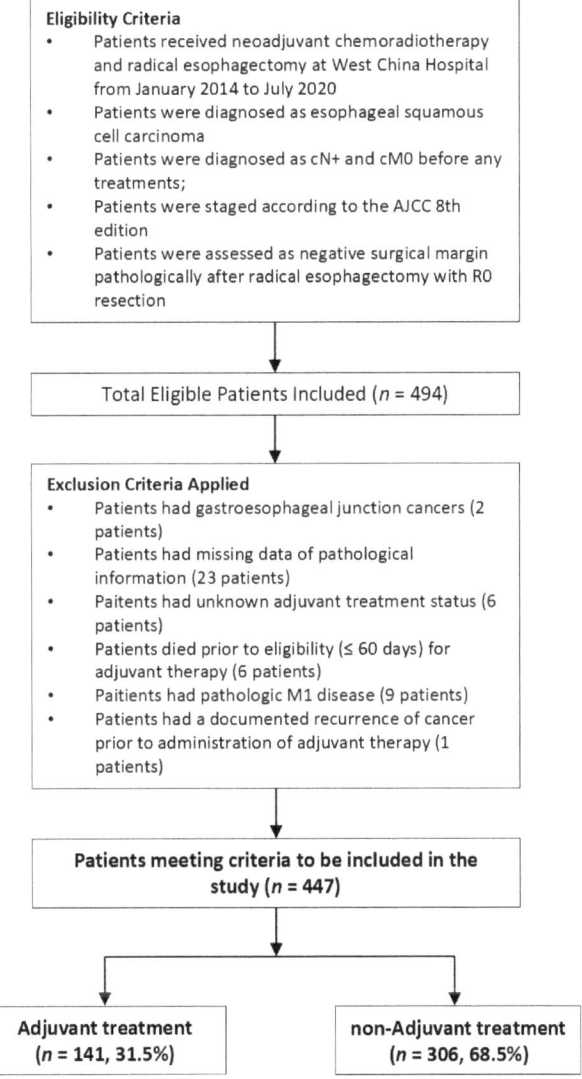

Figure 1. CONSORT diagram.

Patients were divided into adjuvant and non-adjuvant therapy groups for the log-rank test and Cox regression analysis. Demographic characteristics, comorbidities, operative data, postoperative complications, and pathological information were collected for all patients. Patients were followed up every 3 months for the first 2 years, and every 6 months thereafter. Neck and abdominal ultrasound, chest computerized tomography (CT), gastroscopy, and blood tests were performed on the basis of patient's symptoms during follow-up. The patient status (including death and survival), the tumor status (including tumor recurrence and metastasis), and the patient loss of follow-up were all documented. Our follow-ups were implemented via telephone or outpatient department visit. The last follow-up was conducted on 1 January 2022.

2.2. Neoadjuvant Therapy

The selection of neoadjuvant therapy depended on the preoperative clinical stage of the ESCC patients. For patients with cN1-3 and/or cT4a-b, neoadjuvant chemoradiotherapy was routinely administered. The chemotherapeutic drugs were selected according to National Comprehensive Cancer Network (NCCN) Guidelines for esophageal and esophagogastric junction cancers and previous publications [2,9,10]. Neoadjuvant chemoradiotherapy included two cycles of chemotherapy with sequential or concurrent radiotherapy. The neoadjuvant chemoradiotherapy treatment cycle was 21 days (treatment during weeks 1 and 4). Paclitaxel (China Shiyao Pharmaceutical Group Co., Ltd., Shijiazhuang, China) in a dose of 175 mg/m^2 (day 1) or carboplatin (Qilu Pharmaceutical Group Co., Ltd., Jinan, China) in a dose of area under the concentration–time curve 5 (day 1), with a combination of cisplatin (Qilu Pharmaceutical Group Co., Ltd., Jinan, China) in the amount of 75 mg/m^2/24 h (days 1–2 or days 1–3), was given intravenously. Patients received concurrent radiation up to a total dose of 40–50.4 gray (Gy), delivered in 1.8–2.0 Gy fractions, beginning on day 1 of the first chemotherapy cycle (week 1) and ending at the completion of the second chemotherapy cycle (week 4). Sequential radiation to the same doses was arranged after the end of the second chemotherapy cycle. Intensity-modulated radiotherapy technique was used to perform radiotherapy in all patients. We referred to the Ryan scoring system to score tumor regression grades (TRGs) [11]. TRGs 0–3 are defined as follows: TRG 0: complete response (no viable cancer cells), TRG 1: near complete response (rare small groups of cancer cells), TRG 2: partial response (residual cancer with evident tumor regression), and TRG 3: poor or no response (extensive residual cancer with no evident tumor regression). Three pathologists reexamined the results of the pathological sections, and the final TRG had to be agreed upon by two or more pathologists. The strategy of neoadjuvant chemoradiotherapy is showed in Table S1.

2.3. Surgical Procedure and Pathology

McKeown esophagectomy with cervical anastomoses or Ivor Lewis esophagectomy with thoracic anastomoses combined with radical lymph node dissection was performed in a standardized manner. The gastric conduit was used to reconstruct the upper digestive tract during esophagectomy. The lymph nodes were then separated by surgeons from the dissected peri-esophagus and esophagus tissues. Specimens were sent to the pathology department for further analysis where representative sections of the tumor and periesophageal tissues were taken for sufficient pathologic evaluation and staging.

2.4. Adjuvant Therapy

In our institution, each patient was evaluated by a multidisciplinary team by whom adjuvant therapy selection was determined. The final decision was left up to the patients' preference. The adjuvant chemotherapeutic regimens were selected according to the NCCN Guidelines for esophageal and esophagogastric junction cancers and previous publications [2,9,12]. Generally, the chemotherapy regimens included 5-fluorouracil and cisplatin, repeated twice every 3 weeks. 5-fluorouracil in a dose of 800 mg/m^2 was given by continuous infusion on days 1 through 5. Cisplatin in a dose of 80 mg/m^2 was administered by intravenous drip infusion for 2 h on day 1. An intensity-modulated radiotherapy technique was used to administer radiotherapy with a total dose of 45 to 50.4 Gy (1.8–2.0 Gy/d). Combined chemoradiotherapy included giving radiotherapy from the first day of the first chemotherapy cycle. Two cycle of Tislelizumab (200 mg, D1),

Sintilimab (200 mg, D1), or Pembrolizumab (200 mg, D1) administered by intravenous injection combined with radiotherapy was implemented for patients undergoing adjuvant immune radiotherapy. The immunotherapy was repeated twice every 3 weeks. Typically, adjuvant therapy is administered 4 to 6 weeks after esophagectomy based on NCCN Guideline [2,12]. The strategy for adjuvant therapy is showed in Table S2.

2.5. Statistical Analysis

Pearson's chi-square test was used to compare categorical variables expressed as frequencies. Kaplan-Meier curves were used to analyze overall survival (OS) and disease-free survival (DFS), and the log-rank test was employed to determine statistical significance between the adjuvant and non-adjuvant therapy groups. A Cox regression model was used to determine variables independently associated with OS and DFS for patients undergoing neoadjuvant therapy and esophagectomy. Variables were selected for multivariate Cox regression model entry if $p < 0.05$ on univariate analysis. In addition, hazard ratios with 95% confidence intervals (CI) were reported, and we assessed whether the treatment effect differed in certain subgroups by testing the treatment-by-subgroup interaction effect with the use of Cox models via univariate analysis. All tests were two-sided and $p < 0.05$ was considered to be statistically significant. All statistical analyses were implemented with R (version 3.5.3). SPSS version 27.0 software (SPSS Inc. Chicago, IL, USA) was used to perform propensity score matching. The confounding factors including gender, age, smoke history, tumor length, neoadjuvant treated tumor, node, and metastases (ypTNM) stage, neoadjuvant treated tumor (ypT) status, ypN status, tumor differentiation, lymphovascular invasion, peripheral nerve invasion, and tumor regression grade were employed to develop the propensity score matching. The nearest-neighbor method with a caliper width of 0.02 was used to match the selected cases from two groups at a ratio of 1:1.

3. Results

3.1. Patient Characteristics

After application of the inclusion and exclusion criteria, 447 patients with cN+ and cM0 following neoadjuvant chemoradiotherapy and radical esophagectomy were available for analysis. Demographic characteristics, comorbidities, operative data, postoperative complications, and pathological information of the included patients are displayed in Table 1. The median tumor length was 3 cm, which was used as the cut-off value. A complete response (TRG 0) was reported in 150 (33.6%) patients, a near complete response (TRG 1) in 73 (16.3%) patients, a partial response (TRG 2) in 170 (38.0%) patients, and a poor or non-response (TRG 3) in 68 (13.4%) patients. Adjuvant therapy was performed in 141 (31.5%) patients. Of these, 49 (34.8%) received adjuvant chemotherapy, 15 (10.6%) received adjuvant radiotherapy alone, 40 (28.4%) received chemoradiotherapy, and 37 (26.2%) received immuno-radiotherapy. A total of 306 (68.5%) patients received no adjuvant therapy. Patients receiving adjuvant therapy were more likely to have a younger age, a history of smoking, an upper tumor site, a poorer tumor stage, more positive lymph nodes, advanced stage, increased lymphovascular and peripheral nerve invasion, and poorer response to neoadjuvant therapy. Due to the heterogeneity between the two groups, propensity score matching was used to balance the baseline characteristics between the adjuvant group and the non-adjuvant group. After propensity score matching, there were 120 patients remaining in each group and the patients were adjusted for all the potential confounding factors (Table 1). After propensity score matching, there were 38 (31.7%) patients receiving adjuvant chemotherapy, 13 (10.8%) receiving adjuvant radiotherapy alone, 35 (29.2%) receiving chemoradiotherapy, and 34 (28.3%) receiving immuno-radiotherapy.

Table 1. Baseline characteristics of the patients.

Variable	No. (%) (n = 447)	Before Propensity Score Match			After Propensity Score Match		
		Non-Adjuvant Therapy (n = 306)	Adjuvant Therapy (n = 141)	p-Value	Non-Adjuvant Therapy (n = 120)	Adjuvant Therapy (n = 120)	p-Value
Gender				0.155			0.701
Male	359 (80.3%)	274 (79.9%)	121 (85.8%)		106 (88.3%)	103 (85.8%)	
Female	88 (19.7%)	69 (20.1%)	20 (14.2%)		14 (11.6%)	17 (14.2%)	
Age (year)				0.004			0.331
≤65	287 (64.2%)	183 (59.8%)	104 (73.8%)		78 (65.0%)	86 (71.7%)	
>65	160 (35.8%)	123 (40.2%)	37 (26.2%)		42 (35.0%)	34 (28.3%)	
Smoke				0.014			0.155
Yes	230 (51.5%)	145 (47.4%)	85 (60.3%)		58 (48.3%)	70 (58.3%)	
No	217 (48.5%)	161 (52.6%)	56 (39.7%)		62 (51.7%)	50 (41.7%)	
Alcohol consumption				0.837			0.517
Yes	187 (41.8%)	127 (41.5%)	60 (42.6%)		52 (43.3%)	57 (47.5%)	
No	260 (58.2%)	179 (58.5%)	81 (57.4%)		68 (56.7%)	63 (52.5%)	
Hypertension				0.895			0.869
Yes	80 (17.9%)	54 (17.6%)	26 (18.4%)		23 (19.2%)	22 (18.3%)	
No	367 (82.1%)	252 (82.4%)	115 (81.6%)		97 (80.8%)	98 (81.7%)	
Cardiovascular disease (n = 444)				0.450			0.518
Yes	19 (4.3%)	15 (4.9%)	4 (2.9%)		6 (5.0%)	4 (3.3%)	
No	425 (95.7%)	290 (95.1%))	135 (97.1%)		114 (95.0%)	116 (96.7%)	
Cerebrovascular disease (n = 442)				0.443			0.999
Yes	7 (1.6%)	6 (2.0%)	1 (0.7%)		1 (0.8%)	1 (0.8%)	
No	435 (98.4%)	298 (98.0%)	137 (99.3%)		119 (99.2%)	119 (99.2%)	
Chronic liver disease (n = 434)				0.853			0.999
Yes	37 (8.5%)	25 (8.3%)	12 (9.0%)		10 (8.3%)	10 (8.3%)	
No	397 (91.5%)	275 (91.7%)	122 (91.0%)		110 (91.7%)	110 (91.7%)	
COPD (n = 444)				0.533			0.554
Yes	28 (6.3%)	21 (6.9%)	7 (5.0%)		7 (5.8%)	5 (4.2%)	
No	416 (93.7%)	284 (93.1%)	132 (95.0%)		113 (94.2%)	115 (95.8%)	
Arrhythmia (n = 446)				0.515			0.651
Yes	10 (2.2%)	8 (2.6%)	2 (1.4%)		3 (2.5%)	2 (1.7%)	
No	436 (97.8%)	297 (97.4%)	139 (98.6%)		117 (97.5%)	118 (98.3%)	
Tumor site				0.046			0.383
Upper	61 (13.6%)	34 (11.1%)	27 (19.1%)		11 (9.2%)	18 (15.0%)	
Middle	229 (51.2%)	160 (52.3%)	69 (48.9%)		63 (52.5%)	59 (49.2%)	
Lower	157 (35.1%)	112 (36.6%)	45 (31.9%)		46 (38.3%)	43 (35.8%)	
Tumor length (cm)				0.001			0.694
≤3	289 (64.7%)	216 (70.6%)	73 (51.8%)		72 (60.0%)	69 (57.5%)	
>3	158 (35.3%)	90 (29.4%)	68 (48.2%)		48 (40.0%)	51 (42.5%)	
ypTNM				0.000			0.160
I	219 (49.0%)	174 (56.9%)	45 (31.9%)		57 (47.5%)	43 (35.8%)	
II	64 (14.3%)	40 (13.1%)	24 (17.0%)		19 (15.8%)	22 (18.3%)	
IIIA	55 (12.3%)	34 (11.1%)	21 (14.9%)		9 (7.5%)	18 (15.0%)	
IIIB	96 (21.5%)	50 (16.3%)	46 (32.6%)		29 (24.2%)	34 (28.3%)	
IVA	13 (2.9%)	8 (2.6%)	5 (3.5%)		6 (5.0%)	3 (2.5%)	
ypT				0.001			0.493
Tis	2 (0.4%)	2 (0.6%)	0 (0.0%)		0 (0.0%)	0 (0.0%)	
T0	161 (36.0%)	127 (41.5%)	34 (24.1%)		42 (35.0%)	32 (26.6%)	
T1	64 (14.3%)	44 (14.4%)	20 (14.2%)		12 (10.0%)	17 (14.2%)	
T2	65 (14.5%)	44 (14.4%)	21 (14.9%)		19 (15.8%)	20 (16.7%)	
T3	155 (34.5%)	89 (28.8%)	66 (46.8%)		47 (39.2%)	51 (42.5%)	
ypN				0.001			0.304
N0	284 (63.5%)	214 (69.9%)	70 (49.6%)		76 (63.3%)	66 (55.0%)	
N1	112 (25.1%)	67 (21.9%)	45 (31.9%)		26 (21.7%)	34 (28.3%)	
N2	39 (8.7%)	18 (5.9%)	21 (14.9%)		12 (10.0%)	17 (14.2%)	
N3	12 (2.7%)	8 (2.6%)	5 (3.5%)		6 (5.0%)	3 (2.5%)	
Tumor differentiation				0.000			0.116
G1	13 (2.9%)	10 (3.3%)	3 (2.1%)		5 (4.2%)	2 (1.7%)	
G2	108 (24.2%)	73 (23.9%)	35 (24.8%)		35 (29.2%)	25 (20.8%)	
G3	138 (30.9%)	77 (25.2%)	61 (43.3%)		37 (30.8%)	53 (44.2%)	
Gx	188 (42.1%)	146 (47.7%)	42 (29.8%)		43 (35.8%)	40 (33.3%)	

Table 1. Cont.

Variable	No. (%) (n = 447)	Before Propensity Score Match			After Propensity Score Match		
		Non-Adjuvant Therapy (n = 306)	Adjuvant Therapy (n = 141)	p-Value	Non-Adjuvant Therapy (n = 120)	Adjuvant Therapy (n = 120)	p-Value
Lymphovascular invasion				0.001			0.336
Yes	42 (9.4%)	19 (6.2%)	23 (16.3%)		13 (10.8%)	18 (15.0%)	
No	405 (90.6%)	287 (93.8%)	118 (83.7%)		107 (89.2%)	102 (85.0%)	
Peripheral nerve invasion				0.002			0.525
Yes	80 (17.9%)	43 (14.1%)	37 (26.2%)		23 (19.2%)	27 (22.5%)	
No	367 (82.1%)	263 (85.9%)	104 (73.8%)		97 (80.8%)	93 (77.5%)	
Surgical type				0.198			0.678
Open surgery	45 (10.1%)	27 (8.8%)	18 (12.8%)		14 (11.7%)	12 (10.0%)	
Video-assisted Thoracoscopic Surgery	402 (89.9%)	279 (91.2%)	123 (87.2%)		106 (88.3%)	108 (90.0%)	
Anastomotic method				0.285			0.313
Stapled anastomosis	16 (3.6%)	9 (2.9%)	7 (5.0%)		3 (2.5%)	6 (5.0%)	
Hand-sewn anastomosis	431 (96.4%)	297 (97.1%)	134 (95.0%)		117 (97.5%)	114 (95.0%)	
Complications (Clavien-Dindo)				0.606			0.619
Grade I	73 (16.3%)	47 (15.4%)	26 (18.4%)		17 (41.2%)	22 (18.3%)	
Grade II	149 (33.3%)	104 (34.0%)	45 (31.9%)		40 (33.3%)	39 (32.5%)	
Grade III	29 (6.5%)	21 (6.9%)	8 (5.7%)		12 (10.0%)	8 (6.7%)	
Grade IV	7 (1.6%)	6 (2.0%)	1 (0.7%)		2 (1.7%)	1 (0.8%)	
Tumor regression grade				0.000			0.451
TRG 0	150 (33.6%)	120 (39.2%)	30 (21.3%)		39 (32.5%)	28 (23.3%)	
TRG 1	73 (16.3%)	55 (18.0%)	18 (12.8%)		15 (12.5%)	17 (41.2%)	
TRG 2	170 (38.0%)	101 (33.0%)	69 (48.9%)		51 (42.5%)	56 (46.7%)	
TRG 3	54 (12.1%)	30 (9.8%)	24 (17.0%)		15 (12.5%)	19 (15.8%)	

Pearson's chi-squared test was used to compare categorical variables expressed as frequencies. An independent-sample Student's t-test was used to compare continuous variables. COPD, chronic obstructive pulmonary disease; ypTNM, neoadjuvant-treated TNM; ypT, neoadjuvant-treated tumor stage; ypN, neoadjuvant-treated node stage; TRG, tumor regression grade.

3.2. Survival Analysis

The median follow-up time was 13.4 months (interquartile range 6.7–24.47 months) for the overall cohort, 13.38 months (6.8–24.39 months) for those who received adjuvant therapy, and 13.43 months (6.3–25.3 months) for those who did not. After propensity score matching, patients that received adjuvant therapy had a shorter post-resection OS compared to patients not receiving adjuvant therapy (log-rank, OS: $p = 0.046$ (Figure 2a)). Meanwhile, patients receiving adjuvant therapy also had a shorter post-resection DFS compared with patients not receiving adjuvant therapy (log-rank, DFS: $p < 0.001$ (Figure 2a)).

Subgroup survival analysis was performed stratified by the ypN stage (Figure 3). Among the patients with ypN1–3, there was no significant difference in OS between the adjuvant and non-adjuvant groups ($p = 0.500$) (Figure 3a). Meanwhile, no significant difference was found in DFS for patients with ypN1–3 ($p = 0.400$) (Figure 3b). When comparing the OS between the two groups in patients with ypN0, the adjuvant therapy group had a significantly shorter OS when compared with non-adjuvant therapy group ($p = 0.001$) (Figure 3c). Meanwhile, for ypN0 patients the adjuvant therapy group also had a significantly shorter DFS compared to the non-adjuvant therapy group ($p < 0.001$) (Figure 3d).

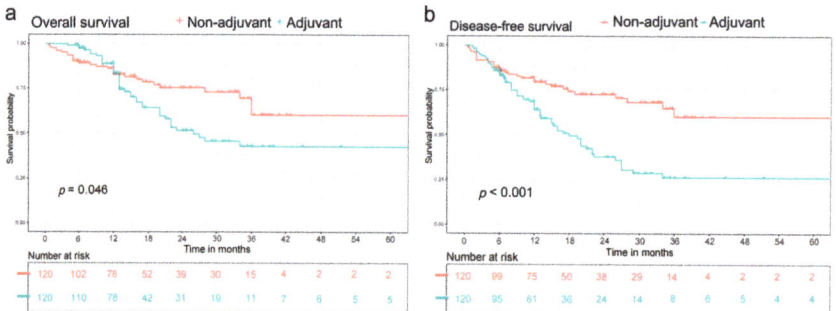

Figure 2. After propensity score matching, Kaplan-Meier curves were used to analyze overall survival (OS) and disease-free survival (DFS), and the log-rank test was employed to determine statistical significance between the two groups. (**a**) Comparison of OS between patients receiving and not receiving adjuvant therapy. Patients receiving adjuvant therapy had a shorter post-resection OS compared with patients not receiving adjuvant therapy (log-rank, OS: $p = 0.046$) (**b**) Comparison of DFS between patients receiving and not receiving adjuvant therapy. Patients receiving adjuvant therapy also had a shorter post-resection DFS compared with patients not receiving adjuvant therapy (log-rank, DFS: $p < 0.001$).

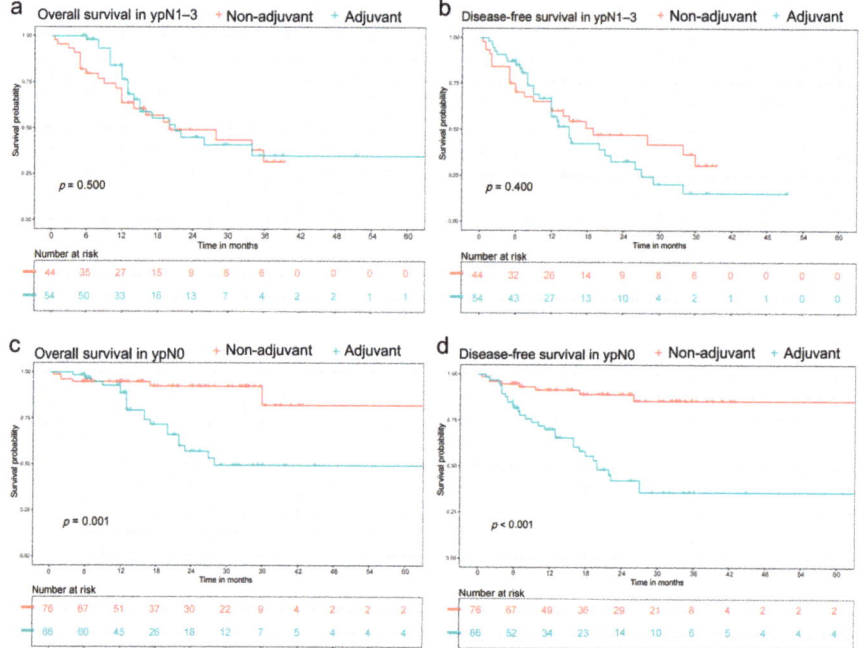

Figure 3. After propensity score matching, Kaplan-Meier curves were used to analyze overall survival (OS) and disease-free survival (DFS), and the log-rank test was employed to determine statistical significance between groups. Subgroup survival analysis were performed stratified by the neoadjuvant treated node (ypN) stage (**a**) In the patients with ypN1–3, there was no significant difference in OS between two groups ($p = 0.500$) (**b**) In the patients with ypN1–3, there was no significant difference in DFS between two groups ($p = 0.400$) (**c**) In the patients with ypN0, the adjuvant therapy group yielded a significantly shorter OS compared with non-adjuvant therapy group ($p = 0.001$) (**d**) In the patients with ypN0, the adjuvant therapy group yielded a significantly shorter DFS compared with non-adjuvant therapy group ($p < 0.001$).

3.3. Cox Regression Analysis

There were 13 variables included in the univariate Cox regression model (Table S3). Eight variables were selected for multivariate Cox regression model entry due to $p < 0.05$ on univariate analysis (Table 2). The results of Cox regression analysis on OS shows that only the ypTNM stage was an independent prognostic factor for OS in patients undergoing neoadjuvant therapy and esophagectomy. However, receiving adjuvant therapy was not an independent prognostic factor for OS (hazard ratio (HR): 1.270, 95% CI: 0.846–1.906, $p = 0.249$). The results of the Cox regression analysis on DFS show that ypTNM stage and adjuvant therapy were independent prognostic factors for DFS patients undergoing neoadjuvant therapy and esophagectomy. Meanwhile, receiving adjuvant therapy was a significantly unfavorably independent prognostic factor for DFS (HR: 2.061, 95% CI: 1.436–2.958, $p < 0.001$).

Table 2. Cox regression model for variables independently associated with adjuvant therapy status for patients with positive nodal disease after neoadjuvant chemoradiotherapy and radical esophagectomy. Ten variables were selected for multivariate Cox regression model entry due to $p < 0.05$ in univariate analysis.

Multivariate Analyses	Overall Survival			Progression-Free Survival		
	HR	95% CI of HR	p-Value	HR	95% CI of HR	p-Value
Gender						
Male versus female	1.034	0.533–2.005	0.921	1.004	0.562–1.794	0.990
Smoke						
Yes versus no	1.505	0.917–2.467	0.106	1.490	0.961–1.924	0.075
Tumor length						
>3 cm versus ≤3 cm	1.486	0.989–2.234	0.056	1.346	0.941–1.924	0.103
ypTNM						
III-IV versus I-II	2.720	1.741–4.249	0.000	2.079	1.411–3.065	0.000
Lymphovascular invasion						
Yes versus no	1.095	0.626–1.915	1.095	1.324	0.819–2.140	0.251
Peripheral nerve invasion						
Yes versus no	0.912	0.558–1.490	0.712	1.409	0.919–2.159	0.115
Tumor regression grade						
TRG 3/2 versus TRG 1/0	1.358	0.839–2.198	0.212	1.074	0.703–1.640	0.743
Adjuvant Therapy						
Yes versus no	1.270	0.846–1.906	0.249	2.061	1.436–2.958	0.000

Cox regression model was used to determine variables independently associated with OS and DFS for patients undergoing neoadjuvant therapy and esophagectomy. ypTNM, neoadjuvant treated TNM; TRG, tumor regression grade.

3.4. Subgroup Analysis by Forest Plot

Figure 4 shows the hazard ratios with 95% CIs for the OS outcome in prespecified subgroups. According to the results of the overall analysis, adjuvant therapy was not a prognostic factor for OS (HR: 1.613, 95% CI: 0.999–2.604, $p = 0.051$). However, adjuvant therapy was an unfavorable prognostic factor for DFS (HR: 2.353, 95% CI: 1.535–3.607, $p < 0.001$). In subgroup analysis, for patients with ypN0, adjuvant therapy was an unfavorable factor for OS (HR: 4.274, 95% CI: 1.714–10.654, $p = 0.002$) and DFS (HR: 5.425, 95% CI: 2.490–11.820, $p < 0.001$). Nevertheless, for patients with ypN1–3, adjuvant therapy was not a prognostic factor for OS (HR: 0.818, 95% CI: 0.452–1.480, $p = 0.506$) or DFS (HR: 1.252, 95% CI: 0.734–2.137, $p = 0.410$). Table 3 contains brief information on the outcomes of prior high-quality publications and the present study.

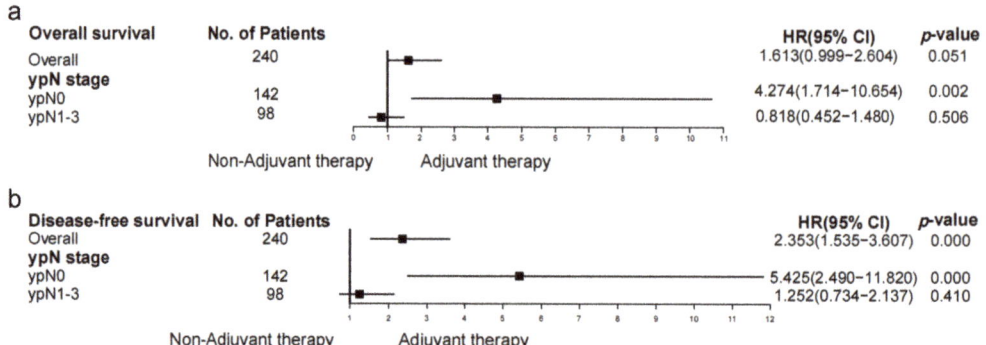

Figure 4. Subgroup analysis with Cox regression model. (**a**) Hazard ratios with 95% CI for the overall survival in prespecified subgroups. For patients with ypN0, adjuvant therapy is an unfavorable factor for OS (HR: 4.274, 95% CI: 1.714–10.654, p = 0.002). For patients with ypN1–3, adjuvant therapy is not a prognostic factor for OS (HR: 0.818, 95% CI: 0.452–1.480, p = 0.506). (**b**) Hazard ratios with 95% CI for the disease-free survival in prespecified subgroups. For patients with ypN0, adjuvant therapy is an unfavorable factor for DFS (HR: 5.425, 95% CI: 2.490–11.820, p < 0.001). For patients with ypN1–3, adjuvant therapy is not a prognostic factor for DFS (HR: 1.252, 95% CI: 0.734–2.137, p = 0.410).

Table 3. Previous publications evaluating the therapeutic value of adjuvant therapy following neoadjuvant therapy and esophagectomy.

Study	Year	Design	Sample Size	Histological Type	ypN Stage	Hazard Ratio	p Value
Burt BM, et al. [7]	2017	Retrospective cohort study based on NCDB	3592	EAC, ESCC	Any	0.93 (ypN0)	Not significant
						0.7 (ypN1–3)	Significant
Samson P, et al. [6]	2018	Retrospective cohort study based on NCDB	3100	EAC, ESCC	+	0.69	<0.001
Mokdad AA, et al. [5]	2018	Retrospective cohort study based on NCDB	10,086	Gastroesophageal adenocarcinoma	Any	0.79 0.68 (ypN0) 0.86 (ypN1–3)	<0.001 Significant Significant
Drake J, et al. [13]	2019	Retrospective cohort study based on NCDB	2046	EAC	+	0.839	0.0311
Semenkovich TR, et al. [14]	2019	Multicenter retrospective cohort study	1082	EAC, ESCC	+	0.76	0.005
Huang Z, et al. [15]	2019	Retrospective cohort study	228	ESCC	Any	1.498	0.052
The present study	2022	Retrospective cohort study	447	ESCC	Any	1.613 4.274 (ypN0) 0.818 (ypN1–3)	0.051 0.002 0.506

NCDB, National Cancer Database; EAC, esophageal adenocarcinoma; ESCC, esophageal squamous cell carcinoma; ypN, neoadjuvant treated node status.

4. Discussion

In this retrospective study, we evaluated the effectiveness of adjuvant therapy on ESCC patients treated with neoadjuvant therapy and surgery. Concurrent neoadjuvant chemoradiotherapy followed by surgery has been considered as a preferred treatment strategy for patients diagnosed as ESCC in China [16,17]. However, a guideline regarding the use of adjuvant therapy after trimodal therapy in patients with ESCC is still missing. According to NCCN guidelines, the use of adjuvant therapy is recommended for all patients with esophageal adenocarcinoma after trimodal therapy, regardless of the existence of positive lymph nodes and pathologic response [2]. However, on account of different epidemiological characteristics it remains unclear if ESCC patients can benefit from adjuvant therapy. Therefore, we conducted this retrospective study to explore the effect of adjuvant therapy after neoadjuvant chemoradiotherapy and surgery in ESCC patients. Meanwhile, subgroup analysis was performed to precisely stratify the patients undergoing neoadjuvant therapy followed by esophagectomy and to provide clinical evidence that can be utilized to guide the multimodal care of ESCC patients.

Burt et al. [7] first conducted a large-scale retrospective study based on data from the National Cancer Database (NCDB) to investigate the role of adjuvant therapy after trimodal therapy in patients diagnosed as EC. Their study indicated that EC patients with residual nodal disease after treatment with neoadjuvant chemoradiation could benefit from adjuvant chemotherapy. However, this benefit cannot be found in patients with no residual nodal disease. Whereafter, Samson et al. [6] reported a retrospective cohort study based on NCDB data only including patients with pathologic node-positive EC after neoadjuvant chemotherapy. Their study came to the same conclusion as the study reported by Burt et al. [7]. In the same year, Mokdad et al. [5] explored the effect of adjuvant chemotherapy after trimodal therapy in patients with gastroesophageal adenocarcinoma. They concluded that patients with gastroesophageal adenocarcinoma could obtain a survival benefit from adjuvant chemotherapy after trimodal therapy regardless of pathologic node status. In 2019, Drake et al. [13] investigated the effect of adjuvant chemotherapy after neoadjuvant therapy and esophagectomy. Their study only included esophageal adenocarcinoma patients with nodal metastases and concluded with the same findings as the study reported by Mokdad et al. [5]. Thereafter, Semenkovich et al. [14] conducted a multicenter retrospective cohort study including both ESCC and esophageal adenocarcinoma patients with nodal metastases, which showed that the patients with pathologic node-positive EC could benefit from adjuvant therapy after neoadjuvant therapy and surgery. Huang et al. [15] conducted a retrospective cohort study including 228 ESCC patients to investigate the effect of adjuvant therapy after neoadjuvant chemotherapy and surgery in 2019. The results of their study showed no significant difference in OS or DFS between the adjuvant therapy group and the non-adjuvant therapy group after propensity score matching. However, subgroup analysis based on status of nodal metastases were not implemented.

In our study, we only included patients with thoracic ESCC. Meanwhile, propensity score matching was used to eliminate the confounding factors, which makes the results more reliable. The results indicated that patients undergoing adjuvant therapy after trimodal therapy yielded significantly shorter OS and DFS when compared to patients not receiving adjuvant therapy. The results were consistent in patients with pathologic node-negative ESCC. However, for patients with nodal metastases after neoadjuvant chemoradiotherapy, no significant difference was seen between adjuvant therapy groups and no adjuvant therapy group. The results were opposite to the study reported by Matsuura et al. [18]. They conducted a retrospective study enrolling 113 thoracic ESCC patients with three or more pathologic positive lymph nodes. The included patients received neoadjuvant chemotherapy followed by radical surgery. The clinical efficacy of adjuvant chemotherapy was then evaluated. Their study concluded that adjuvant therapy may offer a significantly additional benefit to the prognosis of EC patients who have many positive lymph nodes even after neoadjuvant chemotherapy and surgery. The potential reason for their different results could be that their study only included patients with three or more pathologic positive lymph nodes (ypN2–3). However, the evidence was not irrefutable due to the small study population.

Theoretically, adjuvant therapy is expected to instigate a favorable effect and prolong survival for patients. However, in our institution adjuvant therapy could not prolong survival for patients with ESCC after trimodal therapy, even for patients with pathologic positive lymph nodes (ypN1–3). On the contrary, for ESCC patients with pathologic negative lymph nodes (ypN0), adjuvant therapy could be an unfavorable prognostic factor. There are several potential explanations for these results. Patients who were already treated with preoperative chemoradiotherapy could be insensitive to repeated systemic treatment after surgery [19,20]. Meanwhile, as a systemic treatment, all types of adjuvant therapy may cause adverse systemic effects on patients [21]. Especially for ESCC patients, prolonged fasting or reduce of meal could lead to poor nutritional status, which makes them frailer after receiving adjuvant therapy [22,23]. Moreover, the unfavorable impact of adjuvant therapy on the immune system could further weaken the patient's resistance to the tumor, leading to tumor recurrence after adjuvant therapy [24]. Therefore, adjuvant therapy is not recommended for ESCC patients after trimodal therapy regardless of status of nodal metastases.

There are several limitations present in this study. The retrospective nature of this study design could reduce the reliability of the results. Therefore, propensity score matching was used in this study to eliminate the selection bias of included patients. Meanwhile, the sample size is small because of the single-center setting. More participants will be employed in our future study.

5. Conclusions

The results of our study indicate that adjuvant therapy after neoadjuvant chemoradiotherapy and surgery could reduce the OS and DFS in patients with ESCC. Meanwhile, adjuvant therapy is an independently unfavorably prognostic factor for DFS. Therefore, adjuvant therapy is not recommended for ESCC patients after neoadjuvant chemoradiotherapy and esophagectomy, especially patients with node-negative after neoadjuvant therapy. A large-scale well-designed prospective study will be needed to confirm these results.

Supplementary Materials: The following supporting information can be downloaded at: https://www.mdpi.com/article/10.3390/cancers14153721/s1, Table S1: Treatment protocol of neoadjuvant therapy; Table S2: Treatment protocol of adjuvant therapy. Table S3. Univariate Cox regression model was used to determine variables associated with overall survival and disease-free survival for patients undergoing neoadjuvant therapy and esophagectomy.

Author Contributions: Conceptualization, X.L.; methodology, S.L.; software, X.L.; validation, X.L., S.L. and Y.Y. (Yushang Yang); formal analysis, J.Z.; investigation, X.L., P.F.; resources, Y.Y. (Yong Yuan), H.Z.; data curation, Q.S.; writing—original draft preparation, X.L., X.X.; writing—review and editing, X.L., Y.Y. (Yong Yuan); visualization, X.L.; supervision, X.L.; project administration, X.L.; funding acquisition, Y.Y. (Yong Yuan). All authors have read and agreed to the published version of the manuscript.

Funding: This work was supported by the National Natural Science Foundation of China (81970481), the Sichuan Science and Technology Program (2022YFS0048), key projects of Sichuan Provincial Department of Science and Technology (22ZDY1959), and the 1.3.5 project for disciplines of excellence, West China Hospital, Sichuan University (2020HXFH047, ZYJC18010 and 20HXJS005).

Institutional Review Board Statement: This study was approved by the Institutional Review Board of West China Hospital, Sichuan University at April 2021 (2022-636).

Informed Consent Statement: Informed consent was obtained from all subjects involved in the study.

Data Availability Statement: The datasets generated during and/or analyzed during the current study are available from the corresponding author on reasonable request.

Conflicts of Interest: The authors declare no conflict of interest.

References

1. Siegel, R.L.; Miller, K.D.; Fuchs, H.E.; Jemal, A. Cancer statistics, 2022. *CA Cancer J. Clin.* **2022**, *72*, 7–33. [CrossRef] [PubMed]
2. Ajani, J.A.; D'Amico, T.A.; Bentrem, D.J.; Chao, J.; Corvera, C.; Das, P.; Denlinger, C.S.; Enzinger, P.C.; Fanta, P.; Farjah, F.; et al. Esophageal and Esophagogastric Junction Cancers, Version 2.2019, NCCN Clinical Practice Guidelines in Oncology. *J. Natl. Compr. Cancer Netw.* **2019**, *17*, 855–883. [CrossRef]
3. Sung, H.; Ferlay, J.; Siegel, R.L.; Laversanne, M.; Soerjomataram, I.; Jemal, A.; Bray, F. Global Cancer Statistics 2020: GLOBOCAN Estimates of Incidence and Mortality Worldwide for 36 Cancers in 185 Countries. *CA Cancer J. Clin.* **2021**, *71*, 209–249. [CrossRef] [PubMed]

4. Lee, Y.; Samarasinghe, Y.; Lee, M.H.; Thiru, L.; Shargall, Y.; Finley, C.; Hanna, W.; Levine, O.; Juergens, R.; Agzarian, J. Role of Adjuvant Therapy in Esophageal Cancer Patients after Neoadjuvant Therapy and Esophagectomy: A Systematic Review and Meta-analysis. *Ann. Surg.* **2022**, *275*, 91–98. [CrossRef] [PubMed]
5. Mokdad, A.A.; Yopp, A.C.; Polanco, P.M.; Mansour, J.C.; Reznik, S.I.; Heitjan, D.F.; Choti, M.A.; Minter, R.R.; Wang, S.C.; Porembka, M.R. Adjuvant Chemotherapy vs. Postoperative Observation Following Preoperative Chemoradiotherapy and Resection in Gastroesophageal Cancer: A Propensity Score-Matched Analysis. *JAMA Oncol.* **2018**, *4*, 31–38. [CrossRef] [PubMed]
6. Samson, P.; Puri, V.; Lockhart, A.C.; Robinson, C.; Broderick, S.; Patterson, G.A.; Meyers, B.; Crabtree, T. Adjuvant chemotherapy for patients with pathologic node-positive esophageal cancer after induction chemotherapy is associated with improved survival. *J. Thorac. Cardiovasc. Surg.* **2018**, *156*, 1725–1735. [CrossRef] [PubMed]
7. Burt, B.M.; Groth, S.S.; Sada, Y.H.; Farjah, F.; Cornwell, L.; Sugarbaker, D.J.; Massarweh, N.N. Utility of Adjuvant Chemotherapy after Neoadjuvant Chemoradiation and Esophagectomy for Esophageal Cancer. *Ann. Surg.* **2017**, *266*, 297–304. [CrossRef]
8. Sudo, N.; Ichikawa, H.; Muneoka, Y.; Hanyu, T.; Kano, Y.; Ishikawa, T.; Hirose, Y.; Miura, K.; Shimada, Y.; Nagahashi, M.; et al. Clinical Utility of ypTNM Stage Grouping in the 8th Edition of the American Joint Committee on Cancer TNM Staging System for Esophageal Squamous Cell Carcinoma. *Ann. Surg. Oncol.* **2021**, *28*, 650–660. [CrossRef] [PubMed]
9. Ando, N.; Kato, H.; Igaki, H.; Shinoda, M.; Ozawa, S.; Shimizu, H.; Nakamura, T.; Yabusaki, H.; Aoyama, N.; Kurita, A.; et al. A randomized trial comparing postoperative adjuvant chemotherapy with cisplatin and 5-fluorouracil versus preoperative chemotherapy for localized advanced squamous cell carcinoma of the thoracic esophagus (JCOG9907). *Ann. Surg. Oncol.* **2012**, *19*, 68–74. [CrossRef]
10. Smyth, E.C.; Cunningham, D. Adjuvant Chemotherapy Following Neoadjuvant Chemotherapy Plus Surgery for Patients after Gastroesophageal Cancer-Is There Room for Improvement? *JAMA Oncol.* **2018**, *4*, 38–39. [CrossRef]
11. Takeda, F.R.; Tustumi, F.; de Almeida Obregon, C.; Yogolare, G.G.; Navarro, Y.P.; Segatelli, V.; Sallum, R.A.A.; Junior, U.R.; Cecconello, I. Prognostic Value of Tumor Regression Grade Based on Ryan Score in Squamous Cell Carcinoma and Adenocarcinoma of Esophagus. *Ann. Surg. Oncol.* **2020**, *27*, 1241–1247. [CrossRef]
12. Ajani, J.A.; D'Amico, T.A.; Almhanna, K.; Bentrem, D.J.; Besh, S.; Chao, J.; Das, P.; Denlinger, C.; Fanta, P.; Fuchs, C.S.; et al. Esophageal and esophagogastric junction cancers, version 1.2015. *J. Natl. Compr. Cancer Netw.* **2015**, *13*, 194–227. [CrossRef] [PubMed]
13. Drake, J.; Tauer, K.; Portnoy, D.; Weksler, B. Adjuvant chemotherapy is associated with improved survival in patients with nodal metastases after neoadjuvant therapy and esophagectomy. *J. Thorac. Dis.* **2019**, *11*, 2546–2554. [CrossRef]
14. Semenkovich, T.R.; Subramanian, M.; Yan, Y.; Hofstetter, W.L.; Correa, A.M.; Cassivi, S.D.; Inra, M.L.; Stiles, B.M.; Altorki, N.K.; Chang, A.C.; et al. Adjuvant Therapy for Node-Positive Esophageal Cancer after Induction and Surgery: A Multisite Study. *Ann. Thorac. Surg.* **2019**, *108*, 828–836. [CrossRef] [PubMed]
15. Huang, Z.; Li, S.; Yang, X.; Lu, F.; Huang, M.; Zhang, S.; Xiong, Y.; Zhang, P.; Si, J.; Ma, Y.; et al. Long-term survival of patients with locally advanced esophageal squamous cell carcinoma receiving esophagectomy following neoadjuvant chemotherapy: A cohort study. *Cancer Manag. Res.* **2019**, *11*, 1299–1308. [CrossRef] [PubMed]
16. Pasquali, S.; Yim, G.; Vohra, R.S.; Mocellin, S.; Nyanhongo, D.; Marriott, P.; Geh, J.I.; Griffiths, E.A. Survival after Neoadjuvant and Adjuvant Treatments Compared to Surgery Alone for Resectable Esophageal Carcinoma: A Network Meta-analysis. *Ann. Surg.* **2017**, *265*, 481–491. [CrossRef] [PubMed]
17. Chen, Y.; Hao, D.; Wu, X.; Xing, W.; Yang, Y.; He, C.; Wang, W.; Liu, J.; Wang, J. Neoadjuvant versus adjuvant chemoradiation for stage II-III esophageal squamous cell carcinoma: A single institution experience. *Dis. Esophagus* **2017**, *30*, 1–7. [CrossRef] [PubMed]
18. Matsuura, N.; Yamasaki, M.; Yamashita, K.; Tanaka, K.; Makino, T.; Saito, T.; Yamamoto, K.; Takahashi, T.; Kurokawa, Y.; Motoori, M.; et al. The role of adjuvant chemotherapy in esophageal cancer patients after neoadjuvant chemotherapy plus surgery. *Esophagus* **2021**, *18*, 559–565. [CrossRef]
19. Ji, Y.; Du, X.; Zhu, W.; Yang, Y.; Ma, J.; Zhang, L.; Li, J.; Tao, H.; Xia, J.; Yang, H.; et al. Efficacy of Concurrent Chemoradiotherapy after S-1 vs. Radiotherapy Alone for Older Patients after Esophageal Cancer: A Multicenter Randomized Phase 3 Clinical Trial. *JAMA Oncol.* **2021**, *7*, 1459–1466. [CrossRef] [PubMed]
20. Cheraghi, A.; Barahman, M.; Hariri, R.; Nikoofar, A.; Fadavi, P. Comparison of the Pathological Response and Adverse Effects of Oxaliplatin and Capecitabine versus Paclitaxel and Carboplatin in the Neoadjuvant Chemoradiotherapy Treatment Approach for Esophageal and Gastroesophageal Junction Cancer: A Randomized Control Trial Study. *Med. J. Islamic Repub. Iran* **2021**, *35*, 140. [CrossRef]
21. Noordman, B.J.; Verdam, M.G.E.; Lagarde, S.M.; Shapiro, J.; Hulshof, M.; van Berge Henegouwen, M.I.; Wijnhoven, B.P.L.; Nieuwenhuijzen, G.A.P.; Bonenkamp, J.J.; Cuesta, M.A.; et al. Impact of neoadjuvant chemoradiotherapy on health-related quality of life in long-term survivors of esophageal or junctional cancer: Results from the randomized CROSS trial. *Ann. Oncol.* **2018**, *29*, 445–451. [CrossRef] [PubMed]
22. Elliott, J.A.; Docherty, N.G.; Eckhardt, H.G.; Doyle, S.L.; Guinan, E.M.; Ravi, N.; Reynolds, J.V.; Roux, C.W.L. Weight Loss, Satiety, and the Postprandial Gut Hormone Response after Esophagectomy: A Prospective Study. *Ann. Surg.* **2017**, *266*, 82–90. [CrossRef] [PubMed]

23. Kubo, Y.; Miyata, H.; Sugimura, K.; Shinno, N.; Asukai, K.; Hasegawa, S.; Yanagimoto, Y.; Yamada, D.; Yamamoto, K.; Nishimura, J.; et al. Prognostic Implication of Postoperative Weight Loss after Esophagectomy for Esophageal Squamous Cell Cancer. *Ann. Surg. Oncol.* **2021**, *28*, 184–193. [CrossRef] [PubMed]
24. Park, S.Y.; Kim, D.J.; Suh, J.W.; Byun, G.E. Risk Factors for Weight Loss 1 Year after Esophagectomy and Gastric Pull-up for Esophageal Cancer. *J. Gastrointest. Surg.* **2018**, *22*, 1137–1143. [CrossRef] [PubMed]

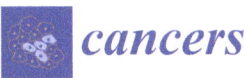

Article

Effect of Pre-Existing Sarcopenia on Oncological Outcomes for Oral Cavity Squamous Cell Carcinoma Undergoing Curative Surgery: A Propensity Score-Matched, Nationwide, Population-Based Cohort Study

Yu-Hsiang Tsai [1,†], Wan-Ming Chen [2,†], Ming-Chih Chen [2], Ben-Chang Shia [2,3], Szu-Yuan Wu [2,3,4,5,6,7,8,9,10,*] and Chun-Chi Huang [1,*]

1. Department of Otorhinolaryngology, Lo-Hsu Medical Foundation, Lotung Poh-Ai Hospital, Yilan 265, Taiwan; b101098034@tmu.edu.tw
2. Graduate Institute of Business Administration, College of Management, Fu Jen Catholic University, Taipei 242062, Taiwan; daisywanmingchen@gmail.com (W.-M.C.); 081438@mail.fju.edu.tw (M.-C.C.); 025674@mail.fju.edu.tw (B.-C.S.)
3. Artificial Intelligence Development Center, Fu Jen Catholic University, Taipei 242062, Taiwan
4. Department of Food Nutrition and Health Biotechnology, College of Medical and Health Science, Asia University, Taichung 41354, Taiwan
5. Division of Radiation Oncology, Lo-Hsu Medical Foundation, Lotung Poh-Ai Hospital, Yilan 265, Taiwan
6. Big Data Center, Lo-Hsu Medical Foundation, Lotung Poh-Ai Hospital, Yilan 265, Taiwan
7. Department of Healthcare Administration, College of Medical and Health Science, Asia University, Taichung 41354, Taiwan
8. Cancer Center, Lo-Hsu Medical Foundation, Lotung Poh-Ai Hospital, Yilan 265, Taiwan
9. Centers for Regional Anesthesia and Pain Medicine, Taipei Municipal Wan Fang Hospital, Taipei Medical University, Taipei 116081, Taiwan
10. Department of Management, College of Management, Fo Guang University, Yilan 262307, Taiwan
* Correspondence: szuyuanwu5399@gmail.com (S.-Y.W.); b8301054@gmail.com (C.-C.H.)
† These authors contributed equally to this work.

Simple Summary: Although sarcopenia during cancer diagnosis is an independent prognostic factor for poor overall survival in patients with various cancers, whether pre-existing sarcopenia is an independent risk factor for oral cavity squamous cell carcinoma (OCSCC) remains unclear. Therefore, we conducted a head-to-head propensity score matching (PSM) study to estimate the oncological outcomes of pre-existing sarcopenia in patients with OCSCC undergoing curative surgery. Both univariate and multivariate Cox regression analyses indicated that pre-existing sarcopenia was associated with poor survival than nonsarcopenia. Old age, male sex, advanced pT, advanced pN, differentiation grade II–III, margin-positive cancer, lymphovascular invasion, and CCI ≥ 1 were significant poor prognostic factors for survival in the patients with OCSCC undergoing curative surgery.

Abstract: Purpose: The effect of pre-existing sarcopenia on patients with oral cavity squamous cell carcinoma (OCSCC) remains unknown. Therefore, we designed a propensity score-matched population-based cohort study to compare the oncological outcomes of patients with OCSCC undergoing curative surgery with and without sarcopenia. Patients and Methods: We included patients with OCSCC undergoing curative surgery and categorized them into two groups according to the presence or absence of pre-existing sarcopenia. Patients in both the groups were matched at a ratio of 2:1. Results: The matching process yielded 16,294 patients (10,855 and 5439 without and with pre-existing sarcopenia, respectively). In multivariate Cox regression analyses, the adjusted hazard ratio (aHR, 95% confidence interval [CI]) of all-cause mortality for OCSCC with and without pre-existing sarcopenia was 1.15 (1.11–1.21, $p < 0.0001$). Furthermore, the aHRs (95% CIs) of locoregional recurrence and distant metastasis for OCSCC with and without pre-existing sarcopenia were 1.07 (1.03–1.18, $p = 0.0020$) and 1.07 (1.03–1.20, $p = 0.0148$), respectively. Conclusions: Pre-existing sarcopenia might be a significant poor prognostic factor for overall survival, locoregional recurrence, and distant metastasis for patients with OCSCC undergoing curative surgery. In susceptible patients

Citation: Tsai, Y.-H.; Chen, W.-M.; Chen, M.-C.; Shia, B.-C.; Wu, S.-Y.; Huang, C.-C. Effect of Pre-Existing Sarcopenia on Oncological Outcomes for Oral Cavity Squamous Cell Carcinoma Undergoing Curative Surgery: A Propensity Score-Matched, Nationwide, Population-Based Cohort Study. *Cancers* 2022, 14, 3246. https://doi.org/10.3390/cancers14133246

Academic Editors: Carlo Lajolo, Gaetano Paludetti and Romeo Patini

Received: 1 June 2022
Accepted: 26 June 2022
Published: 1 July 2022

Publisher's Note: MDPI stays neutral with regard to jurisdictional claims in published maps and institutional affiliations.

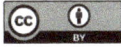

Copyright: © 2022 by the authors. Licensee MDPI, Basel, Switzerland. This article is an open access article distributed under the terms and conditions of the Creative Commons Attribution (CC BY) license (https://creativecommons.org/licenses/by/4.0/).

at a risk of OCSCC, sarcopenia prevention measures should be encouraged, such as exercise and early nutrition intervention.

Keywords: sarcopenia; nonsarcopenia; OCSCC; survival; prognosis

1. Introduction

Head and neck cancer (HNC) is the third most common cancer and the fifth leading cause of cancer deaths in men in Taiwan [1] because of betel nut chewing, cigarette smoking, and alcohol use [2–10]. The median age of patients with HNC in Taiwan is 55 years, indicating that they are an economically active population [1–10]; thus, improving their survival is essential. In Taiwan, the oral cavity squamous cell carcinoma (OCSCC) subtype accounts for more than 80% of HNC, whereas in Western countries, most HNCs are oropharyngeal cancers [2–10]. This difference is likely due to the habit of betel nut chewing in Taiwan [8–10]. Moreover, there are 377,713 new cases and 177,757 new deaths per year for oral cancer in the world based on the last updated GLOBOCAN (IARC, WHO) report in 2020 [11]. Despite advancements in therapeutics [8–10], the survival rate of HNC in Taiwan has remained dismal [1]. From the perspective of preventive medicine, if a prognostic factor for survival in patients with OCSCC can be corrected before cancer diagnosis, the factor should be screened and corrected for improving survival in OCSCC.

Sarcopenia, characterized by the loss of muscle mass, strength, and performance [12–14], can occur not only in overweight and underweight individuals but also in those with normal weight [15]. Unlike cachexia, sarcopenia does not require the presence of an underlying illness [16]. In addition, although most people with cachexia are sarcopenic, most individuals with sarcopenia are not considered cachectic [16]. Sarcopenia is associated with increased functional impairment, disability, fall, and mortality rates [17]. The causes of sarcopenia are multifactorial and include disuse, endocrine function alteration, chronic diseases, inflammation, insulin resistance, and nutritional deficiencies [14]. Therefore, sarcopenia and cancer cachexia-related sarcopenia are distinct conditions. Pre-existing sarcopenia can be prevented, whereas cancer-related sarcopenia cannot be prevented but can be treated.

Sarcopenia is associated with increased mortality for most cancers, except hormone-related cancers (endometrial, breast, ovarian, and prostate cancers) and hematopoietic cancers [18–21], thus making it a major prognostic factor for poor overall survival and mortality in patients with cancer [18–21]. Sarcopenia-related cancer mortality might be a consequence of treatment-related toxicity [22,23]. However, whether pre-existing sarcopenia is an independent risk factor for different cancers, including OCSCC, remains unclear. A propensity score matching (PSM)-based design can resolve this issue by maintaining balance among the confounding factors of the case and control groups—all in the absence of bias [24–26]. Moreover, PSM is currently the recommended standard tool for estimating the effects of covariates in studies where any potential bias may exist [24–26]. Therefore, we conducted a head-to-head PSM study to estimate the oncological outcomes of pre-existing sarcopenia in patients with OCSCC undergoing curative surgery.

2. Patients and Methods

2.1. Study Population

We selected patients with OCSCC who had undergone curative surgery—tumor resection and neck dissection—between 1 January 2007 and 31 December 2017 from the Taiwan Cancer Registry Database (TCRD). The follow-up period was from the index date (i.e., date of surgery) to 31 December 2018. The types and indications of neck dissection were as follows: supraomohyoid neck dissection for clinically N0 tumors [27], modified neck dissection for ipsilateral clinically positive nodes [28], and bilateral neck dissection for contralateral metastases or tumors cross the midline [29]. Adjuvant treatments indicated for patients with OCSCC were based on the National Comprehensive Cancer Network (NCCN) guidelines and patients' tolerance [30]. The TCRD contains detailed cancer-related data of patients, including the clinical stage, cigarette smoking habit, treatment modalities, pathologic data, and grade of differentiation [5,8–10,31]. The study protocols were reviewed and approved by the Institutional Review Board of Tzu-Chi Medical Foundation (IRB109-015-B).

The diagnoses of the enrolled patients were confirmed after reviewing their pathological data, and patients who were newly diagnosed as having OCSCC were confirmed to have no other cancers or distant metastasis (DM). All patients with OCSCC underwent curative-intent surgery. The inclusion criteria were as follows: being aged ≥20 years, having a diagnosis of pathologic stage I–IVB OCSCC without metastasis according to the American Joint Committee on Cancer criteria (AJCC, 7th edition), and undergoing tumor resection and neck dissection. Patients were excluded if they had a history of other cancers before the index date, an unknown pathological stage, missing sex data, unclear differentiation of tumor grade, or a nonsquamous cell carcinoma pathologic type.

2.2. Interventions/Exposures

Our definition of sarcopenia is according to the previous study from the Taiwan NHIRD [32]. In order to diminish the selection bias of the definition of sarcopenia, we only recorded the sarcopenia from the rehabilitation specialists, orthopedics, or family physicians. We have also added the sensitivity analysis of the recorded sarcopenia from the rehabilitation specialists, orthopedics, and family physician with/without other specialties (including endocrinology department) (Supplementary Table S2). In Taiwan, the coding of sarcopenia was based on a previous Taiwan study [33]; sarcopenia was defined as the skeletal muscle mass index (SMI) of 2 standard deviations (SDs) or more below the normal sex-specific means for young persons. Patients diagnosed as having sarcopenia after OCSCC diagnosis and those with sarcopenia diagnosed within 1 year before OCSCC diagnosis (excluding cancer treatment-related and cancer cachexia-related sarcopenia) were excluded. We also supplied the sensitivity analysis for the comparison of washout time intervals of one year and two years (Supplementary Table S1).

2.3. Comparisons

We categorized the patients into two groups depending on whether they had sarcopenia before OCSCC diagnosis: Group 1 (nonsarcopenic OCSCC) and Group 2 (pre-existing sarcopenic OCSCC). In addition, we estimated oncological outcomes (all-cause mortality, locoregional recurrence [LRR], and DM) associated with sarcopenia. Comorbidity was assessed using the Charlson comorbidity index (CCI) [6,34]. Only comorbidities which appeared 12 months before the index date were included and they were coded and classified according to the International Classification of Diseases, Ninth Revision, Clinical Modification (ICD-9-CM) or International Classification of Diseases, Tenth Revision, Clinical Modification (ICD-10-CM) codes at the first admission or after >2 appearances of a diagnostic code at outpatient visits.

2.4. Outcomes

The oncologic outcomes were defined as all-cause death, LRR, and DM according to the previous oncologic studies [35–37]. All-cause mortality was the primary endpoint in both the groups. The secondary endpoints were LRR and DM.

2.5. Design Setting

To reduce the effects of potential confounders when comparing all-cause mortality between patients without and with sarcopenia, we performed 2:1 PSM with a caliper of 0.2 for the following variables: age, sex, years of diagnosis, AJCC pathologic stages, pathologic tumor stages (pT), pathologic nodal stage (pN), differentiation grade, surgical margin, lymphovascular invasion (LVI), adjuvant treatments, CCI scores, cigarette smoking, alcohol use, and betel nut chewing. These variables are potential prognostic factors for all-cause mortality for patients with OCSCC undergoing curative surgery. A Cox proportional hazards model was used to regress all-cause mortality in patients with OCSCC with a robust sandwich estimator used to account for clustering within matched sets [38]. Potential confounding factors for all-cause mortality for OCSCC were controlled in the PSM (Table 1). After well-matched PSM, the actual real-world data can indicate the oncological outcomes of pre-existing sarcopenia in patients with OCSCC undergoing curative surgery.

Table 1. Characteristics of patients with oral cavity squamous cell carcinoma with and without pre-existing sarcopenia (After propensity score matching 1:2).

	Nonsarcopenia N = 10,855		Sarcopenia N = 5439		p Value
	N	%	N	%	
Age (mean ± SD)	55.79 ± 10.89		55.44 ± 11.14		0.2384
Age, median (IQR), years	55.00 (48.00, 63.00)		55.00 (48.00, 63.00)		0.9929
Age groups					0.5057
<50 years	3061	28.20%	1492	27.43%	
50–60 years	3930	36.20%	1969	36.20%	
≥60 years	3864	35.60%	1978	36.37%	
Sex					0.1720
Male	9803	90.31%	4875	89.63%	
Female	1052	9.69%	564	10.37%	
Years of diagnosis					0.3349
2007–2010	2264	20.86%	1149	21.13%	
2011–2014	4612	42.49%	2246	41.29%	
2015–2017	3979	36.66%	2044	37.58%	
AJCC pathologic stage					0.9995
I	2279	21.00%	1142	21.00%	
II	1492	13.74%	747	13.73%	
III	1281	11.80%	642	11.80%	
IVA	5304	48.86%	2658	48.87%	
IVB	499	4.60%	250	4.60%	
AJCC pathologic stage T					0.9899
pT1	107	0.99%	56	1.03%	
pT2	3186	29.35%	1595	29.33%	
pT3	3270	30.12%	1637	30.10%	
pT4A	989	9.11%	497	9.14%	
pT4B	3303	30.43%	1654	30.41%	
AJCC pathologic stage N					0.9979
pN0	5117	47.14%	2572	47.29%	
pN1	1560	14.37%	779	14.32%	
pN2	3745	34.50%	1872	34.42%	
pN3	433	3.99%	216	3.97%	

Table 1. Cont.

	Nonsarcopenia N = 10,855		Sarcopenia N = 5439		p Value
	N	%	N	%	
Differentiation					0.9526
I	2253	20.76%	1130	20.78%	
II	6272	57.78%	3140	57.73%	
III	2330	21.46%	1169	21.49%	
Surgical margin	10,855		5439		0.9467
Negative	9078	83.63%	4539	83.45%	
Positive	1777	16.37%	900	16.55%	
Lymphovascular invasion					0.9705
No	4962	45.71%	2481	45.62%	
YES	5893	54.29%	2958	54.38%	
Adjuvant treatments					0.2968
No adjuvant	2129	19.61%	1080	19.86%	
Adjuvant RT	1452	13.38%	779	14.32%	
Adjuvant sequential CT and RT	2149	19.80%	1097	20.17%	
Adjuvant CT	322	2.97%	164	3.02%	
Adjuvant CCRT	4803	44.25%	2319	42.64%	
Adjuvant RT dose (Gy), mean	63.08 ± 15.48		63.77 ± 15.34		0.1691
Median (IQR, Q1, Q3)	66.00 (60.00, 70.00)		66.00 (60.00, 70.00)		0.1414
Adjuvant chemotherapy with cumulative platinum dose (mg), mean	542.11 ± 413.46		541.16 ± 414.90		0.9082
Median	450.00 (300.00, 650.00)		450.00 (300.00, 650.00)		0.1630
CCI scores					
Mean (SD)	0.70 ± 1.11		0.73 ± 1.13		0.2747
CCI scores					0.3813
0	7032	64.78%	3448	63.39%	
≥1	3823	35.22%	1991	36.61%	
Cigarette smoking	7590	69.92%	3794	69.76%	0.9891
Alcohol use	6299	58.03%	3144	57.80%	0.8910
Betel nut chewing	6624	61.02%	3310	60.86%	0.8872
Outcomes					
Median follow-up, y (mean ± SD)	3.87 ± 3.03		3.46 ± 2.90		<0.0001
Median follow-up, y (IQR, Q1, Q3)	3.11 (1.28, 5.81)		2.65 (1.00, 5.18)		<0.0001
All-cause mortality	10,855		5439		0.0039
No	5445	50.16%	2598	47.77%	
YES	5410	49.84%	2841	52.23%	
Metastasis					<0.0001
No	9086	83.70%	4515	83.01%	
YES	1769	16.30%	924	16.99%	

Table 1. Cont.

	Nonsarcopenia N = 10,855		Sarcopenia N = 5439		p Value
	N	%	N	%	
Locoregional recurrence					0.0030
No	9152	84.31%	4569	84.00%	
YES	1703	15.69%	870	16.00%	

RT, radiotherapy; CCRT, concurrent chemoradiotherapy; CCI, Charlson comorbidity index; SD, standard deviation; IQR, interquartile range; AJCC, American Joint Committee on Cancer; y, years old; N, numbers; Gy, Gray; pT, pathologic tumor stages; pN, pathologic nodal stages.

2.6. Statistical Analysis

The aforementioned variables might be independent prognostic factors for all-cause mortality with residual imbalance after PSM [39,40]. Therefore, multivariate Cox regression analyses were performed to calculate hazard ratios (HRs) to determine whether pre-existing sarcopenia is an independent predictor of all-cause mortality.

After adjustment for confounders, all statistical analyses were performed using SAS version 9.4 (SAS Institute, Cary, NC, USA). In a two-tailed Wald test, $p < 0.05$ was considered significant. OS, LRR, and DM were estimated using the Kaplan–Meier method and between-group differences were compared using the stratified log-rank test (stratified according to matched sets) [41].

3. Results

3.1. Study Cohorts before and after PSM

We identified 45,219 patients with OCSCC undergoing curative surgery (39,775 without and 5445 [12.04%] with pre-existing sarcopenia) before PSM (Supplementary Table S1). Compared with the patients without pre-existing sarcopenia, those with sarcopenia were older; were predominantly women; had higher CCI scores; more likely received the diagnosis in 2015–2017; had more advanced pT and pN stages; had more poor differentiation, margin positivity, and LVI-positive tumors; and received more adjuvant concurrent chemoradiotherapy (CCRT), higher radiotherapy (RT) doses, and higher cumulative platinum doses. PSM yielded 16,294 patients (10,855 without and 5439 with sarcopenia) who were eligible for further analysis and their characteristics are summarized in Table 1. Age, sex, years of diagnosis, cancer subtypes, AJCC pathological stages, pT, pN, differentiation, surgical margin, lymphovascular invasion, adjuvant treatments, CCI scores, cigarette smoking, alcohol use, and betel nut chewing were balanced between the cohorts (all $p > 0.05$). After PSM, the crude all-cause mortality, LRR, and DM were significantly higher in the patients with sarcopenia than in those without sarcopenia (Table 1).

3.2. Cox Proportional Hazard Models of All-Cause Mortality

According to multivariate Cox regression analysis, pre-existing sarcopenia was a significant predictor of all-cause mortality (Table 2). Both univariate and multivariate Cox regression analyses indicated that sarcopenia was associated with poorer OS than nonsarcopenia. The HR for the univariate model was similar to that for the multivariate Cox regression analysis. Old age, male sex, advanced pT, advanced pN, differentiation grade II/III, margin positivity, LVI positivity, and CCI ≥ 1 were significantly poor prognostic factors for OS in the patients with OCSCC. In multivariate Cox regression analyses, the adjusted hazard ratio (aHRs, 95% confidence interval [CI]) of all-cause mortality for OCSCC with and without pre-existing sarcopenia was 1.14 (1.10–1.19, $p < 0.0001$). The aHRs (95% CIs) of mortality for male sex, age 50–59 years, age ≥ 60 years, pT2, pT3, pT4A, pT4B, pN1, pN2, pN3, differentiation grades II and III, margin positivity, LVI positivity, CCI ≥ 1, cigarette smoking, alcohol use, and betel nut chewing compared with female sex, age < 50 years, pT1, pN0, differentiation grade I, margin negativity, LVI negativity, CCI = 0, no cigarette smoking, no alcohol use, no betel nut chewing were 1.28 (1.20–1.39), 1.14 (1.07–1.19), 1.25 (1.19–1.33), 1.05 (1.01–1.31), 1.31 (1.05–1.63), 1.66 (1.33–2.11), 1.72 (1.39–2.17), 1.11 (1.04–1.24), 1.21 (1.05–1.41), 2.03 (1.72–2.71), 1.18 (1.12–1.23), 1.21 (1.12–1.31), 1.23 (1.18–1.33), 1.59 (1.38–1.87), 1.19 (1.13–1.26), 1.10 (1.04–1.22), 1.08 (1.03–1.23), and 1.09 (1.02–1.30), respectively.

Table 2. Univariable and multivariable Cox proportional regression model for all-cause mortality of the propensity score-matched groups of patients with oral cavity squamous cell carcinoma with and without pre-existing sarcopenia.

	Crude HR (95% CI)		p Value	Adjusted HR * (95% CI)		p Value
Sarcopenia						
Nonsarcopenia (Ref.)	1			1		
Sarcopenia	1.18	(1.12, 1.24)	<0.0001	1.15	(1.11, 1.21)	<0.0001
Sex						
Female (Ref.)	1			1		
Male	1.36	(1.28, 1.44)	<0.0001	1.28	(1.20, 1.39)	<0.0001
Age						
<50 years (Ref.)	1			1		
50–60 years	1.06	(1.04, 1.16)	0.0430	1.14	(1.07, 1.19)	0.0021
≥60 years	1.14	(1.12, 1.22)	<0.0001	1.25	(1.19, 1.33)	<0.0001
Years of diagnosis						
2007–2010 (Ref.)	1			1		
2011–2014	0.90	(0.84, 1.06)	0.6420	0.91	(0.89, 1.08)	0.4268
2015–2017	0.77	(0.72, 1.09)	0.6664	0.83	(0.79, 1.09)	0.2332
AJCC pathologic T						
pT1 (Ref.)	1			1		
pT2	0.94	(1.04, 1.21)	0.2361	1.05	(1.01, 1.31)	0.0380
pT3	1.14	(0.92, 1.46)	0.1412	1.31	(1.05, 1.63)	0.0113
pT4A	1.64	(1.31, 2.01)	<0.0001	1.66	(1.33, 2.11)	<0.0001
pT4B	1.71	(1.37, 2.13)	<0.0001	1.72	(1.39, 2.17)	<0.0001
AJCC pathologic N						
pN0 (Ref.)	1			1		
pN1	1.51	(1.42, 1.64)	<0.0001	1.11	(1.04, 1.24)	0.0002
pN2	2.37	(2.14, 2.58)	<0.0001	1.21	(1.05, 1.41)	0.0023
pN3	3.89	(3.31, 5.03)	<0.0001	2.03	(1.72, 2.71)	<0.0001
Differentiation						
I (Ref.)	1			1		
II	1.41	(1.35, 1.43)	<0.0001	1.18	(1.12, 1.23)	<0.0001
III	1.67	(1.54, 1.80)	<0.0001	1.21	(1.12, 1.31)	<0.0001
Surgical margin						
Negative (Ref.)	1			1		
Positive	1.50	(1.42, 1.61)	<0.0001	1.23	(1.18, 1.33)	<0.0001

Table 2. Cont.

	Crude HR (95% CI)		p Value	Adjusted HR * (95% CI)		p Value
Lymphovascular invasion						
No	1			1		
Yes	2.16	(2.04, 2.29)	<0.0001	1.59	(1.38, 1.87)	<0.0001
Adjuvant treatments						
No adjuvant treatments (Ref.)						
Adjuvant RT	1.05	(0.82, 1.44)	0.3530	1.04	(0.92, 1.45)	0.6012
Adjuvant sequential CT and RT	1.13	(0.69, 1.84)	0.5731	1.10	(0.72, 1.82)	0.7531
Adjuvant CT	1.10	(0.67, 1.44)	0.4310	1.07	(0.79, 1.45)	0.7405
Adjuvant CCRT	1.15	(0.62, 1.91)	0.1320	1.09	(0.79, 1.31)	0.3302
CCI ≥1 (Ref. CCI = 0)	1.21	(1.18, 1.29)	<0.0001	1.19	(1.13, 1.26)	<0.0001
Cigarette smoking (Ref. no use)	1.13	(1.03, 1.34)	<0.0001	1.10	(1.04, 1.22)	<0.0001
Alcohol use (Ref. no use)	1.16	(1.08, 1.39)	<0.0001	1.08	(1.03, 1.23)	<0.0001
Betel nut chewing (Ref. no use)	1.11	(1.03, 1.41)	<0.0001	1.09	(1.02, 1.30)	<0.0001

RT, radiotherapy; CCRT, concurrent chemoradiotherapy; CCI, Charlson comorbidity index; AJCC, American Joint Committee on Cancer; y, years old; pT, pathologic tumor stages; pN, pathologic nodal stages; Ref., reference group; CI, confidence interval; HR, hazard ratio. * All the aforementioned variables in Table 2 were used in multivariate analysis.

3.3. Cox Proportional Hazard Models of LRR and DM

Both univariate and multivariate Cox regression analyses indicated that pre-existing sarcopenia was associated with higher risk of LRR and DM than nonsarcopenia (Tables 3 and 4). In the multivariate Cox regression analysis, the aHRs (95% CIs) of LRR and DM for OCSCC with and without pre-existing sarcopenia were 1.07 (1.03–1.18, p = 0.0020) and 1.07 (1.03–1.20, p = 0.0148), respectively. In addition, poor prognostic factors for LRR and DM were similar with those of mortality, except old age and CCI scores. The multivariable Cox model revealed that male sex, advanced pT, advanced pN, differentiation grade II–III, margin positivity, LVI positivity, cigarette smoking use, alcohol use, and betel nut chewing use were independent poor prognostic factors for LRR and DM (Tables 3 and 4).

Table 3. Univariable and multivariable Cox proportional regression model for locoregional recurrence of the propensity score-matched groups of patients with oral cavity squamous cell carcinoma with and without pre-existing sarcopenia.

	Crude HR (95% CI)		p Value	Adjusted HR (95% CI)		p Value
Sarcopenia						
Nonsarcopenia (Ref.)	1			1		
Sarcopenia	1.08	(1.04, 1.15)	0.0061	1.07	(1.03, 1.18)	0.0020
Sex						
Female (Ref.)	1			1		
Male	1.51	(1.37, 1.70)	<0.0001	1.46	(1.30, 1.64)	<0.0001
Age						

Table 3. Cont.

	Crude HR (95% CI)		p Value	Adjusted HR (95% CI)		p Value
<50 years (Ref.)	1			1		
50–60 years	0.97	(0.90, 1.07)	0.6451	0.96	(0.90, 1.05)	0.6530
≥60 years	0.88	(0.82, 1.03)	0.3510	0.92	(0.80, 1.11)	0.2035
Years of diagnosis						
2007–2010 (Ref.)	1			1		
2011–2014	0.87	(0.50, 1.15)	0.3751	0.88	(0.52, 1.19)	0.3292
2015–2017	0.89	(0.62, 1.10)	0.2307	0.91	(0.61, 1.09)	0.2211
AJCC pathologic T						
pT1 (Ref.)	1			1		
pT2	1.11	(0.86, 1.44)	0.4421	1.51	(1.15, 2.01)	0.0017
pT3	1.08	(0.83, 1.42)	0.6248	1.38	(1.05, 1.85)	0.0064
pT4A	1.03	(0.88, 1.31)	0.5462	1.21	(1.05, 1.64)	0.0110
pT4B	1.08	(0.89, 1.34)	0.6286	1.17	(1.08, 1.55)	0.0089
AJCC pathologic N						
pN0 (Ref.)	1			1		
pN1	1.13	(1.06, 1.23)	0.0012	1.12	(1.04, 1.30)	0.0017
pN2	1.04	(1.02, 1.11)	0.0269	1.17	(1.05, 1.25)	0.0002
pN3	1.13	(1.04, 1.29)	0.0006	1.21	(1.11, 1.88)	0.0008
Differentiation						
I (Ref.)	1			1		
II	1.09	(1.03, 1.16)	0.0105	1.06	(1.01, 1.14)	0.0147
III	1.13	(0.86, 1.05)	0.0962	1.12	(1.03, 1.20)	0.0188
Surgical margin						
Negative (Ref.)	1			1		
Positive	1.21	(1.18, 1.33)	<0.0001	1.20	(1.11, 1.33)	<0.0001
Lymphovascular invasion						
No						
Yes	1.08	(1.04, 1.15)	0.0022	1.30	(1.07, 1.66)	0.0011
Adjuvant treatments						
No adjuvant treatments (Ref.)						
Adjuvant RT	0.99	(0.94, 1.06)	0.7440	1.01	(0.94, 1.05)	0.7624
Adjuvant sequential CT and RT	0.97	(0.93, 1.04)	0.4545	1.00	(0.96, 1.09)	0.7827
Adjuvant CT	1.03	(0.95, 1.08)	0.7632	1.04	(0.96, 1.12)	0.2424
Adjuvant CCRT	1.11	(0.98, 1.26)	0.0922	1.09	(0.96, 1.24)	0.1145
CCI ≥1 (Ref. CCI = 0)	0.96	(0.91, 1.06)	0.3596	0.98	(0.92, 1.05)	0.8620
Cigarette smoking (Ref. no use)	1.08	(1.01, 1.22)	0.0085	1.07	(1.00, 120)	0.0431
Alcohol use (Ref. no use)	1.11	(1.03, 1.19)	0.0020	1.06	(1.01, 1.13)	0.0338
Betel nut chewing (Ref. no use)	1.31	(1.12, 1.45)	<0.0001	1.19	(1.10, 1.38)	<0.0001

RT, radiotherapy; CCRT, concurrent chemoradiotherapy; CCI, Charlson comorbidity index; AJCC, American Joint Committee on Cancer; y, years old; pT, pathologic tumor stages; pN, pathologic nodal stages; Ref., reference group; CI, confidence interval; HR, hazard ratio.

Table 4. Univariable and multivariable Cox proportional regression model for distant metastasis of the propensity score-matched groups of patients with oral cavity squamous cell carcinoma with and without pre-existing sarcopenia.

	Crude HR (95% CI)		p Value	Adjusted HR (95% CI)		p Value
Sarcopenia						
Nonsarcopenia (Ref.)	1			1		
Sarcopenia	1.08	(1.02, 1.15)	0.0342	1.07	(1.03, 1.20)	0.01482
Sex						
Female (Ref.)	1			1		
Male	1.72	(1.54, 1.91)	<0.0001	1.60	(1.45, 1.80)	<0.0001
Age						
<50 years (Ref.)	1			1		
50–60 years	0.93	(0.88, 1.12)	0.1793	0.98	(0.93, 1.07)	0.8381
≥60 years	0.80	(0.64, 1.09)	0.5402	0.82	(0.79, 1.07)	0.4429
Years of diagnosis						
2007–2010 (Ref.)	1			1		
2011–2014	0.98	(0.92, 1.09)	0.7552	1.03	(0.96, 1.11)	0.2075
2015–2017	1.01	(0.94, 1.12)	0.8335	1.14	(0.90, 1.19)	0.6418
AJCC pathologic T						
pT1 (Ref.)	1			1		
pT2	1.26	(0.88, 1.80)	0.1719	2.32	(1.64, 3.40)	<0.0001
pT3	1.59	(1.12, 2.28)	0.0072	2.37	(1.64, 3.34)	<0.0001
pT4A	1.71	(1.22, 2.67)	0.0001	2.44	(1.60, 3.35)	<0.0001
pT4B	1.76	(1.25, 2.49)	0.0018	2.11	(1.51, 3.33)	<0.0001
AJCC pathologic N						
pN0 (Ref.)	1			1		
pN1	1.47	(1.32, 1.65)	<0.0001	1.26	(1.14, 1.95)	<0.0001
pN2	1.80	(1.64, 1.92)	<0.0001	1.41	(1.23, 1.50)	<0.0001
pN3	2.29	(1.53, 3.42)	<0.0001	1.51	(1.22, 1.72)	<0.0001
Differentiation						
I (WD) (Ref.)	1			1		
II (moderately differentiated)	1.31	(1.21, 1.42)	<0.0001	1.08	(1.04, 1.19)	0.0110
III	1.39	(1.30, 1.58)	<0.0001	1.14	(1.08, 1.25)	0.0066
Surgical margin						
Negative (Ref.)	1			1		
Positive	1.42	(1.30, 1.56)	<0.0001	1.17	(1.07, 1.28)	0.0003
Lymphovascular invasion						
No						
Yes	1.65	(1.54, 1.79)	<0.0001	1.31	(1.10, 1.63)	0.0073
Adjuvant treatments						
No adjuvant treatments (Ref.)						

Table 4. Cont.

	Crude HR (95% CI)		p Value	Adjusted HR (95% CI)		p Value
Adjuvant RT	0.96	(0.91, 1.02)	0.3243	1.02	(0.98, 1.13)	0.0755
Adjuvant sequential CT and RT	0.86	(0.78, 0.91)	<0.0001	0.94	(0.86, 1.04)	0.1688
Adjuvant CT	0.83	(0.79, 0.88)	<0.0001	0.97	(0.92, 1.05)	0.3443
Adjuvant CCRT	0.89	(0.81, 0.93)	<0.0001	1.02	(0.94, 1.09)	0.3468
CCI ≥ 1 (Ref. CCI = 0)	0.88	(0.77, 1.05)	0.1312	1.06	(0.92, 1.23)	0.2503
Cigarette smoking (Ref. no use)	1.04	(0.93, 1.20)	0.0923	1.06	(1.01, 123)	0.0207
Alcohol use (Ref. no use)	1.01	(0.91, 1.27)	0.0791	1.04	(1.00, 1.22)	0.0441
Betel nut chewing (Ref. no use)	1.07	(0.89, 1.33)	0.1201	1.04	(1.08, 1.31)	0.0363

RT, radiotherapy; CCRT, concurrent chemoradiotherapy; CCI, Charlson comorbidity index; AJCC, American Joint Committee on Cancer; y, years old; pT, pathologic tumor stages; pN, pathologic nodal stages; Ref., reference group; CI, confidence interval; HR, hazard ratio.

3.4. Kaplan–Meier Curves of Overall Survival, LRR, and DM

Figure 1 and Supplementary Figures S1 and S2 present survival curves for OS, LRR, and DM plotted using the Kaplan–Meier method for the PSM sarcopenia and nonsarcopenia OCSCC groups who underwent curative surgery. The OS curve for nonsarcopenic OCSCC was higher than that for sarcopenic OCSCC (Figure 1, $p < 0.001$). The 5-year OS was 56.03% and 48.93% for the patients with OCSCC without and with pre-existing sarcopenia, respectively. Moreover, the cumulative LRR and DM rates were significantly higher for sarcopenic OCSCC than nonsarcopenic OCSCC in the log-rank test (Supplementary Figures S1 and S2, p values were all <0.0001 for LRR and DM, respectively).

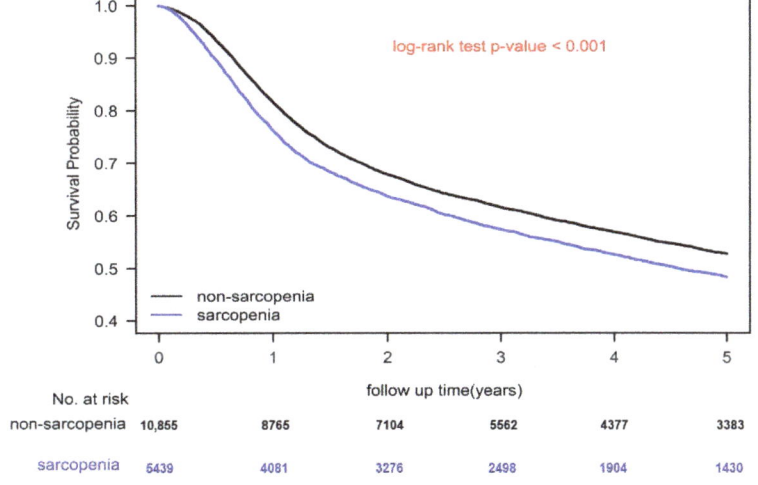

Figure 1. Kaplan–Meier overall survival curves for the propensity score-matched sarcopenia and nonsarcopenia groups (controls).

4. Discussion

Sarcopenia is an independent prognostic factor for poor survival in patients with HNC undergoing surgery, RT, or CCRT [20,42–47]. However, these studies included heterogeneous definitions of sarcopenia, inconsistent treatments for HNCs, different HNC subtypes, inhomogeneous HNC stages, very small sample sizes, and inconsistent cancer subtypes including oropharyngeal, hypopharyngeal, oral cavity, and laryngeal cancers [20,42–47]. None of these studies differentiated between sarcopenia as pre-existing or that related to cancer cachexia. Accordingly, their result that sarcopenia is a poor prognostic factor for survival outcomes might be due to cancer-related cachexia-induced sarcopenia or cancer treatment-related sarcopenia instead of pre-existing sarcopenia [20,42–47]. However, sarcopenia is different from cancer cachexia [14,16,17]. The causes of sarcopenia are multifactorial [14] and include muscle disuse, changes in endocrine function, chronic diseases, inflammation, insulin resistance, and nutritional deficiencies; many of these conditions can be detected early on and corrected through measures such as exercise or nutrition to prevent sarcopenia progression [48–51]. Therefore, we estimated the oncological outcomes of pre-existing sarcopenia in the patients with OCSCC undergoing curative surgery to determine the effect of pre-existing sarcopenia on OCSCC. To our knowledge, this is the first head-to-head PSM, largest, and longest follow-up study evaluating the effect of pre-existing sarcopenia on patients with OCSCC undergoing curative surgery. Our data indicated that pre-existing sarcopenia is an independent poor prognostic factor for mortality, LRR, and DM.

The definition of sarcopenia has been inconsistent in previous studies [20,42–47]. In patients with HNC receiving RT or CCRT, sarcopenia has been reported to be associated with poor OS and disease-free survival outcomes [42–45,47]. Only one report including patients with HNC receiving surgical excision demonstrated that sarcopenia appears to be a significant negative predictor of long-term OS in patients with HNC undergoing major surgery [43]. Stone et al. defined sarcopenia by using cross-sectional abdominal imaging performed within 45 days prior to surgery [43]. However, this definition precluded the differentiation of pre-existing sarcopenia from cancer cachexia-related sarcopenia [43]. This renders any results on the effect of sarcopenia unclear [43] and does not affect clinical practice in patients with HNC because cachexia is a well-known poor prognostic factor for OS in HNCs [52,53]. Our study is the first to present a clear definition of pre-existing sarcopenia (diagnosed ≥1 year before the diagnosis of OCSCC) in a homogenous group of patients with the same subtype of HNC (OCSCC) undergoing curative surgery. Therefore, our finding that pre-existing sarcopenia is the poor prognostic factor for OS, LRR, and DM might encourage the implementation of early screening for sarcopenia and intervention such as resistance exercise, protein supplementation, and vitamin D for patients at a high risk of OCSCC (betel nut chewing, cigarette smoking, or alcohol abuse) [48–51]. These valuable outcomes would provide references for the health government to establish health policies to correct, interrupt, or prevent the progression of pre-existing sarcopenia, particularly in the susceptible population.

Performing a randomized controlled trial (RCT) to evaluate oncological outcomes in patients with OCSCC undergoing curative surgery with and without pre-existing sarcopenia is difficult because sarcopenia cannot be treated using a tangible intervention [54]. Traditionally, striking a balance among the confounding factors of mortality in patients with OCSCC with and without sarcopenia (i.e., the case and control groups, respectively)—a main requirement of the RCT design—is impossible [54]. Although the main advantage of the PSM methodology is the more precise estimation of the covariate effect, PSM cannot control for factors not accounted for in the model. Moreover, PSM is predicated on an explicit selection bias of those who could be matched; in other words, individuals who could not be matched are not part of the scope of inference.

In the current study, our multivariable Cox regression analysis results indicated that age ≥ 50 years, male sex, advanced pT, advanced pN, differentiation grade II–III, margin positivity, LVI positivity, CCI ≥ 1, cigarette smoking, alcohol use, and betel nut chewing are significant poor prognostic factors for mortality—corroborating the results of previous studies (Table 2 and Figure 1) [1–10,31,55–59]. Moreover, male sex, advanced pT, advanced pN, differentiation grade II-III, margin positivity, LVI positivity, cigarette smoking, alcohol use, and betel nut chewing were the poor independent prognostic factors for LRR and DM in patients with OCSCC undergoing curative surgery (Tables 3 and 4 and Supplementary Figures S1 and S2). Age > 50 years was associated with the risk of mortality in patients with HNC undergoing curative surgery, consistent with our results [3,31]. In Taiwan, male sex and high CCI scores are known poor prognostic factors for OS in patients with HNC undergoing curative surgery [3,31,59]. Our data indicated that advanced pT/pN, margin positivity, and LVI positivity are associated with an increase in all-cause mortality, LRR, and DM, consistent with previous studies and NCCN guidelines [3,30,55–57]. In our multivariable analysis, poor prognostic factors for oncological outcomes for patients with OCSCC undergoing curative surgery were similar to those reported in previous studies [1–10,30,31,55–59]. Pre-existing sarcopenia was the only independent poor prognostic factor for OS, LRR, and DM for OCSCC that was never reported in previous studies. Although cancer cachexia is a well-known poor prognostic factor for survival in HNC [52,53], ours is the first study to establish pre-existing sarcopenia as an independent prognostic factor for OCSCC.

The mechanism through which pre-existing sarcopenia serves as a poor prognostic factor for OS, LRR, and DM might be associated with multiple factors including the metabolic processes of insulin resistance and systemic inflammation [14,16,17]. Patients with sarcopenia might have systemic inflammation that reduces liver cytochrome activities and drug clearance and metabolic processes, leading to a poor therapeutic effect [60]. In addition, inflammation by sarcopenia can cause a decrease in skeletal muscle density. A decreased muscle density is related to intramuscular lipid accumulation and favored by systemic inflammation, thus leading to a vicious cycle [60]. Therefore, early intervention to break this cycle is critical in patients with sarcopenia [48–51]. According to an epidemiological study in Taiwan, the incidence of oral cancer was 123-fold higher in patients who smoked, consumed alcohol, and chewed betel quid than in abstainers [2]. Patients with sarcopenia with risk factors for OCSCC [60] are the susceptible population for poor OS. Early screening for and treatment of sarcopenia for the susceptible population might improve survival outcomes in case they develop OCSCC.

This study has several limitations. First, the cohort derived from an Asian population in Taiwan. Although no evidence indicating a significant difference in survival of OCSCC between Asian and non-Asian populations has been reported, the current results should be cautiously extrapolated to non-Asian populations. Second, this study was performed on a big database and thus it is a real challenge to rule out an ecological bias (attributed to confounding or risk factors). PSM cannot control for factors not accounted for in the model and is predicated on an explicit selection bias of the variables that were matched. Third, patients with antecedents of other cancers were excluded. The field cancerization theory is well accepted on this anatomical area, i.e., a patient with oral cancer has a higher risk to develop future aerodigestive carcinomas (and vice versa) [4,61,62]. However, the primary endpoint in the current study is the all-cause death between sarcopenia and nonsarcopenia OCSCC, OCSCC patients combined with other cancers will have higher mortality attributed to more aggressive treatments or more advanced stages on the other cancers, whatever synchronous or metachronous cancers [4,61,62]. In order to decrease the bias of all-cause death from the other cancers in the OCSCC patients, patients with antecedents of other cancers were excluded. Fourth, the diagnoses of all comorbid conditions were based on *ICD-9-CM* or *ICD-10-CM* codes in this study. Nevertheless, the Taiwan Cancer Registry Administration reviews charts and interviews of beneficiaries in the TCRD to verify the accuracy of the diagnoses, and it audits hospitals with outlier chargers or practices and subsequently heavily penalizes them if it identifies any malpractice or discrepancies. However, to obtain precise population specificity and disease occurrence data, a large-scale RCT carefully comparing patients with OCSCC with or without sarcopenia is warranted, but such RCTs may be difficult to execute.

Despite these limitations, a major strength of our study is the use of a nationwide population-based registry with detailed baseline information. The TCRD is linked with Taiwan's National Cause of Death Database; thus, in the current study, we could perform a lifelong follow-up for most patients. Moreover, this study is the first, largest, and longest follow-up comparative cohort study to estimate the primary endpoint of OS in patients with OCSCC with and without pre-existing sarcopenia undergoing curative surgery. The covariates between the two groups were homogenous and any bias between the two groups was removed through PSM (Table 1). Considering the magnitude and statistical significance of the observed effects in the current study, the limitations are unlikely to have affected our conclusions.

5. Conclusions

Our results indicate that pre-existing sarcopenia is a significantly poor prognostic factor for OS, LRR, and DM in patients with OCSCC undergoing curative surgery. Individuals with a high risk of OCSCC, such as those who have a habit of betel nut chewing, alcohol, or smoking, should be screened for sarcopenia and intervention in terms of exercise and nutrition should be promoted.

Supplementary Materials: The following supporting information can be downloaded at: https://www.mdpi.com/article/10.3390/cancers14133246/s1, Figure S1: Kaplan–Meier overall cumulative locoregional recurrence curves for the propensity score–matched sarcopenia and nonsarcopenia groups (controls); Figure S2: Kaplan–Meier overall cumulative distant metastasis curves for the propensity score–matched sarcopenia and nonsarcopenia groups (controls); Table S1: Sensitivity analysis of washout time-intervals of one year and two years for definition of preexisting sarcopenia; Table S2: Sensitivity analysis of preexisting sarcopenia recorded by special specialties and all specialties.

Author Contributions: Conception and Design: Y.-H.T., W.-M.C., M.-C.C., B.-C.S., C.-C.H. and S.-Y.W.; Collection and Assembly of Data: Y.-H.T., C.-C.H. and S.-Y.W.; Data Analysis and Interpretation: W.-M.C., B.-C.S. and S.-Y.W.; Administrative Support: S.-Y.W.; Manuscript Writing: Y.-H.T., C.-C.H. and S.-Y.W.; Final Approval of Manuscript: All authors. All authors have read and agreed to the published version of the manuscript.

Funding: Lo-Hsu Medical Foundation, LotungPoh-Ai Hospital, supports Szu-Yuan Wu's work (Funding Number: 10908, 10909, 11001, 11002, 11003, 11006).

Institutional Review Board Statement: The study protocols were reviewed and approved by the Institutional Review Board of Tzu-Chi Medical Foundation (IRB109-015-B).

Informed Consent Statement: Not applicable.

Data Availability Statement: The data sets supporting the study conclusions are included in the manuscript. We used data from the National Health Insurance Research Database and Taiwan Cancer Registry database. The authors confirm that, for approved reasons, some access restrictions apply to the data underlying the findings. The data used in this study cannot be made available in the manuscript, the supplementary files, or in a public repository due to the Personal Information Protection Act executed by Taiwan's government, starting in 2012. Requests for data can be sent as a formal proposal to obtain approval from the ethics review committee of the appropriate governmental department in Taiwan. Specifically, links regarding contact info for which data requests may be sent to are as follows: http://nhird.nhri.org.tw/en/Data_Subsets.html#S3 and http://nhis.nhri.org.tw/point.html (accessed on 5 February 2021).

Conflicts of Interest: The authors declare no conflict of interest.

Abbreviations

RT, radiotherapy; CCRT, concurrent chemoradiotherapy; CCI, Charlson comorbidity index; SD, standard deviation; IQR, interquartile range; AJCC, American Joint Committee on Cancer; y, years old; N, numbers; Gy, Gray; pT, pathologic tumor stages; pN, pathologic nodal stages; CI, confidence interval; HR, hazard ratio; OCSCC, oral cavity squamous cell carcinoma; PSM, propensity score matching; LRR, locoregional recurrence; DM, distant metastasis; HNCs, head and neck cancers; TCRD, Taiwan Cancer Registry Database; NCCN, National Comprehensive Cancer Network; AJCC, American Joint Committee on Cancer criteria; ICD-9-CM, International Classification of Diseases, Ninth Revision, Clinical Modification; ICD-10-CM, International Classification of Diseases, Tenth Revision, Clinical Modification; CCI, Charlson comorbidity index; LVI, lymphovascular invasion; RCT, randomized controlled trial.

References

1. Health Promotion Administration, Ministry of Health and Welfare. *Taiwan Cancer Registry Annual Report*; Health Promotion Administration, Ministry of Health and Welfare: Taipei, Taiwan, 2020.
2. Ko, Y.C.; Huang, Y.L.; Lee, C.H.; Chen, M.J.; Lin, L.M.; Tsai, C.C. Betel quid chewing, cigarette smoking and alcohol consumption related to oral cancer in Taiwan. *J. Oral Pathol. Med.* **1995**, *24*, 450–453. [CrossRef] [PubMed]
3. Chang, J.H.; Wu, C.C.; Yuan, K.S.; Wu, A.T.H.; Wu, S.Y. Locoregionally recurrent head and neck squamous cell carcinoma: Incidence, survival, prognostic factors, and treatment outcomes. *Oncotarget* **2017**, *8*, 55600–55612. [CrossRef]
4. Chen, J.H.; Yen, Y.C.; Chen, T.M.; Yuan, K.S.; Lee, F.P.; Lin, K.C.; Lai, M.T.; Wu, C.C.; Chang, C.L.; Wu, S.Y. Survival prognostic factors for metachronous second primary head and neck squamous cell carcinoma. *Cancer Med.* **2017**, *6*, 142–153. [CrossRef] [PubMed]
5. Chang, C.L.; Yuan, K.S.; Wu, S.Y. High-dose or low-dose cisplatin concurrent with radiotherapy in locally advanced head and neck squamous cell cancer. *Head Neck* **2017**, *39*, 1364–1370. [CrossRef] [PubMed]
6. Chen, J.H.; Yen, Y.C.; Yang, H.C.; Liu, S.H.; Yuan, S.P.; Wu, L.L.; Lee, F.P.; Lin, K.C.; Lai, M.T.; Wu, C.C.; et al. Curative-Intent Aggressive Treatment Improves Survival in Elderly Patients with Locally Advanced Head and Neck Squamous Cell Carcinoma and High Comorbidity Index. *Medicine* **2016**, *95*, e3268. [CrossRef]
7. Wu, S.Y.; Wu, A.T.; Liu, S.H. MicroRNA-17-5p regulated apoptosis-related protein expression and radiosensitivity in oral squamous cell carcinoma caused by betel nut chewing. *Oncotarget* **2016**, *7*, 51482–51493. [CrossRef]
8. Liu, W.C.; Liu, H.E.; Kao, Y.W.; Qin, L.; Lin, K.C.; Fang, C.Y.; Tsai, L.L.; Shia, B.C.; Wu, S.Y. Definitive intensity-modulated radiotherapy or surgery for early oral cavity squamous cell carcinoma: Propensity-score-matched, nationwide, population-based cohort study. *Head Neck* **2020**, *43*, 1142–1152. [CrossRef]
9. Lin, K.C.; Chen, T.M.; Yuan, K.S.; Wu, A.T.H.; Wu, S.Y. Assessment of Predictive Scoring System for 90-Day Mortality among Patients with Locally Advanced Head and Neck Squamous Cell Carcinoma Who Have Completed Concurrent Chemoradiotherapy. *JAMA Netw. Open* **2020**, *3*, e1920671. [CrossRef]
10. Liu, W.C.; Liu, H.E.; Kao, Y.W.; Qin, L.; Lin, K.C.; Fang, C.Y.; Tsai, L.L.; Shia, B.C.; Wu, S.Y. Definitive radiotherapy or surgery for early oral squamous cell carcinoma in old and very old patients: A propensity-score-matched, nationwide, population-based cohort study. *Radiother. Oncol.* **2020**, *152*, 214–221. [CrossRef]
11. Sung, H.; Ferlay, J.; Siegel, R.L.; Laversanne, M.; Soerjomataram, I.; Jemal, A.; Bray, F. Global Cancer Statistics 2020: GLOBOCAN Estimates of Incidence and Mortality Worldwide for 36 Cancers in 185 Countries. *CA Cancer J. Clin.* **2021**, *71*, 209–249. [CrossRef]
12. Roubenoff, R. Origins and clinical relevance of sarcopenia. *Can. J. Appl. Physiol.* **2001**, *26*, 78–89. [CrossRef] [PubMed]
13. Cruz-Jentoft, A.J.; Baeyens, J.P.; Bauer, J.M.; Boirie, Y.; Cederholm, T.; Landi, F.; Martin, F.C.; Michel, J.P.; Rolland, Y.; Schneider, S.M.; et al. Sarcopenia: European consensus on definition and diagnosis: Report of the European Working Group on Sarcopenia in Older People. *Age Ageing* **2010**, *39*, 412–423. [CrossRef] [PubMed]
14. Janssen, I. The epidemiology of sarcopenia. *Clin. Geriatr. Med.* **2011**, *27*, 355–363. [CrossRef] [PubMed]
15. Lindle, R.S.; Metter, E.J.; Lynch, N.A.; Fleg, J.L.; Fozard, J.L.; Tobin, J.; Roy, T.A.; Hurley, B.F. Age and gender comparisons of muscle strength in 654 women and men aged 20–93 yr. *J. Appl. Physiol.* **1997**, *83*, 1581–1587. [CrossRef]
16. Muscaritoli, M.; Anker, S.D.; Argiles, J.; Aversa, Z.; Bauer, J.M.; Biolo, G.; Boirie, Y.; Bosaeus, I.; Cederholm, T.; Costelli, P.; et al. Consensus definition of sarcopenia, cachexia and pre-cachexia: Joint document elaborated by Special Interest Groups (SIG) "cachexia-anorexia in chronic wasting diseases" and "nutrition in geriatrics". *Clin. Nutr.* **2010**, *29*, 154–159. [CrossRef]
17. Janssen, I. Influence of sarcopenia on the development of physical disability: The Cardiovascular Health Study. *J. Am. Geriatr. Soc.* **2006**, *54*, 56–62. [CrossRef]
18. Shachar, S.S.; Williams, G.R.; Muss, H.B.; Nishijima, T.F. Prognostic value of sarcopenia in adults with solid tumours: A meta-analysis and systematic review. *Eur. J. Cancer* **2016**, *57*, 58–67. [CrossRef]
19. Buentzel, J.; Heinz, J.; Bleckmann, A.; Bauer, C.; Rover, C.; Bohnenberger, H.; Saha, S.; Hinterthaner, M.; Baraki, H.; Kutschka, I.; et al. Sarcopenia as Prognostic Factor in Lung Cancer Patients: A Systematic Review and Meta-analysis. *Anticancer Res.* **2019**, *39*, 4603–4612. [CrossRef]
20. Hua, X.; Liu, S.; Liao, J.F.; Wen, W.; Long, Z.Q.; Lu, Z.J.; Guo, L.; Lin, H.X. When the Loss Costs Too Much: A Systematic Review and Meta-Analysis of Sarcopenia in Head and Neck Cancer. *Front. Oncol.* **2019**, *9*, 1561. [CrossRef]

21. Au, P.C.; Li, H.L.; Lee, G.K.; Li, G.H.; Chan, M.; Cheung, B.M.; Wong, I.C.; Lee, V.H.; Mok, J.; Yip, B.H.; et al. Sarcopenia and mortality in cancer: A meta-analysis. *Osteoporos Sarcopenia* **2021**, *7*, S28–S33. [CrossRef]
22. Xu, Y.Y.; Zhou, X.L.; Yu, C.H.; Wang, W.W.; Ji, F.Z.; He, D.C.; Zhu, W.G.; Tong, Y.S. Association of Sarcopenia with Toxicity and Survival in Postoperative Recurrent Esophageal Squamous Cell Carcinoma Patients Receiving Chemoradiotherapy. *Front. Oncol.* **2021**, *11*, 655071. [CrossRef] [PubMed]
23. Hua, X.; Liao, J.F.; Huang, X.; Huang, H.Y.; Wen, W.; Long, Z.Q.; Guo, L.; Yuan, Z.Y.; Lin, H.X. Sarcopenia is associated with higher toxicity and poor prognosis of nasopharyngeal carcinoma. *Ther. Adv. Med. Oncol.* **2020**, *12*, 1758835920947612. [CrossRef] [PubMed]
24. Austin, P.C. A comparison of 12 algorithms for matching on the propensity score. *Stat. Med.* **2014**, *33*, 1057–1069. [CrossRef]
25. Austin, P.C. An Introduction to Propensity Score Methods for Reducing the Effects of Confounding in Observational Studies. *Multivar. Behav. Res.* **2011**, *46*, 399–424. [CrossRef] [PubMed]
26. Austin, P.C. Balance diagnostics for comparing the distribution of baseline covariates between treatment groups in propensity-score matched samples. *Stat. Med.* **2009**, *28*, 3083–3107. [CrossRef]
27. Dias, F.L.; Lima, R.A.; Kligerman, J.; Farias, T.P.; Soares, J.R.; Manfro, G.; Sa, G.M. Relevance of skip metastases for squamous cell carcinoma of the oral tongue and the floor of the mouth. *Otolaryngol. Head Neck Surg.* **2006**, *134*, 460–465. [CrossRef]
28. Byers, R.M.; Weber, R.S.; Andrews, T.; McGill, D.; Kare, R.; Wolf, P. Frequency and therapeutic implications of "skip metastases" in the neck from squamous carcinoma of the oral tongue. *Head Neck* **1997**, *19*, 14–19. [CrossRef]
29. Capote-Moreno, A.; Naval, L.; Munoz-Guerra, M.F.; Sastre, J.; Rodriguez-Campo, F.J. Prognostic factors influencing contralateral neck lymph node metastases in oral and oropharyngeal carcinoma. *J. Oral Maxillofac. Surg.* **2010**, *68*, 268–275. [CrossRef]
30. NCCN Clinical Practice Guidelines in Oncology: Head and Neck Cancer. Available online: https://www.nccn.org/professionals/physician_gls/pdf/head-and-neck.pdf (accessed on 22 April 2022).
31. Qin, L.; Chen, T.-M.; Kao, Y.-W.; Lin, K.-C.; Yuan, K.S.-P.; Wu, A.T.H.; Shia, B.-C.; Wu, S.-Y. Predicting 90-Day Mortality in Locoregionally Advanced Head and Neck Squamous Cell Carcinoma after Curative Surgery. *Cancers* **2018**, *10*, 392. [CrossRef]
32. Sun, M.Y.; Chang, C.L.; Lu, C.Y.; Wu, S.Y.; Zhang, J.Q. Sarcopenia as an Independent Risk Factor for Specific Cancers: A Propensity Score-Matched Asian Population-Based Cohort Study. *Nutrients* **2022**, *14*, 1910. [CrossRef]
33. Chien, M.Y.; Huang, T.Y.; Wu, Y.T. Prevalence of sarcopenia estimated using a bioelectrical impedance analysis prediction equation in community-dwelling elderly people in Taiwan. *J. Am. Geriatr. Soc.* **2008**, *56*, 1710–1715. [CrossRef] [PubMed]
34. Charlson, M.; Szatrowski, T.P.; Peterson, J.; Gold, J. Validation of a combined comorbidity index. *J. Clin. Epidemiol.* **1994**, *47*, 1245–1251. [CrossRef]
35. Wu, S.Y.; Chang, S.C.; Chen, C.I.; Huang, C.C. Oncologic Outcomes of Radical Prostatectomy and High-Dose Intensity-Modulated Radiotherapy with Androgen-Deprivation Therapy for Relatively Young Patients with Unfavorable Intermediate-Risk Prostate Adenocarcinoma. *Cancers* **2021**, *13*, 1517. [CrossRef] [PubMed]
36. Shih, H.J.; Chang, S.C.; Hsu, C.H.; Lin, Y.C.; Hung, C.H.; Wu, S.Y. Comparison of Clinical Outcomes of Radical Prostatectomy versus IMRT with Long-Term Hormone Therapy for Relatively Young Patients with High- to Very High-Risk Localized Prostate Cancer. *Cancers* **2021**, *13*, 5986. [CrossRef]
37. Zhang, J.; Lu, C.Y.; Qin, L.; Chen, H.M.; Wu, S.Y. Breast-conserving surgery with or without irradiation in women with invasive ductal carcinoma of the breast receiving preoperative systemic therapy: A cohort study. *Breast* **2020**, *54*, 139–147. [CrossRef]
38. Austin, P.C. The performance of different propensity score methods for estimating marginal hazard ratios. *Stat. Med.* **2013**, *32*, 2837–2849. [CrossRef]
39. Nguyen, T.L.; Collins, G.S.; Spence, J.; Daures, J.P.; Devereaux, P.J.; Landais, P.; Le Manach, Y. Double-adjustment in propensity score matching analysis: Choosing a threshold for considering residual imbalance. *BMC Med. Res. Methodol.* **2017**, *17*, 78. [CrossRef]
40. Zhang, Z.; Kim, H.J.; Lonjon, G.; Zhu, Y.; written on behalf of AME Big-Data Clinical Trial Collaborative Group. Balance diagnostics after propensity score matching. *Ann. Transl. Med.* **2019**, *7*, 16. [CrossRef]
41. Austin, P.C. The use of propensity score methods with survival or time-to-event outcomes: Reporting measures of effect similar to those used in randomized experiments. *Stat. Med.* **2014**, *33*, 1242–1258. [CrossRef]
42. Thureau, S.; Lebret, L.; Lequesne, J.; Cabourg, M.; Dandoy, S.; Gouley, C.; Lefebvre, L.; Mallet, R.; Mihailescu, S.D.; Moldovan, C.; et al. Prospective Evaluation of Sarcopenia in Head and Neck Cancer Patients Treated with Radiotherapy or Radiochemotherapy. *Cancers* **2021**, *13*, 753. [CrossRef]
43. Stone, L.; Olson, B.; Mowery, A.; Krasnow, S.; Jiang, A.; Li, R.; Schindler, J.; Wax, M.K.; Andersen, P.; Marks, D.; et al. Association Between Sarcopenia and Mortality in Patients Undergoing Surgical Excision of Head and Neck Cancer. *JAMA Otolaryngol. Head Neck Surg.* **2019**, *145*, 647–654. [CrossRef] [PubMed]
44. van Rijn-Dekker, M.I.; van den Bosch, L.; van den Hoek, J.G.M.; Bijl, H.P.; van Aken, E.S.M.; van der Hoorn, A.; Oosting, S.F.; Halmos, G.B.; Witjes, M.J.H.; van der Laan, H.P.; et al. Impact of sarcopenia on survival and late toxicity in head and neck cancer patients treated with radiotherapy. *Radiother. Oncol.* **2020**, *147*, 103–110. [CrossRef] [PubMed]
45. Takenaka, Y.; Takemoto, N.; Oya, R.; Inohara, H. Prognostic impact of sarcopenia in patients with head and neck cancer treated with surgery or radiation: A meta-analysis. *PLoS ONE* **2021**, *16*, e0259288. [CrossRef] [PubMed]
46. Findlay, M.; White, K.; Stapleton, N.; Bauer, J. Is sarcopenia a predictor of prognosis for patients undergoing radiotherapy for head and neck cancer? A meta-analysis. *Clin. Nutr.* **2021**, *40*, 1711–1718. [CrossRef] [PubMed]

47. Chargi, N.; Bril, S.I.; Emmelot-Vonk, M.H.; de Bree, R. Sarcopenia is a prognostic factor for overall survival in elderly patients with head-and-neck cancer. *Eur. Arch. Otorhinolaryngol.* **2019**, *276*, 1475–1486. [CrossRef]
48. Yamada, M.; Kimura, Y.; Ishiyama, D.; Nishio, N.; Otobe, Y.; Tanaka, T.; Ohji, S.; Koyama, S.; Sato, A.; Suzuki, M.; et al. Synergistic effect of bodyweight resistance exercise and protein supplementation on skeletal muscle in sarcopenic or dynapenic older adults. *Geriatr. Gerontol. Int.* **2019**, *19*, 429–437. [CrossRef]
49. Morley, J.E.; Argiles, J.M.; Evans, W.J.; Bhasin, S.; Cella, D.; Deutz, N.E.; Doehner, W.; Fearon, K.C.; Ferrucci, L.; Hellerstein, M.K.; et al. Nutritional recommendations for the management of sarcopenia. *J. Am. Med. Dir. Assoc.* **2010**, *11*, 391–396. [CrossRef]
50. Gkekas, N.K.; Anagnostis, P.; Paraschou, V.; Stamiris, D.; Dellis, S.; Kenanidis, E.; Potoupnis, M.; Tsiridis, E.; Goulis, D.G. The effect of vitamin D plus protein supplementation on sarcopenia: A systematic review and meta-analysis of randomized controlled trials. *Maturitas* **2021**, *145*, 56–63. [CrossRef]
51. Phu, S.; Boersma, D.; Duque, G. Exercise and Sarcopenia. *J. Clin. Densitom.* **2015**, *18*, 488–492. [CrossRef]
52. Matsuzuka, T.; Kiyota, N.; Mizusawa, J.; Akimoto, T.; Fujii, M.; Hasegawa, Y.; Iwae, S.; Monden, N.; Matsuura, K.; Onozawa, Y.; et al. Clinical impact of cachexia in unresectable locally advanced head and neck cancer: Supplementary analysis of a phase II trial (JCOG0706-S2). *Jpn. J. Clin. Oncol.* **2019**, *49*, 37–41. [CrossRef]
53. Hayashi, N.; Sato, Y.; Fujiwara, Y.; Fukuda, N.; Wang, X.; Nakano, K.; Urasaki, T.; Ohmoto, A.; Ono, M.; Tomomatsu, J.; et al. Clinical Impact of Cachexia in Head and Neck Cancer Patients Who Received Chemoradiotherapy. *Cancer Manag. Res.* **2021**, *13*, 8377–8385. [CrossRef] [PubMed]
54. Deaton, A.; Cartwright, N. Understanding and misunderstanding randomized controlled trials. *Soc. Sci. Med.* **2018**, *210*, 2–21. [CrossRef] [PubMed]
55. Bernier, J.; Cooper, J.S.; Pajak, T.F.; van Glabbeke, M.; Bourhis, J.; Forastiere, A.; Ozsahin, E.M.; Jacobs, J.R.; Jassem, J.; Ang, K.K.; et al. Defining risk levels in locally advanced head and neck cancers: A comparative analysis of concurrent postoperative radiation plus chemotherapy trials of the EORTC (#22931) and RTOG (# 9501). *Head Neck* **2005**, *27*, 843–850. [CrossRef] [PubMed]
56. Bernier, J.; Domenge, C.; Ozsahin, M.; Matuszewska, K.; Lefebvre, J.L.; Greiner, R.H.; Giralt, J.; Maingon, P.; Rolland, F.; Bolla, M.; et al. Postoperative irradiation with or without concomitant chemotherapy for locally advanced head and neck cancer. *N. Engl. J. Med.* **2004**, *350*, 1945–1952. [CrossRef] [PubMed]
57. Cooper, J.S.; Pajak, T.F.; Forastiere, A.A.; Jacobs, J.; Campbell, B.H.; Saxman, S.B.; Kish, J.A.; Kim, H.E.; Cmelak, A.J.; Rotman, M.; et al. Postoperative concurrent radiotherapy and chemotherapy for high-risk squamous-cell carcinoma of the head and neck. *N. Engl. J. Med.* **2004**, *350*, 1937–1944. [CrossRef]
58. Lee, L.Y.; Lin, C.Y.; Cheng, N.M.; Tsai, C.Y.; Hsueh, C.; Fan, K.H.; Wang, H.M.; Hsieh, C.H.; Ng, S.H.; Yeh, C.H.; et al. Poor tumor differentiation is an independent adverse prognostic variable in patients with locally advanced oral cavity cancer–Comparison with pathological risk factors according to the NCCN guidelines. *Cancer Med.* **2021**, *10*, 6627–6641. [CrossRef]
59. Shia, B.C.; Qin, L.; Lin, K.C.; Fang, C.Y.; Tsai, L.L.; Kao, Y.W.; Wu, S.Y. Outcomes for Elderly Patients Aged 70 to 80 Years or Older with Locally Advanced Oral Cavity Squamous Cell Carcinoma: A Propensity Score-Matched, Nationwide, Oldest Old Patient-Based Cohort Study. *Cancers* **2020**, *12*, 258. [CrossRef]
60. Antoun, S.; Borget, I.; Lanoy, E. Impact of sarcopenia on the prognosis and treatment toxicities in patients diagnosed with cancer. *Curr. Opin. Support. Palliat. Care* **2013**, *7*, 383–389. [CrossRef]
61. Liao, C.T.; Wallace, C.G.; Lee, L.Y.; Hsueh, C.; Lin, C.Y.; Fan, K.H.; Wang, H.M.; Ng, S.H.; Lin, C.H.; Tsao, C.K.; et al. Clinical evidence of field cancerization in patients with oral cavity cancer in a betel quid chewing area. *Oral Oncol.* **2014**, *50*, 721–731. [CrossRef]
62. Liao, C.T.; Kang, C.J.; Chang, J.T.; Wang, H.M.; Ng, S.H.; Hsueh, C.; Lee, L.Y.; Lin, C.H.; Cheng, A.J.; Chen, I.H.; et al. Survival of second and multiple primary tumors in patients with oral cavity squamous cell carcinoma in the betel quid chewing area. *Oral Oncol.* **2007**, *43*, 811–819. [CrossRef]

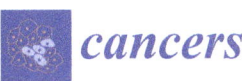

Article

Oral Health Status in Patients with Head and Neck Cancer before Radiotherapy: Baseline Description of an Observational Prospective Study

Cosimo Rupe [1], Alessia Basco [1], Anna Schiavelli [1,*], Alessandra Cassano [2], Francesco Micciche' [3], Jacopo Galli [4], Massimo Cordaro [1] and Carlo Lajolo [1,†]

1. Head and Neck Department, Fondazione Policlinico Universitario A. Gemelli—IRCCS, School of Dentistry, Università Cattolica del Sacro Cuore, Largo A. Gemelli, 8, 00168 Rome, Italy; cosimorupe@gmail.com (C.R.); alessiabasco19@gmail.com (A.B.); massimo.cordaro@policlinicogemelli.it (M.C.); carlo.lajolo@policlinicogemelli.it (C.L.)
2. Department of Medical Oncology, Fondazione Policlinico Universitario A. Gemelli—IRCCS, Institute of Radiology, Università Cattolica del Sacro Cuore, Largo A. Gemelli, 8, 00168 Rome, Italy; alessandra.cassano@policlinicogemelli.it
3. Department of Radiation Oncology, Fondazione Policlinico Universitario A. Gemelli—IRCCS, Institute of Radiology, Università Cattolica del Sacro Cuore, Largo A. Gemelli, 8, 00168 Rome, Italy; francesco.micciche@policlinicogemelli.it
4. Head and Neck Department, Fondazione Policlinico Universitario A. Gemelli—IRCCS, Institute of Otolaryngology, Università Cattolica del Sacro Cuore, Largo A. Gemelli, 8, 00168 Rome, Italy; jacopo.galli@policlinicogemelli.it
* Correspondence: anna.schiavelli@gmail.com
† On behalf of the multidisciplinary Head and Neck Tumor Board of the Fondazione Policlinico Universitario A. Gemelli—IRCCS.

Simple Summary: Patients with head and neck cancer (HNC) are often considered as a group with compromised oral conditions, but this idea is not sufficiently supported by data in the literature. This study examined the oral condition—specifically the presence of caries and periodontal disease—of a cohort of patients with HNC waiting to start radiation therapy treatment and possible correlations between oral health, different types of HNC and various risk factors. The results confirm that the oral status of many patients with HNC is poor even before radiotherapy treatments and that smoking habit and tumor site are associated with poor oral health. These findings underline the importance of a dentist within a head and neck tumor board (TB), so that oral health can be restored as soon as possible.

Abstract: (1) Background: The general hypothesis that HNC patients show compromised oral health (OH) is generally accepted, but it is not evidence-based. The objective of this baseline report of a prospective observational study was to describe the oral health of a cohort of patients with HNC at the time of dental evaluation prior to radiotherapy (RT). (2) Materials and Methods: Two hundred and thirteen patients affected by HNC who had received an indication for RT were examined with the support of orthopantomography (OPT). The DMFt of all included subjects, their periodontal status and the grade of mouth opening were recorded. (3) Results: A total of 195 patients were ultimately included: 146/195 patients (74.9%) showed poor OH (defined as having a DMFt score ≥ 13 and severe periodontitis). The following clinical characteristics were correlated with poor oral health in the univariate analysis: tumor site, smoking habit and age of the patients (in decades); χ^2 test, $p < 0.05$. (4) Conclusions: This study confirms that the OH of HNC patients is often compromised even before the beginning of cancer treatment and, consequently, highlights how important it is to promptly schedule a dental evaluation at the moment of diagnosis of the cancer.

Keywords: head and neck cancer; oral status; periodontitis; dental caries; DMFt

1. Introduction

The head and neck region is an anatomical heterogeneous area that can give rise to a variety of malignancies and show different risk factors, prognoses and treatments. Head and neck cancers (HNCs) represent the seventh most common malignancy worldwide [1].

The general hypothesis that HNC patients show a high prevalence of caries and periodontitis and, therefore, compromised oral health (OH) even before cancer therapy (i.e., radiotherapy, RT) is generally accepted, but it is not evidence-based. In fact, it is possible to highlight a lack of clinical data about the OH of these patients before oncological treatments.

Several studies reported that the majority of HNC patients did not attend any dental visit during the year preceding the cancer diagnosis and that many of these patients consulted a dental specialist only in cases of acute pain or other urgencies [2–4]. The overlapping of some risk factors—the most important being smoking habit—might be another possible explanation for the compromised conditions of HNC patients. Tobacco smoking is considered the main risk factor for the majority of HNCs and one of the main risk factors for the onset and progression of periodontitis and for its response to treatment [5–8]; furthermore, hyposalivation following prolonged exposure to tobacco smoking could increase the risk of caries development [9,10].

Furthermore, especially when RT is performed, preserving OH becomes crucial in the multidisciplinary management of these patients, since RT increases the risk of developing dental caries, leading to tooth loss, a well-known risk factor for major complications such as osteoradionecrosis [11–13].

Considering this, it is easy to imagine that HNC patients have a higher probability of developing dental diseases. Nevertheless, data available from the literature are scarce, often inaccurate or incomplete, and many articles do not stratify the statistical analysis according to the primary location of the cancer. The present study is the first report of a prospective protocol aiming to evaluate the OH of an HNC cohort undergoing RT.

The primary objective of this cross-sectional study was to describe the OH conditions of a cohort of HNC patients evaluated during the dental visit preceding RT. The secondary objective was to identify a correlation between the clinical characteristics of the patients and their OH status.

2. Materials and Methods

This study was conducted according to the Declaration of Helsinki, and all patients signed an informed consent form. The protocol was approved by the Ethics Committee of the Università Cattolica del Sacro Cuore (Ref. 22858/18) and was registered at ClinicalTrials.gov (ID: NCT04009161).

Patients affected by HNC attending the Oral Medicine, Head and Neck Department—Fondazione Policlinico Universitario A. Gemelli—IRCSS, between March 2017 and September 2021 were consecutively recruited in this study.

The following inclusion criteria were considered: HNC diagnosis and indication for RT.

The exclusion criteria were the impossibility of accurately evaluating OH conditions (i.e., outcomes of oncologic surgery incompatible with the dental procedures to diagnose caries and periodontitis) and patients having already received RT in the head and neck region.

All patients were visited prior to RT, with the support of an orthopantomograph (OPT). Firstly, anagraphic and anamnestic data were carefully recorded, particularly focusing on the oncologic history of the patient and on exposure to risk factors for oncologic and dental diseases.

Subsequently, the clinical evaluation of the following parameters was performed: presence of dental caries and DMFt score, periodontal health, maximal mouth opening (MMO).

The DMFt index is the key measure of caries experience in dental epidemiology [14]. It sums the number of decayed teeth, missing teeth due to caries and filled teeth in the permanent dentition. An examination for dental caries in permanent teeth is performed, examining 32 teeth. The permanent dentition status of each tooth (crown and root) is recorded as a score, where 0 corresponds to a tooth that shows no evidence of treated or untreated caries, and 1 corresponds to the case of tooth decay (treated or untreated) or a missing tooth (due to caries) [15].

The diagnosis of caries was performed through the clinical examination with the help of a dental explorer and a mouth mirror and, when in doubt, with the support of an intraoral radiograph (periapical or bitewing), performed with the help of film holders (Dentsply Sirona, Rome, IT). A bitewing radiograph was performed in every case in which visual inspection of the interproximal tooth surface was not possible. Nevertheless, when a diagnosis of an endodontic or periodontal lesion had to be performed, a periapical radiograph was taken. Caries involving the dentine were considered in the DMFt score (ICDAS™ code 3 and higher) [16–18].

Clinical evaluation of periodontitis was performed according to international standards [19]. A full-mouth periodontal examination was performed by the same operator (L.C.), with more than ten years of experience in periodontology, using an NCP15 periodontal probe and collecting the following data (six sites for each tooth): periodontal probing depth (PPD), the distance between the tip of the periodontal probe and the gingival margin; gingival recession (REC), the distance between the gingival margin and the cementoenamel junction; clinical attachment loss (CAL) for each assessed site; furcation involvement (FI), according to the Hamp classification [20]; number of tooth losses due to periodontitis; tooth mobility; full-mouth plaque score (FMPS) [21]; and full-mouth bleeding score (FMBS) [22].

After data collection, the periodontal cases were staged according to the diagnostic criteria of the 2017 classification: $CAL \geq 2$ mm affecting two nonadjacent teeth, buccal or oral $CAL \geq 3$ mm and $PPD > 3$ mm affecting two or more teeth were the diagnostic criteria to define a periodontitis case. Interdental CAL from 3 to 4 mm was the parameter which shifted the diagnosis to stage II periodontitis, while more severe CAL or at least one tooth lost due to periodontitis was the criterion which determined the shift to stage III or IV periodontitis. The differential diagnosis between stage III and IV periodontitis was driven by the following parameters: tooth loss due to periodontitis ≥ 5, masticatory dysfunction due to secondary occlusal trauma, bite collapse, drifting or flaring, which were the diagnostic criteria for stage IV periodontitis [19]. The clinical charts of the patients visited before 2017 were rescreened to stage the periodontal cases according to the abovementioned classification. OPT was used as a support to complete the diagnosis and staging of periodontitis; in case of uncertainty, an intraoral radiograph was performed, compatible with the outcomes of the major oncologic surgery.

The M parameter (teeth missed due to caries), as well as the number of teeth lost due to periodontitis, was evaluated by analysing old radiographic exams provided by the patients. In case old radiographic exams were unavailable, the patients were asked about the reason for previous teeth extractions.

The MMO was defined as the greatest distance (mm) between the incisal edge of the maxillary central incisor and the incisal edge of the mandibular central incisor and was measured by using a modified vernier caliper [23]. The MMO of the edentulous patients was measured by removing every removable prosthesis, and the edentulous ridges were used as reference points.

The following variables were recorded: sex, age, risk factors (smoking, diabetes), previous or scheduled oncological treatment (chemotherapy and surgery), site, histological type and stage of the tumor, DMFt, stage of periodontitis and MMO.

The oral health (OH) parameter was defined as a dichotomous variable, and DMFt and periodontal staging were used to define OH status, defined as "poor" in cases of $DMFt \geq 13$ and/or stage III or IV periodontitis and as "good" only in cases of lower values of each of these variables. The DMFt score of 13 was chosen as a cut-off defining good OH, since it has been reported to be the mean value of DMFt in non-developing countries [24,25]. Stage III and IV periodontitis were chosen as cut-off values, since they define "severe" periodontitis, according to the 2017 classification [19].

STROBE guidelines were followed to write this paper (Table S1).

Statistical Analysis

The sample size was calculated according to the simple causal sampling formula. Considering a DMFt ≥ 13 and/or stage III or IV periodontitis as predictive of poor OH, and setting the possible prevalence of poor OH at 85% and a desired precision of 5%, 195 patients were included in the final sample.

Qualitative variables were described using absolute and percent frequencies, whereas quantitative variables were summarized either as the mean and standard deviation (SD), if normally distributed, or as the median, otherwise.

The following variables were evaluated as absolute values and reclassified in ranges. DMFt was reclassified according to the established cut-off defining a poor OH condition: DMFt ≥13; periodontitis was reclassified into three categories: absence of periodontitis, stage I or II periodontitis and stage III or IV periodontitis; MMO was reclassified according to the reduced mouth opening cut-off: MMO ≤ 25 mm [26,27]. DMFt and periodontal staging were used to define OH status as either "poor" or "good", as described in the Materials and Methods section.

Correlation analysis between the OH parameters (DMFt and periodontitis) and the clinical characteristics of the patients was performed. The Kolmogorov–Smirnov test was performed to evaluate the normal distribution of the quantitative variables. The Mann–Whitney U test and Kruskal–Wallis test were performed to compare continuous variables with nonparametric distributions, whereas parametric variables were analyzed using ANOVA. Pearson's χ^2 test and Fisher's exact test were used to compare discontinuous variables. A logistic regression model was built to evaluate factors affecting the probability of the main outcome variable ("poor OH").

The statistical analysis was stratified according to the following variables: tumor site; patient age (by decade); and smoking habit.

Univariate analysis was performed to determine risk factors associated with poor OH (as defined in the Materials and Methods section), and the risk factors were introduced in a stepwise logistic regression analysis to identify independent predictors of poor OH. All statistical analyses were performed using IBM SPSS Statistics software (IBM Corp. Released 2017. IBM SPSS Statistics for Apple, Version 25.0 Armonk, NY, USA: IBM Corp).

3. Results

3.1. General Characteristics of the Population

Two hundred and thirteen patients were consecutively assessed and enrolled, while eighteen patients were excluded, since they did not fulfil the inclusion criteria (their clinical conditions did not allow clinical evaluation). The final sample included 195 patients (67 female and 128 male subjects), with a mean age of 60.4 years (SD: 12.4; range: 22–92). The mean time between the cancer diagnosis and the dental evaluation was 37.2 days (SD: 12.02; range: 15–64).

The general characteristics of the population are presented in Table 1. It is worth mentioning that the studied population represents a sample of a HNC population, reflecting the heterogeneous characteristics and risk factors for each malignancy.

Table 1. General characteristics of the population and correlation with OH.

		Total Sample	Good OH	Poor OH	Significance
Gender	Men	128 (65.6%)	26	102	χ^2 Test—$p < 0.05$
	Women	67 (34.4%)	23	44	
Age	Mean (range; SD)	60.4 (22–92; 12.4)	50.4 (22–86; 13.4)	63.7 (40–92; 10)	Pearson's Correlation Analysis—$p < 0.05$

Table 1. Cont.

		Total Sample	Good OH	Poor OH	Significance
Gender	Men	128 (65.6%)	26	102	χ2 Test—$p < 0.05$
	Women	67 (34.4%)	23	44	
	<40	9 (4.6%)	9	0	
	40–49	26 (13.4%)	14	12	
	50–59	50 (25.6%)	13	37	
	60–69	65 (33.3%)	11	54	
	70–79	37 (19.0%)	0	37	
	>80	8 (4.1%)	2	6	
Tumor Type	SCC	173 (88.7%)	44	129	-
	Other types	22 (11.3%)	5	17	
Tumor Stage	Stage I	13 (6.7%)	3	10	-
	Stage II	31 (15.9%)	12	19	
	Stage III	49 (25.1%)	9	40	
	Stage IV	102 (52.3%)	25	77	
Tumor Site	Hypopharynx	6 (3.1%)	2	4	χ2 Test—$p < 0.05$
	Larynx	44 (22.6%)	6	38	
	Oral cavity	41 (21%)	9	32	
	Oropharynx	49 (25.1%)	13	36	
	Rhinopharynx	23 (11.8%)	13	10	
	Salivary glands	15 (7.7%)	2	13	
	Other sites	17 (8.7%)	4	13	
Smoking	Smokers	125 (64.1%)	22	103	χ2 Test—$p < 0.05$
	No smokers	70 (35.9%)	27	43	
Diabetes	Yes	11 (5.6%)	2	9	-
	No	184 (94.4%)	47	137	
Surgery [a]	Performed	86 (44.1%)	17	69	-
	Not performed	109 (55.9%)	32	77	
Chemotherapy	Scheduled	104 (53.3%)	30	74	-
	Not scheduled	91 (46.7%)	19	72	
	Total	195 (100%)	49	146	

[a] Major oncologic surgery (i.e., fibula free flap for mandible reconstruction, glossectomy). SCC: squamous cell carcinoma.

3.1.1. Oral Health

The clinical and radiographic evaluation showed that 8/195 (4.1%) subjects were totally edentulous, 115/195 (59%) showed a DMFt score ≥ of 13 and 150/195 (76.9%) were affected by periodontitis. Among these 150 patients, 107 (71.3%) showed stage III or IV periodontitis. Only 3/195 patients had a DMFt score = 0 (1.53%), while the median DMFt score was 16.91 (range: 0–32; SD: 9.1). A total of 146 patients out of 195 (74.9%) showed poor OH. The results describing the oral health of the studied population are reported in Table 2.

Table 2. Oral health parameters of the studied population and correlation with OH. SD: standard deviation.

		Total	Good OH	Poor OH	Significance
Edentulism	Edentulous patients	8 (4.1%)	0	8	-
	Non-edentulous patients	187 (95.9%)	49	138	
		195 (100%)			
Periodontitis	Affected patients	150 (76.9%)	16	134	χ2 Test—$p < 0.05$
	Non-affected patients	45 (23.1%)	33	12	
		195 (100%)			
Periodontal Staging	Stage I	21 (14%)	9	12	χ2 Test—$p < 0.05$
	Stage II	22 (14.7%)	7	15	
	Stage III	42 (28%)	0	42	
	Stage IV	65 (43.3%)	0	65	
		150 (100%)			
Periodontal Grading	Grade A	40 (26.7%)	5	35	-
	Grade B	66 (44%)	10	56	
	Grade C	44 (29.3%)	4	40	
		150 (100%)			
DMFt	Median (range)	16 (0–32)	8 (0–13)	20 (0–32)	Pearson's Correlation Analysis—$p < 0.05$
DMFt ≥ 13	No	80 (41.0%)	49	31	χ2 Test—$p < 0.05$
	Yes	115 (59.0%)	0	115	
		195 (100%)			
Mouth Opening	Mean (range; SD)	38.8 (12–63; 10.1)	38.6 (12–54; 11.1)	39.1 (12–63; 9.8)	-
	<20 mm	21 (10.8%)	7	14	
	≥20 mm	174 (89.2%)	42	132	
		195 (100%)			
		195 (100%)	49	146	

3.1.2. Tumor Localization and OH Conditions

Patients with different tumor sites showed different OH conditions (χ2 test, $p <0.05$), with the larynx being associated with poor OH (86.4% of the cases) and the rhinopharynx being associated with good OH conditions (56.5%). The prevalence of DMFt ≥ 13 was higher in salivary gland (80%) and laryngeal (75%) patients than in patients with other tumor sites (χ2 test, $p < 0.05$). The subjects affected by laryngeal tumors also had a high prevalence of stage III or IV periodontitis, although this association was not statistically significant. The results of the statistical analysis, stratified according to the localization of the tumor, are reported in Table 3.

3.1.3. Smoking and OH Conditions

Smoking habit was correlated with the diagnosis of periodontitis: 74.8% of severe periodontal patients (stage III or IV) were smokers or former smokers (χ2 test, $p < 0.05$). The habit of smoking was also correlated with DMFt ≥ 13 (71.3%; χ2 test, $p < 0.05$) and poor OH (70.5%; χ2 test, $p < 0.05$). Multiple logistic regression analysis confirmed that smoking habit was a risk factor for severe periodontitis (OR = 4.78; 95% CI = 2.01–11.36; $p < 0.05$), for DMFt ≥ 13 (OR = 2.30; 95% CI = 1.19–4.44; $p < 0.05$) and, therefore, for poor OH (OR = 3.27; 95% CI = 1.46–7.33; $p < 0.05$). The results of the analysis, stratified according to smoking habit, are reported in Table 4, and Figures 1–3.

Table 3. General and oral health characteristics of the studied population, according to the localization of the tumor.

		Larynx 44	Oral Cavity 41	Oropharynx 49	Rhinopharynx 23	Salivary Glands 15	Other Sites 23	Total Sample 195	Significance
Gender	Male	35 (27.3%)	23 (18%)	38 (29.7%)	11 (8.6%)	9 (7%)	12 (9.4%)	128 (100%)	χ2 Test— $p < 0.05$
	Female	9 (13.4%)	18 (26.9%)	11 (16.4%)	12 (17.9%)	6 (9%)	11 (16.4%)	67 (100%)	
Age	<40	0 (0%)	2 (22.2%)	0 (0%)	4 (44.4%)	1 (11.1%)	2 (22.2%)	9 (100%)	Pearson's Correlation Analysis— $p < 0.05$
	40–49	6 (23.1%)	5 (19.2%)	6 (23.1%)	4 (15.4%)	1 (3.8%)	4 (15.4%)	26 (100%)	
	50–59	12 (24%)	11 (22%)	14 (28%)	4 (8%)	4 (8%)	5 (10%)	50 (100%)	
	60–69	15 (23.1%)	12 (18.5%)	21 (32.3%)	9 (13.8%)	2 (3%)	6 (9.3%)	65 (100%)	
	70–79	11 (29.7%)	7 (18.9%)	8 (21.6%)	2 (5.4%)	4 (10.9%)	5 (13.5%)	37 (100%)	
	>80	0 (0%)	4 (50%)	0 (0%)	0 (0%)	3 (37.5%)	1 (12.5%)	8 (100%)	
Tumor Type	SCC	44 (25.4%)	39 (22.5%)	47 (27.1%)	22 (12.7%)	3 (1.7%)	18 (10.4%)	173 (100%)	-
	Other types	0 (0%)	2 (9.1%)	2 (9.1%)	1 (4.5%)	12 (54.4%)	5 (22.7%)	22 (100%)	
Tumor Stage	Stage I	3 (23%)	1 (7.7%)	4 (30.8%)	1 (7.7%)	2 (15.4%)	2 (15.4%)	13 (100%)	-
	Stage II	9 (29%)	3 (9.7%)	6 (19.4%)	6 (19.4%)	6 (19.4%)	1 (3.2%)	31 (100%)	
	Stage III	9 (18.4%)	8 (16.3%)	16 (32.6%)	7 (14.4%)	3 (6.1%)	6 (12.2%)	49 (100%)	
	Stage IV	23 (22.6%)	29 (28.4%)	23 (22.6%)	9 (8.8%)	4 (3.9%)	14 (13.7%)	102 (100%)	
Chemotherapy	Scheduled	15 (14.4%)	18 (17.4%)	38 (36.5%)	17 (16.3%)	4 (3.8%)	12 (11.6%)	104 (100%)	χ2 Test— $p < 0.05$
	Not scheduled	29 (31.9%)	23 (25.4%)	11 (12%)	6 (6.7%)	11 (12%)	11 (12%)	91 (100%)	
Surgery	Performed	19 (22.1%)	35 (40.7%)	6 (7%)	3 (3.5%)	13 (15.1%)	10 (11.6%)	86 (100%)	χ2 Test— $p < 0.05$
	Not performed	25 (23%)	6 (5.5%)	43 (39.4%)	20 (18.3%)	2 (1.9%)	13 (11.9%)	109 (100%)	
Smoking	Yes	38 (30.4%)	25 (20%)	34 (27.2%)	10 (8%)	6 (4.8%)	12 (9.6%)	125 (100%)	χ2 Test— $p < 0.05$
	No	6 (8.6%)	16 (22.9%)	15 (21.4%)	13 (18.6%)	9 (12.9%)	11 (15.6%)	70 (100%)	
Edentulism	Yes	3 (37.5%)	2 (25%)	1 (12.5%)	0 (0%)	2 (25%)	0 (0%)	8 (100%)	-
	No	41 (22%)	39 (20.8%)	48 (25.7%)	23 (12.3%)	13 (6.9%)	23 (12.3%)	187 (100%)	
Periodontitis	Not affected	6 (13.3%)	10 (22.2%)	9 (20%)	11 (24.5%)	3 (6.7%)	6 (13.3%)	45 (100%)	-
	Stage I and II	8 (18.7%)	6 (13.9%)	15 (34.9%)	5 (11.7%)	3 (6.9%)	6 (13.9%)	43 (100%)	
	Stage III and IV	30 (28%)	25 (23.4%)	25 (23.4%)	7 (6.5%)	9 (8.4%)	11 (10.3%)	107 (100%)	
DMFt	Median	21	15	16	10	19	14	16	-
DMFt ≥ 13	No	11 (13.8%)	18 (22.5%)	22 (27.5%)	15 (18.8%)	3 (3.7%)	11 (13.7%)	80 (100%)	χ2 Test— $p < 0.05$
	Yes	33 (28.7%)	23 (20%)	27 (23.5%)	8 (7%)	12 (10.4%)	12 (10.4%)	115 (100%)	
Mouth Opening (mm)	<25	3 (14.3%)	7 (33.3%)	6 (28.6%)	1 (4.8%)	2 (9.5%)	2 (9.5%)	21 (100%)	-
	≥ 25	41 (23.6%)	34 (19.5%)	43 (24.7%)	22 (12.6%)	13 (7.5%)	21 (12.1%)	174 (100%)	
Oral Health	Good	6 (12.2%)	9 (18.5%)	13 (26.5%)	13 (26.5%)	2 (4.1%)	6 (12.2%)	49 (100%)	χ2 Test— $p < 0.05$
	Poor	38 (26%)	32 (21.9%)	36 (24.7%)	10 (6.8%)	13 (8.9%)	17 (11.7%)	146 (100%)	

Table 4. General and oral health characteristics of the studied population, according to the habit of smoking.

		Smokers 125	Non-Smokers 70	Total Sample 195	Significance
Gender	Male	92 (71.9%)	36 (28.1%)	128 (100%)	χ2 Test—p < 0.05
	Female	33 (49.2%)	34 (50.8%)	67 (100%)	
Age	<40	4 (44.4%)	5 (55.6%)	9 (100%)	-
	40–49	16 (61.5%)	10 (38.5%)	26 (100%)	
	50–59	34 (68%)	16 (32%)	50 (100%)	
	60–69	43 (66.2%)	22 (33.8%)	65 (100%)	
	70–79	24 (64.9%)	13 (35.1%)	37 (100%)	
	>80	4 (50%)	4 (50%)	8 (100%)	
Tumor Type	SCC	115 (66.5%)	58 (33.5%)	173 (100%)	
	Other types	10 (45.6%)	12 (54.5%)	22 (100%)	
Tumor Site	Larynx	38 (86.3%)	6 (13.7%)	44 (100%)	χ2 Test—p < 0.05
	Oral cavity	25 (61%)	16 (39%)	41 (100%)	
	Oropharynx	34 (69.4%)	15 (30.6%)	49 (100%)	
	Rhinopharynx	10 (43.5%)	13 (56.5%)	23 (100%)	
	Salivary glands	6 (40%)	9 (60%)	15 (100%)	
	Other sites	12 (52.2%)	11 (47.8%)	23 (100%)	
Tumor Stage	Stage I	7 (53.8%)	6 (46.2%)	13 (100%)	
	Stage II	15 (48.4%)	16 (51.6%)	31 (100%)	
	Stage III	29 (59.2%)	20 (40.8%)	49 (100%)	
	Stage IV	74 (72.6%)	28 (27.4%)	102 (100%)	
Chemotherapy	Scheduled	68 (65.4%)	36 (34.6%)	104 (100%)	
	Not scheduled	57 (62.6%)	34 (37.4%)	91 (100%)	
Surgery	Performed	52 (60.5%)	34 (39.5%)	86 (100%)	
	Not performed	73 (67%)	36 (33%)	109 (100%)	
Edentulism	Yes	4 (50%)	4 (50%)	8 (100%)	
	No	121 (64.7%)	66 (35.3%)	187 (100%)	
Periodontitis	Not affected	19 (42.2%)	26 (57.8%)	45 (100%)	χ2 Test—p < 0.05
	Stage I and II	26 (60.5%)	17 (39.5%)	43 (100%)	
	Stage III and IV	80 (74.8%)	27 (25.2%)	107 (100%)	
DMFt	Mean	17.8	15.3	16.9	
	Median	18	13	16	
DMFt ≥ 13	No	43 (53.8%)	37 (46.2%)	80 (100%)	χ2 Test—p < 0.05
	Yes	82 (71.3%)	33 (28.7%)	115 (100%)	
Mouth Opening (mm)	<25	14 (66.6%)	7 (33.4%)	21 (100%)	
	≥25	111 (63.8%)	63 (36.2%)	174 (100%)	
Oral Health	Good	22 (44.9%)	27 (55.1%)	49 (100%)	χ2 Test—p < 0.05
	Poor	103 (70.5%)	43 (29.5%)	146 (100%)	

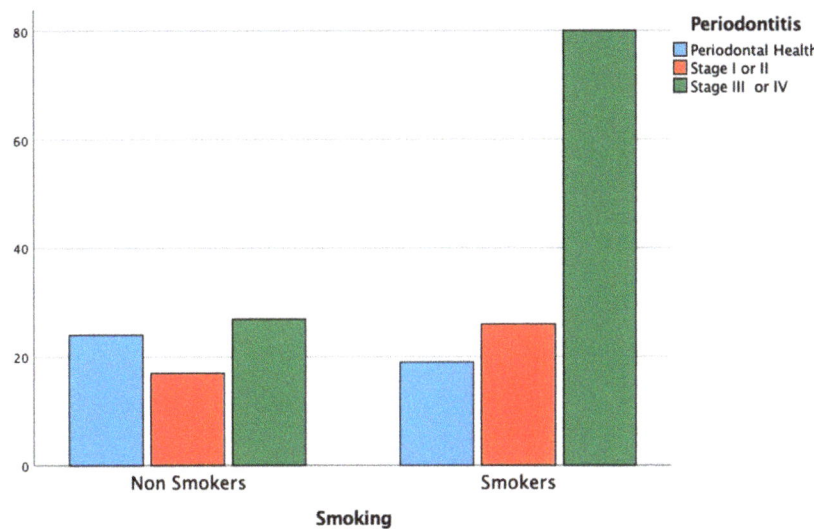

Figure 1. Distribution of periodontitis according to the habit of smoking.

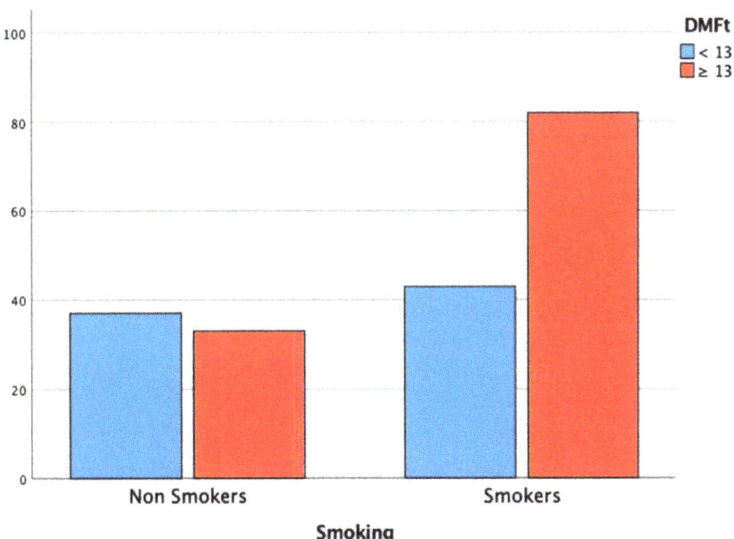

Figure 2. Distribution of DMFt < 13 according to the habit of smoking.

3.1.4. Age and OH Conditions

The cases of severe periodontitis (stages III and IV) were diagnosed only in subjects aged > 40 years, and 93.5% of periodontal patients were older than 49 years (χ^2 test, $p < 0.05$). Additionally, the distribution of high scores of DMFt (13 or higher) was not homogeneous (χ^2 test, $p < 0.05$): DMFt scores of ≥ 13 were only found among subjects aged > 40 years, with a peak in the 70–79 years decade (86.4% of the subjects who were allocated to this decade) and in the > 80 years category (75%). Consequently, poor OH conditions were more prevalent among the elderly population, with a peak in subjects aged > 70 years (95.6% of subjects being older than 70 years). All edentulous patients in the studied population were older than 60 years (χ^2 test, $p < 0.05$). Multiple logistic regression analysis showed that age (in decades) was a risk factor for periodontitis (stage I and II periodontitis: OR 1.73, 95% CI = 1.15–2.61; stage III and IV periodontitis: OR 3.30, 95% CI = 2.17–5.00; $p < 0.05$); for DMFt $\geq$ 13 (OR = 2.07; 95% CI = 1.53–2.79; $p < 0.05$); and for poor OH (OR = 2.98; 95% CI = 2.01–4.41; $p < 0.05$). The results of the analysis, stratified according to age, are reported in Table 5, and Figures 4–6.

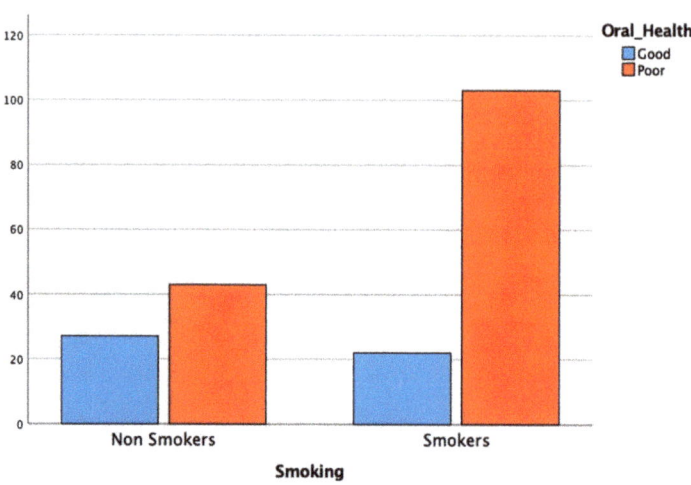

Figure 3. Distribution OH status according to the habit of smoking.

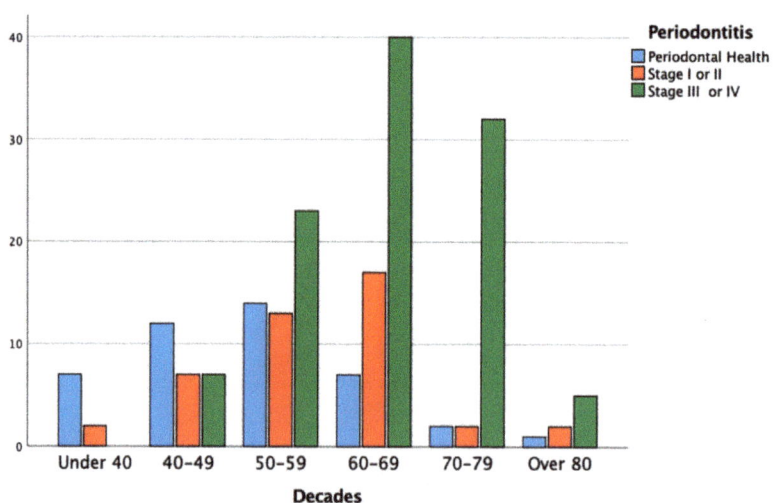

Figure 4. Distribution of periodontitis according to age of the patients (in decades).

Table 5. General and oral health characteristics of the studied population, according to the age of the subjects (decades).

		Age of the Subjects						Total Sample	Significance
		<40 9 (4.6%)	40–49 26 (13.3%)	50–59 50 (25.7%)	60–69 65 (33.3%)	70–79 37 (19%)	>80 8 (4.1%)	195 (100%)	
Gender	Male	4 (3.1%)	17 (13.3%)	30 (23.4%)	52 (40.6%)	21 (16.4%)	4 (3.1%)	128 (100%)	
	Female	5 (7.5%)	9 (13.4%)	20 (29.9%)	13 (19.4%)	16 (23.8%)	4 (6%)	67 (100%)	

Table 5. Cont.

		Age of the Subjects						Total Sample	Significance
		<40 9 (4.6%)	40–49 26 (13.3%)	50–59 50 (25.7%)	60–69 65 (33.3%)	70–79 37 (19%)	>80 8 (4.1%)	195 (100%)	
Tumor Type	SCC	6 (3.5%)	25 (14.5%)	44 (25.3%)	60 (34.7%)	32 (18.5%)	6 (3.5%)	173 (100%)	
	Other types	3 (13.7%)	1 (4.5%)	6 (27.3%)	5 (22.7%)	5 (22.7%)	2 (9.1%)	22 (100%)	
Tumor Site	Larynx	0 (0%)	6 (13.7%)	12 (27.2%)	15 (34.1%)	11 (25%)	0 (0%)	44 (100%)	χ2 Test—$p < 0.05$
	Oral cavity	2 (4.9%)	5 (12.2%)	11 (26.8%)	12 (29.4%)	7 (17%)	4 (9.7%)	41 (100%)	
	Oropharynx	0 (0%)	6 (12.2%)	14 (28.6%)	21 (42.9%)	8 (16.3%)	0 (0%)	49 (100%)	
	Rhinopharynx	4 (17.4%)	4 (17.4%)	4 (17.4%)	9 (39.1%)	2 (8.7%)	0 (0%)	23 (100%)	
	Salivary glands	1 (6.7%)	1 (6.6%)	4 (26.7%)	2 (13.3%)	4 (26.7%)	3 (20%)	15 (100%)	
	Other sites	2 (8.7%)	4 (17.4%)	5 (21.7%)	6 (26.9%)	5 (21.7%)	1 (4.3%)	23 (100%)	
Tumor Stage	Stage I	0 (0%)	3 (23.1%)	4 (30.8%)	2 (15.3%)	4 (30.8%)	0 (0%)	13 (100%)	
	Stage II	2 (6.5%)	3 (9.7%)	8 (25.8%)	10 (32.3%)	6 (19.3%)	2 (6.4%)	31 (100%)	
	Stage III	1 (2%)	6 (12.2%)	14 (28.6%)	19 (38.8%)	8 (16.3%)	1 (2%)	49 (100%)	
	Stage IV	6 (5.9%)	14 (13.7%)	24 (23.6%)	34 (33.3%)	19 (18.6%)	5 (4.9%)	102 (100%)	
Chemotherapy	Scheduled	5 (4.8%)	17 (16.4%)	36 (34.6%)	35 (33.7%)	10 (9.6%)	1 (0.9%)	104 (100%)	χ2 Test—$p < 0.05$
	Not scheduled	4 (4.4%)	9 (9.9%)	14 (15.4%)	30 (32.9%)	27 (29.7%)	7 (7.7%)	91 (100%)	
Surgery	Performed	2 (2.4%)	12 (13.9%)	24 (27.9%)	21 (24.4%)	22 (25.6%)	5 (5.8%)	86 (100%)	
	Not performed	7 (6.4%)	14 (12.8%)	26 (23.9%)	44 (40.3%)	15 (13.8%)	3 (2.8%)	109 (100%)	
Smoking	Yes	4 (3.2%)	16 (12.8%)	34 (27.2%)	43 (34.4%)	24 (19.2%)	4 (3.2%)	125 (100%)	
	No	5 (7.1%)	10 (14.3%)	16 (22.9%)	22 (31.4%)	13 (18.6%)	4 (5.7%)	70 (100%)	
Edentulism	Yes	0 (0%)	0 (0%)	0 (0%)	2 (25%)	5 (62.5%)	1 (12.5%)	8 (100%)	χ2 Test—$p < 0.05$
	No	9 (4.8%)	26 (13.9%)	50 (26.7%)	63 (33.7%)	32 (17.1%)	7 (3.7%)	187 (100%)	
Periodontitis	Not affected	7 (15.6%)	12 (26.7%)	15 (33.3%)	8 (17.9%)	2 (4.4%)	1 (2.2%)	45 (100%)	χ2 Test—$p < 0.05$
	Stage I and II	2 (4.7%)	7 (16.4%)	13 (30.2%)	17 (39.5%)	2 (4.6%)	2 (4.6%)	43 (100%)	
	Stage III and IV	0 (0%)	7 (6.5%)	23 (21.5%)	40 (37.4%)	32 (29.9%)	5 (4.7%)	107 (100%)	
DMFt	Median	5	8	16	16	25	23	16	Pearson's Correlation Analysis—$p < 0.05$
DMFt ≥ 13	No	9 (11.3%)	19 (23.8%)	17 (21.2%)	28 (35%)	5 (6.2%)	2 (2.5%)	80 (100%)	χ2 Test—$p < 0.05$
	Yes	0 (0%)	7 (6.1%)	33 (28.7%)	37 (32.2%)	32 (27.9%)	6 (5.2%)	115 (100%)	
Mouth Opening (mm)	<25	2 (9.5%)	3 (14.3%)	9 (42.8%)	4 (19%)	3 (14.3%)	0 (0%)	21 (100%)	-
	≥25	7 (4%)	23 (13.3%)	41 (23.7%)	61 (35%)	34 (19.5%)	8 (4.6%)	174 (100%)	
Oral Health	Good	9 (18.4%)	14 (28.6%)	13 (26.5%)	11 (22.3%)	0 (0%)	2 (4.1%)	49 (100%)	χ2 Test—$p < 0.05$
	Poor	0 (0%)	12 (8.2%)	37 (25.4%)	54 (36.9%)	37 (25.4%)	6 (4.1%)	146 (100%)	

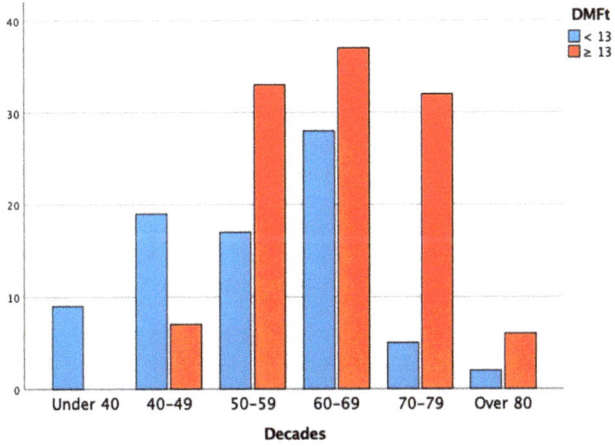

Figure 5. Distribution of DMFt < 13 according to age of the patients (in decades).

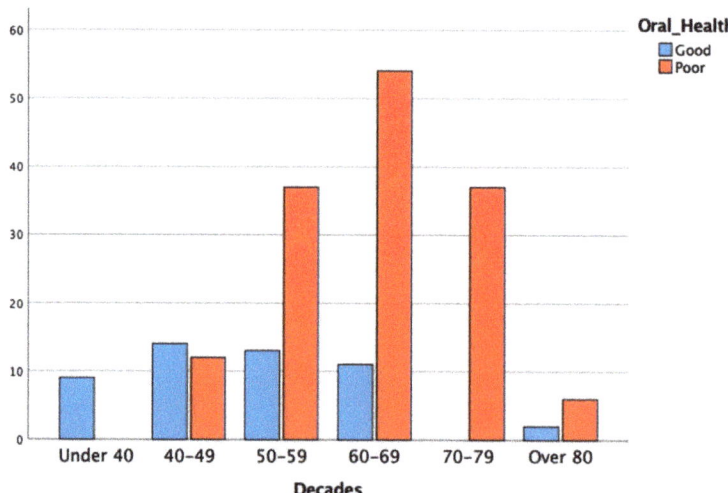

Figure 6. Distribution of OH status according to age of the patients (in decades).

4. Discussion

The role of the dentist in the head and neck tumor board (TB) is becoming increasingly important, especially in the context of modern multidisciplinary management, which places greater emphasis on the quality of life of patients after, or during, cancer therapy. The results of the present work confirm the importance of a dental evaluation prior to RT to prepare a patient for these complex therapies.

Available studies regarding the oral status of subjects with HNC at the time of diagnosis are few and often inaccurate or incomplete [28]. From this lack and from the clinical impressions of many specialists derives the probably correct belief that HNC patients present poor OH. This idea is even more ingrained when it comes to subjects with oral cavity tumors.

The description of the oral status of the cohort of patients with HNC proposed by this study confirms, within the limits of a cross-sectional study, the generally accepted idea that subjects with HNC very often present poor OH, although this is not supported by the current literature.

In particular, the subjects of this cohort presented poor OH (DMFt $\geq$ 13 and/or periodontitis stage III or IV) in 74.9% of cases. The OH conditions were not equally distributed among the different tumor sites ($\chi2$ test, $p < 0.05$): the subjects affected by SCC of the larynx (86.4%), of the salivary glands (86.6%) and of the oral cavity (78%) presented a higher prevalence of poor OH, when compared to the subjects affected by nasopharyngeal cancer (56.5% of nasopharyngeal patients presented DMFt < 13 and absence of severe periodontitis). Nevertheless, in the multivariate analysis, none of the tumor sites were revealed as an independent risk factor for poor OH.

The present work confirms that OH was more compromised the older the subjects were, with a peak (95.6% of cases) at 70 years of age and older (OR = 2.98; 95% CI = 2.01–4.41; $p < 0.05$). Multiple logistic regression analysis also showed that age was an independent risk factor for periodontitis (stage I and II periodontitis: OR 1.73, 95% CI = 1.15–2.61; stage III and IV periodontitis: OR 3.30, 95% CI = 2.17–5.00; $p < 0.05$) and for DMFt $\geq$ 13 (OR = 2.07; 95% CI = 1.53–2.79; $p < 0.05$).

The median DMFt value of the cohort analysed was 16.9. Fifty-nine percent of the included patients (115/195) had DMFt $\geq$ 13. Within the total population, only three subjects had DMFt = 0.

Although it is not possible to compare our results with those of previous works that studied cohorts of HNC patients, mainly due to the heterogenous methodology, some studies that reached similar conclusions can be found, such as those by Critchlow et al., Raskin et al. and Patel et al., who reported mean DMFt values of 19.6, 17.6 and 16.2 in HNC cohorts, respectively [28–30]. On the other hand, other studies (i.e., Jham et al. [31], Tezal et al. [32], Moraes et al. [33] and Kim et al. [34]) reported no significant correlation between HNC cancer and caries experience. Likely, the heterogeneity of the data stems from the different study designs, the criteria used in the different evaluations and the differences among the studied populations (i.e., geographical area, oral hygiene, access to dental care, distribution of different HNCs).

The percentage of subjects with periodontitis included in the present study was high (76.9%, 150/195) compared with epidemiological studies conducted in Europe, in which the prevalence of periodontitis did not exceed 70%, even in older age groups [35].

The classification of periodontitis proposed in 2017 [19] aims to remedy many of the critical issues present in epidemiological studies and to provide a more complete and detailed description of the populations under study. For this reason, in the present work, we chose to classify all cases of periodontitis based on this classification. In fact, if this study had limited itself to adopting the criteria proposed by previous classifications, many of the subjects with poor oral conditions, or a terminal dentition, would not have been included among the cases of severe periodontitis. The new classification, moreover, has made it possible to evaluate the periodontal status with a system based on two parameters (staging and grading) that, combined, provide information on the prognosis of the teeth and the complexity of the treatments required by the individual case. The combination of all this information constitutes a fundamental aid in deciding whether or not to perform extractions before RT.

Studies adopting the criteria proposed by the 2017 classification are very few [36–38], and our present work is the first to use them in a cohort of patients with HNC. Studies that have attempted to investigate a possible correlation between periodontitis and HNC are extremely diverse and often methodologically weak, as highlighted by a recent review [39]. In particular, the majority of studies did not adopt sound criteria to diagnose periodontitis [28,40–50], and only one [33] was based on a clinical evaluation integrated by the collection of truly suitable parameters (PPD and CAL).

Almost all authors who have analysed the OH of HNC patients before RT reported a high prevalence of periodontitis: Bonan et al. [51] reported a 93% prevalence of moderate or severe periodontitis, although cases were evaluated on the basis of a different classification; Moraes et al. [33] found that 80% of patients with oral and oropharyngeal SCC had generalized chronic periodontitis, almost exclusively severe. Although the results reported in the present study cannot be significantly compared with those of previous works because of methodological differences, they confirm that periodontitis, due to still unproven causes, is very common among patients with HNC.

Among the most plausible causes, the high incidence of smokers in these populations could play a key role. The data reported in our present study support this hypothesis; in fact, smokers represented 74.7% of the patients affected by stage III–IV periodontitis (80/107) (OR = 4.78; 95% CI = 2.01–11.36; $p < 0.05$). Statistical analysis showed that smoking also affected caries susceptibility (OR = 2.30; 95% CI = 1.19–4.44; $p < 0.05$) and, consequently, overall OH (OR = 3.27; 95% CI = 1.46–7.33; $p < 0.05$).

Despite the high percentage of patients with poor OH, only 8/195 (4.1%) were completely edentulous. The difference between the data reported by the present work and those of previous studies [4,31,51] may be influenced by the lower proportion of older individuals included in the present study (only 23.1% of patients were >70 years of age).

Interestingly, reduced MMO (<25 mm) did not correlate with the parameters of OH assessment. Reduced MMO is a very frequent clinical finding in HNC cohorts, as it can occur following both oncologic surgery and RT and makes dental care and inspection of the oral cavity particularly difficult, including during cancer follow-up appointments. However, a prospective study aiming to evaluate the correlation between MMO and OH is needed. It is very likely, in fact, that the greater difficulty in oral hygiene procedures, as well as in routine dental therapies and inspection procedures, due to a reduced MMO leads to an increase in the incidence of caries and a worsening of periodontal conditions.

This cross-sectional study has several strengths. The description of the oral status of the cohort is based on validated diagnostic and prognostic criteria, obtained through clinical and radiographic evaluation. Additionally, the reported results open the way to further investigating possible correlations between OH and HNC.

This study does not solely report the prevalence of caries and periodontitis in the analysed population; it proposes, for the first time, a criterion that may allow evaluating the OH of examined patients in a global and objective way. Establishing a cut-off to divide subjects into two groups according to the OH found emphasizes how defining an oral condition as "good" or "poor" is necessary, not only to find the presence or absence of caries and/or periodontitis, but also to quantify severity and to evaluate the two diseases through an integrated system.

Presenting a representative sample from each subsite of HNCs is one of the strengths of this study, as it provides a more specific picture of the OH conditions of patients with different HNCs. However, this also implies a limitation: the analysed sample, including subjects with tumors differing profoundly in risk factors and clinical manifestations, might be inhomogeneous. However, statistical analysis stratified by tumor subsites effectively allows highlighting the different peculiarities of individual HNCs from an OH perspective.

This study also has several limitations, among which, like all studies having evaluated the OH of HNC patients using DMFt as a parameter, is the retrospective attribution of the M parameter. This consideration also applies to the retrospective attribution of the number of teeth lost due to periodontitis. This necessity could lead to overestimating the prevalence of one pathology over another. However, the use of the "OH" parameter allows us to curb the extent of this potential bias, since it integrates the two main variables of interest.

In addition, a possible bias for this study is the lack of a control group, homogeneous to the one studied in terms of age, gender and smoking habits. More studies, with a different design (i.e., case–control studies), are needed to confirm that HNC patients have poorer OH than the general population.

Another parameter rendering the characteristics of the population peculiar is that all included patients had received an indication to undergo RT, since a dental visit is overwhelmingly indicated to prevent unwanted effects of RT. With this study being a real-life monocentric experience, indication for RT was chosen since the treatment of RT patients is the most "demanding", both from oncological and dental points of view. Nevertheless, our study also includes patients that underwent major oncological surgeries. Their inclusion within our sample could have made the observed population more homogeneous in terms of OH variables, making our sample more representative of HNC patients than a population undergoing exclusive RT.

Nevertheless, it could be considered as a selection bias, since patients who underwent a major oncologic surgery often present poorer OH, due to the reduced ability to adequately perform oral hygiene procedures, resulting from surgical procedure-induced anatomic alterations. Nevertheless, the results of our study show that previous oncologic treatment did not have a statistically significant correlation with OH, somehow confirming that this possible bias did not have a great impact. This could be explained by the fact that the dental evaluation was carried out in a time-lapse not exceeding 60 days, an insufficient time frame to significantly influence the parameters analyzed in this study. Notwithstanding, the results of the present work demonstrate how HNC patients present poor OH even prior to RT, which makes their inclusion within a protocol of primary and secondary dental prevention indicated.

5. Conclusions

This work highlights, with a high level of evidence, the number of HNC patients presenting poor OH in the months immediately following their malignancy diagnosis and their consequent need for prevention protocols and highly rigorous dental therapy, considering the increasing number of patients undergoing RT.

With the time window between the dental evaluation and the start of RT being particularly narrow, performing multiple extractions becomes necessary, resulting in further worsening of the periodontitis stage and masticatory function. This can only be avoided by referring the patient to a dental team, who will commence necessary therapies and preventive measures. Moreover, due to the increasing rate of recurrences and second primary tumors, an increasing number of patients receive an indication for RT.

It is important, therefore, that the figure of the dentist be regularly involved in multidisciplinary TBs for the management of head and neck patients to improve patient quality of life as much as possible and to reduce the risk of complications following oncologic treatment.

Supplementary Materials: The following supporting information can be downloaded at: https://www.mdpi.com/article/10.3390/cancers14061411/s1, Table S1: STROBE Statement—Checklist of items that should be included in reports of *cohort studies*.

Author Contributions: Conceptualization, C.L. and C.R.; data curation, C.R. and A.S.; methodology, C.L. and C.R.; formal analysis, C.L. and C.R.; investigation, C.R., A.S. and A.B.; resources, J.G., F.M., M.C. and C.L.; writing—original draft preparation, C.R. and A.S.; writing—review and editing, C.R., C.L. and A.S.; supervision, C.L., A.C., J.G. and M.C.; project administration, C.L., M.C., J.G. and F.M. All authors have read and agreed to the published version of the manuscript.

Funding: This research received no external funding.

Institutional Review Board Statement: This study was conducted in accordance with the Declaration of Helsinki, approved by the Ethics Committee of the Università Cattolica del Sacro Cuore (Ref. 22858/18) and registered at ClinicalTrials.gov (ID: NCT04009161).

Informed Consent Statement: Informed consent was obtained from all subjects involved in the study.

Data Availability Statement: The data presented in this study are available on request from the corresponding author. The data are not publicly available due to privacy.

Acknowledgments: The authors would like to acknowledge the help received from Sunstar Europe S.A., Route de Pallatex 11, P.O. Box 32, 1163 Etoy, Switzerland. (prot. CA-19-0888).

Conflicts of Interest: The authors declare no conflict of interest.

References

1. Sung, H.; Ferlay, J.; Siegel, R.L.; Laversanne, M.; Soerjomataram, I.; Jemal, A.; Bray, F. Global Cancer Statistics 2020: GLOBOCAN Estimates of Incidence and Mortality Worldwide for 36 Cancers in 185 Countries. *CA Cancer J. Clin.* **2021**, *71*, 209–249. [CrossRef] [PubMed]
2. Frydrych, A.; Slack-Smith, L. Dental attendance of oral and oropharyngeal cancer patients in a public hospital in Western Australia. *Aust. Dent. J.* **2011**, *56*, 278–283. [CrossRef] [PubMed]
3. Maier, H.; Zöller, J.; Herrmann, A.; Kreiss, M.; Heller, W.D. Dental Status and Oral Hygiene in Patients with Head and Neck Cancer. *Otolaryngol. Head Neck Surg.* **1993**, *108*, 655–661. [CrossRef] [PubMed]
4. Lockhart, P.B.; Clark, J. Pretherapy dental status of patients with malignant conditions of the head and neck. *Oral Surg. Oral Med. Oral Pathol.* **1994**, *77*, 236–241. [CrossRef]
5. Patel, R.A.; Wilson, R.F.; Palmer, R.M. The Effect of Smoking on Periodontal Bone Regeneration: A Systematic Review and Meta-Analysis. *J. Periodontol.* **2012**, *83*, 143–155. [CrossRef] [PubMed]
6. Papapanou, P.N. Periodontal Diseases: Epidemiology. *Ann. Periodontol.* **1996**, *1*, 1–36. [CrossRef] [PubMed]
7. Bergström, J. Tobacco smoking and chronic destructive periodontal disease. *Odontology* **2004**, *92*, 1–8. [CrossRef]
8. Paulander, J.; Wennström, J.L.; Axelsson, P.; Lindhe, J. Some risk factors for periodontal bone loss in 50-year-old individuals: A 10-year cohort study. *J. Clin. Periodontol.* **2004**, *31*, 489–496. [CrossRef]
9. Reibel, J. Tobacco and oral diseases. Update on the evidence, with recommendations. *Med. Princ. Pract.* **2003**, *12*, 22–32. [CrossRef]
10. Rad, M.; Kakoie, S.; Brojeni, F.N.; Pourdamghan, N. Effect of Long-term Smoking on Whole-mouth Salivary Flow Rate and Oral Health. *J. Dent. Res. Dent. Clin. Dent. Prospect.* **2010**, *4*, 110–114. [CrossRef]
11. Kielbassa, A.M.; Hinkelbein, W.; Hellwig, E.; Meyer-Lückel, H. Radiation-related damage to dentition. *Lancet Oncol.* **2006**, *7*, 326–335. [CrossRef]
12. Berrone, M.; Lajolo, C.; De Corso, E.; Settimi, S.; Rupe, C.; Crosetti, E.; Succo, G. Cooperation between ENT surgeon and dentist in head and neck oncology. *Acta Otorhinolaryngol. Ital.* **2021**, *41*, S124–S137. [CrossRef] [PubMed]

13. Lajolo, C.; Rupe, C.; Gioco, G.; Troiano, G.; Patini, R.; Petruzzi, M.; Micciche, F.; Giuliani, M. Osteoradionecrosis of the Jaws Due to Teeth Extractions during and after Radiotherapy: A Systematic Review. *Cancers* **2021**, *13*, 5798. [CrossRef] [PubMed]
14. Dholam, K.P.; Sharma, M.R.; Gurav, S.V.; Singh, G.P.; Prabhash, K. Oral and dental health status in patients undergoing neoadjuvant chemotherapy for locally advanced head and neck cancer. *Oral Surg. Oral Med. Oral Pathol. Oral Radiol.* **2021**, *132*, 539–548. [CrossRef] [PubMed]
15. Varenne, D.B. World Health Organization. Available online: https://www.who.int/data/gho/indicator-metadata-registry/imr-details/3812#:~{}:text=DMFT%20is%20the%20sum%20of,the%20WHO%20indicator%20age%20groups (accessed on 18 February 2022).
16. American Dental Association. Caries diagnosis and risk assessment, a review of preventive strategies and management. *J. Am. Dent. Assoc.* **1995**, *126*, 1S–24S.
17. Gomez, J.L. Detection and diagnosis of the early caries lesion. *BMC Oral Heal.* **2015**, *15*, S3. [CrossRef] [PubMed]
18. Ismail, A.I.; Pitts, N.B.; Tellez, M.; Authors of the International Caries Classification and Management System (ICCMS). The International Caries Classification and Management System (ICCMS™) An Example of a Caries Management Pathway. *BMC Oral Heal.* **2015**, *15*, S9. [CrossRef]
19. Papapanou, P.; Sanz, M.; Buduneli, N.; Dietrich, T.; Feres, M.; Fine, D.; Flemmig, T.; Garcia, R.; Giannobile, W.; Graziani, F.; et al. Periodontitis: Consensus report of workgroup 2 of the 2017 World Workshop on the Classification of Periodontal and Peri-Implant Diseases and Conditions. *J. Periodontol.* **2018**, *89*, S173–S182. [CrossRef]
20. Hamp, S.; Nyman, S.; Lindhe, J. Periodontal treatment of multirooted teeth. Results after 5 years. *J. Clin. Periodontol.* **1975**, *2*, 126–135. [CrossRef]
21. O'Leary, T.J.; Drake, R.B.; Naylor, J.E. The Plaque Control Record. *J. Periodontol.* **1972**, *43*, 38. [CrossRef] [PubMed]
22. Lang, N.P.; Joss, A.; Tonetti, M.S. Monitoring disease during supportive periodontal treatment by bleeding on probing. *Periodontology 2000* **1996**, *12*, 44–48. [CrossRef] [PubMed]
23. Fatima, J.; Kaul, R.; Jain, P.; Saha, S.; Halder, S.; Sarkar, S. Clinical Measurement of Maximum Mouth Opening in Children of Kolkata and Its Relation with Different Facial Types. *J. Clin. Diagn. Res.* **2016**, *10*, ZC01–ZC05. [CrossRef] [PubMed]
24. WHO. *Oral Health Programme: Global Data on Dental Caries Prevalence (DMFT) in Adults Aged 35–44 Years*; Global Oral Data Bank; Oral Health/Area Profile Programme; World Health Organization: Geneva, Switzerland, 2000.
25. Frencken, J.E.; Sharma, P.; Stenhouse, L.; Green, D.; Laverty, D.; Dietrich, T. Global epidemiology of dental caries and severe periodontitis—A comprehensive review. *J. Clin. Periodontol.* **2017**, *44* (Suppl. 18), S94–S105. [CrossRef] [PubMed]
26. Dijkstra, P.; Huisman, P.; Roodenburg, J. Criteria for trismus in head and neck oncology. *Int. J. Oral Maxillofac. Surg.* **2006**, *35*, 337–342. [CrossRef] [PubMed]
27. Kamstra, J.; Dijkstra, P.; van Leeuwen, M.; Roodenburg, J.; Langendijk, J.A. Mouth opening in patients irradiated for head and neck cancer: A prospective repeated measures study. *Oral Oncol.* **2015**, *51*, 548–555. [CrossRef] [PubMed]
28. Patel, V.; Patel, D.; Browning, T.; Patel, S.; McGurk, M.; Sassoon, I.; Urbano, T.G.; Fenlon, M. Presenting pre-radiotherapy dental status of head and neck cancer patients in the novel radiation era. *Br. Dent. J.* **2020**, *228*, 435–440. [CrossRef]
29. Critchlow, S.B.; Morgan, C.; Leung, T. The oral health status of pre-treatment head and neck cancer patients. *Br. Dent. J.* **2014**, *216*, E1. [CrossRef]
30. Raskin, A.; Ruquet, M.; Weiss-Pelletier, L.; Mancini, J.; Boulogne, O.; Michel, J.; Fakhry, N.; Foletti, J.; Chossegros, C.; Giorgi, R. Upper aerodigestive tract cancer and oral health status before radiotherapy: A cross-sectional study of 154 patients. *J. Stomatol. Oral Maxillofac. Surg.* **2018**, *119*, 2–7. [CrossRef]
31. Jham, B.C.; Reis, P.M.; Miranda, E.L.; Lopes, R.C.; Carvalho, A.; Scheper, M.A.; Freire, A.R. Oral health status of 207 head and neck cancer patients before, during and after radiotherapy. *Clin. Oral Investig.* **2007**, *12*, 19–24. [CrossRef]
32. Tezal, M.; Scannapieco, F.A.; Wactawski-Wende, J.; Meurman, J.H.; Marshall, J.R.; Rojas, I.G.; Stoler, D.L.; Genco, R.J. Dental Caries and Head and Neck Cancers. *JAMA Otolaryngol. Neck Surg.* **2013**, *139*, 1054–1060. [CrossRef]
33. De Moraes, R.C.; Dias, F.L.; Figueredo, C.M.; Fischer, R.G. Association between Chronic Periodontitis and Oral/Oropharyngeal Cancer. *Braz. Dent. J.* **2016**, *27*, 261–266. [CrossRef] [PubMed]
34. Kim, Y.-S.; Jung, Y.-S.; Kim, B.-K.; Kim, E.-K. Oral Health of Korean Patients With Head and Neck Cancer. *J. Cancer Prev.* **2018**, *23*, 77–81. [CrossRef] [PubMed]
35. Mack, F.; Mojon, P.; Budtz-Jorgensen, E.; Kocher, T.; Splieth, C.; Schwahn, C.; Bernhardt, O.; Gesch, D.; Kordass, B.; John, U.; et al. Caries and periodontal disease of the elderly in Pomerania, Germany: Results of the Study of Health in Pomerania. *Gerodontology* **2004**, *21*, 27–36. [CrossRef] [PubMed]
36. Ravidà, A.; Qazi, M.; Troiano, G.; Saleh, M.H.A.; Greenwell, H.; Kornman, K.; Wang, H. Using periodontal staging and grading system as a prognostic factor for future tooth loss: A long-term retrospective study. *J. Periodontol.* **2020**, *91*, 454–461. [CrossRef] [PubMed]
37. Iao, S.; Pei, X.; Ouyang, X.; Liu, J.; Liu, W.; Cao, C. Natural progression of periodontal diseases in Chinese villagers based on the 2018 classification. *J. Periodontol.* **2021**, *92*, 1232–1242. [CrossRef] [PubMed]
38. Graetz, C.; Mann, L.; Krois, J.; Sälzer, S.; Kahl, M.; Springer, C.; Schwendicke, F. Comparison of periodontitis patients' classification in the 2018 versus 1999 classification. *J. Clin. Periodontol.* **2019**, *46*, 908–917. [CrossRef] [PubMed]
39. Gasparoni, L.; Alves, F.; Holzhausen, M.; Pannuti, C.; Serpa, M. Periodontitis as a risk factor for head and neck cancer. *Med. Oral Patol. Oral Cir. Bucal* **2021**, *26*, e430–e436. [CrossRef]

40. Ahmed, R.; Malik, S.; Khan, M.F.; Khattak, M.R. Epidemiologi- cal and clinical correlates of oral squamous cell carcinoma in patients from north-west Pakistan. *J. Pak. Med. Assoc.* **2019**, *69*, 1074–1078.
41. Eliot, M.N.; Michaud, M.S.; Langevin, S.M.; McClean, M.D.; Kelsey, K.T. Periodontal disease and mouthwash use are risk factors for head and neck squamous cell carcinoma. *Cancer Causes Control* **2013**, *24*, 1315–1322. [CrossRef] [PubMed]
42. Divaris, K.; Olshan, A.F.; Smith, J.; Bell, M.E.; Weissler, M.C.; Funkhouser, W.K.; Bradshaw, P.T. Oral health and risk for head and neck squamous cell carcinoma: The Carolina Head and Neck Cancer Study. *Cancer Causes Control* **2010**, *21*, 567–575. [CrossRef]
43. Michaud, D.S.; Liu, Y.; Meyer, M.; Giovannucci, E.; Joshipura, K. Periodontal disease, tooth loss, and cancer risk in male health professionals: A prospective cohort study. *Lancet Oncol.* **2008**, *9*, 550–558. [CrossRef]
44. De Rezende, C.P.; Ramos, M.B.; Daguíla, C.H.; Dedivitis, R.A.; Rapoport, A. Oral Health Changes in Patients with Oral and Oropharyngeal Cancer. *Braz. J. Otorhinolaryngol.* **2008**, *74*, 596–600. [CrossRef]
45. Tezal, M.; Sullivan, M.A.; Reid, M.E.; Marshall, J.R.; Hyland, A.; Loree, T.; Lillis, C.; Hauck, L.; Wactawski-Wende, J.; Scannapieco, F.A. Chronic Periodontitis and the Risk of Tongue Cancer. *Arch. Otolaryngol. Head Neck Surg.* **2007**, *133*, 450–454. [CrossRef] [PubMed]
46. Tezal, M.; Sullivan, M.A.; Hyland, A.; Marshall, J.R.; Stoler, D.; Reid, M.E.; Loree, T.R.; Rigual, N.R.; Merzianu, M.; Hauck, L.; et al. Chronic Periodontitis and the Incidence of Head and Neck Squamous Cell Carcinoma. *Cancer Epidemiol. Biomark. Prev.* **2009**, *18*, 2406–2412. [CrossRef] [PubMed]
47. Shin, Y.; Choung, H.; Lee, J.; Rhyu, I.; Kim, H. Association of Periodontitis with Oral Cancer: A Case-Control Study. *J. Dent. Res.* **2019**, *98*, 526–533. [CrossRef] [PubMed]
48. Moergel, M.; Kämmerer, P.; Kasaj, A.; Armouti, E.; Alshihri, A.; Weyer, V.; Al-Nawas, B. Chronic periodontitis and its possible association with oral squamous cell carcinoma—A retrospective case control study. *Head Face Med.* **2013**, *9*, 39. [CrossRef] [PubMed]
49. Talamini, R.; Vaccarella, S.; Barbone, F.; Tavani, A.; La Vecchia, C.; Herrero, R.; Muñoz, N.; Franceschi, S. Oral hygiene, dentition, sexual habits and risk of oral cancer. *Br. J. Cancer* **2000**, *83*, 1238–1242. [CrossRef] [PubMed]
50. Guha, N.; Boffetta, P.; Wünsch Filho, V.; Eluf Neto, J.; Shangina, O.; Zaridze, D.; Curado, M.P.; Koifman, S.; Matos, E.; Menezes, A.; et al. Oral health and risk of squamous cell carcinoma of the head and neck and esophagus: Results of two multicentric case-control studies. *Am. J. Epidemiol.* **2007**, *166*, 1159–1173. [CrossRef] [PubMed]
51. Bonan, P.R.F.; Lopes, M.A.; Pires, F.R.; De Almeida, O.P. Dental management of low socioeconomic level patients before radiotherapy of the head and neck with special emphasis on the prevention of osteoradionecrosis. *Braz. Dent. J.* **2006**, *17*, 336–342. [CrossRef]

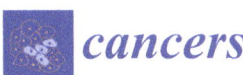

Article

Comparative Analysis of Vascular Mimicry in Head and Neck Squamous Cell Carcinoma: In Vitro and In Vivo Approaches

Roosa Hujanen [1], Rabeia Almahmoudi [1], Tuula Salo [1,2,3,4,5,†] and Abdelhakim Salem [1,2,3,*,†]

1. Department of Oral and Maxillofacial Diseases, Clinicum, University of Helsinki, 00014 Helsinki, Finland; roosa.hujanen@helsinki.fi (R.H.); rabeia.mustafa@helsinki.fi (R.A.); tuula.salo@helsinki.fi (T.S.)
2. Translational Immunology Research Program (TRIMM), Research Program Unit (RPU), University of Helsinki, 00014 Helsinki, Finland
3. Helsinki University Hospital (HUS), 00029 Helsinki, Finland
4. Cancer and Translational Medicine Research Unit, University of Oulu, 90014 Oulu, Finland
5. Department of Pathology, Helsinki University Hospital (HUS), 00029 Helsinki, Finland
* Correspondence: abdelhakim.salem@helsinki.fi
† These authors jointly supervised this work.

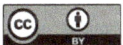

Citation: Hujanen, R.; Almahmoudi, R.; Salo, T.; Salem, A. Comparative Analysis of Vascular Mimicry in Head and Neck Squamous Cell Carcinoma: In Vitro and In Vivo Approaches. *Cancers* **2021**, *13*, 4747. https://doi.org/10.3390/cancers13194747

Academic Editors: Carlo Lajolo, Gaetano Paludetti and Romeo Patini

Received: 17 August 2021
Accepted: 20 September 2021
Published: 23 September 2021

Publisher's Note: MDPI stays neutral with regard to jurisdictional claims in published maps and institutional affiliations.

Copyright: © 2021 by the authors. Licensee MDPI, Basel, Switzerland. This article is an open access article distributed under the terms and conditions of the Creative Commons Attribution (CC BY) license (https://creativecommons.org/licenses/by/4.0/).

Simple Summary: Head and neck squamous cell carcinomas (HNSCCs) are common and among the deadliest neoplasms worldwide, wherein metastasis represents the main cause of the poor survival outcomes. Tumour cells require blood vessels in order to grow and invade the surrounding tissues. Recently, a new phenomenon termed vascular mimicry (VM) was introduced, whereby tumour cells can independently form vessel-like structures to promote their growth and metastasis. VM has been characterized in many solid tumours, including HNSCC. A large body of research evidence shows that patients with positive VM exhibit poor treatment response and dismal survival rates. Thus, VM represents a promising therapeutic and prognostic target in cancer. However, there is limited knowledge regarding the identification of VM in HNSCC (in vitro and in vivo) and what factors may influence such a phenomenon. This study aims to address these limitations, which may facilitate the therapeutic exploitation of VM in HNSCC.

Abstract: Tissue vasculature provides the main conduit for metastasis in solid tumours including head and neck squamous cell carcinoma (HNSCC). Vascular mimicry (VM) is an endothelial cell (EC)-independent neovascularization pattern, whereby tumour cells generate a perfusable vessel-like meshwork. Yet, despite its promising clinical utility, there are limited approaches to better identify VM in HNSCC and what factors may influence such a phenomenon in vitro. Therefore, we employed different staining procedures to assess their utility in identifying VM in tumour sections, wherein mosaic vessels may also be adopted to further assess the VM-competent cell phenotype. Using 13 primary and metastatic HNSCC cell lines in addition to murine- and human-derived matrices, we elucidated the impact of the extracellular matrix, tumour cell type, and density on the formation and morphology of cell-derived tubulogenesis in HNSCC. We then delineated the optimal cell numbers needed to obtain a VM meshwork in vitro, which revealed cell-specific variations and yet consistent expression of the EC marker CD31. Finally, we proposed the zebrafish larvae as a simple and cost-effective model to evaluate VM development in vivo. Taken together, our findings offer a valuable resource for designing future studies that may facilitate the therapeutic exploitation of VM in HNSCC and other tumours.

Keywords: head and neck squamous cell carcinoma; vascular mimicry; Matrigel; Myogel; zebrafish; metastasis

1. Introduction

Head and neck squamous cell carcinoma (HNSCC) includes tumours of the oral cavity, hypopharynx, oropharynx, nasopharynx, and larynx [1]. Overall, HNSCC represents one of the most common cancers worldwide with relatively poor survival outcomes that remain stagnant at around 50% [2]. Such dismal prognosis of HNSCC patients has been largely attributed to tumour cell invasiveness and metastasis [3,4]. Thus, a better understanding of the different mechanisms and patterns underlying tumour cell dissemination could improve the management and survival outcomes of HNSCC patients.

Vascular mimicry (VM; a.k.a. vasculogenic mimicry) is a newly described pattern of tumour-related neoangiogenesis, whereby aggressive tumour cells can form tube-like vascular networks independently of endothelial cells [5,6]. These de novo VM structures were first described in patients with aggressive melanoma. Shortly thereafter, myriad studies have revealed many interesting characteristics of VM in various cancers including HNSCC [7,8]. In addition to satisfying the nutrient need of the primary tumour, VM is believed to provide tumour cells with an alternative route to intravasate and undergo metastasis [9,10]. In this regard, VM was shown to efficiently drive tumour cell metastasis in a polyclonal mouse model of breast cancer [10]. Furthermore, several studies revealed significant association between VM and lymph node metastasis (LNM) and hence worse prognosis in numerous malignancies [11–13]. We showed in a recent meta-analysis study that HNSCC patients with VM^{+ve} tumours had shorter overall survival and worse clinicopathological features, including LNM, compared with the VM^{-ve} group [8].

A vessel-like structure expressing CD31^{-ve}/periodic acid–Schiff (PAS)$^{+ve}$ staining is often considered the "golden" standard to identify VM in histological samples [14]. However, in spite of the spirited debate ignited by this phenomenon, characterizing VM in patient samples has recently drawn criticism for its limitations. On the one hand, such CD31^{-ve}/PAS^{+ve} structures may represent irrelevant glycogen-rich areas rather than true mimetic vessels [14–16]. On the other hand, the mosaic vessels, concurrently expressing endothelial and tumour cell markers, have been overlooked in HNSCC-related studies, which show limited approaches to identify VM both in vitro and in vivo [7,8]. Therefore, we conducted a comprehensive comparative analysis of VM formation in HNSCC using a variety of procedures. We also proposed the zebrafish larvae as a feasible tool to model VM formation in vivo.

2. Materials and Methods

2.1. Patient Samples

This study was approved by the National Supervisory Authority for Welfare and Health (VALVIRA) and the Ethics Committee of the Northern Ostrobothnia Hospital District. Our study comprised patients diagnosed with oral tongue SCC (OTSCC) who had undergone surgery in Oulu University Hospital during the period 1990–2010. Formalin-fixed paraffin-embedded (FFPE) samples ($n = 30$) were obtained from the pathology department of Oulu University Hospital. None of these patients had received other prior treatments.

2.2. CD31 and PAS Double Staining

The FFPE specimens were deparaffinized and rehydrated and subjected to heat-induced antigen retrieval using Micromed T/T Mega Microwave Processing Lab Station (Hacker Instruments & Industries). Non-specific binding was blocked with Dako peroxidase blocking solution S2023 for 15 min (Dako, Glostrup, Denmark), followed by incubation in a 1:100 polyclonal rabbit anti-CD31 antibody (ab28364; Abcam, Cambridge, UK) for 1 h. Sections were then incubated with horseradish peroxidase for 30 min; treated with DAB (Pierce™ DAB Substrate Kit; Thermo Fisher Scientific; Waltham, MA, USA) for 5 min; and incubated with 0.5% freshly made periodic acid for 10 min. Sections were further stained with Schiff solution for 15 min and rinsed under running water for another 15 min. Slides were incubated with Cole's hematoxylin for 6 min and mounted in Mountex (HistoLab, Gothenburg, Sweden). All incubations were conducted at room temperature.

2.3. Double-Labelling Immunofluorescence (IF)

Following deparaffinization and heat-induced antigen retrieval, sections were blocked for 1 h with 10% donkey normal serum (Sigma-Aldrich; St. Louis, MO, USA). Sections were then incubated overnight with a primary antibody solution containing 1:50 polyclonal rabbit anti-CD31 antibody (ab28364, Abcam, Cambridge, UK) and 1:100 monoclonal mouse antihuman pan-cytokeratin (CK) (M3515, Dako, Glostrup, Denmark) at 4 °C. The following day, the sections were incubated in (1) 1:200 donkey anti-mouse Alexa Fluor®-568 or donkey anti-rabbit Alexa Fluor®-488 conjugated secondary antibodies (Vector Laboratories; Burlingame, CA, USA) for 1 h and (2) 4′,6-diamidino-2-phenylindole (DAPI; 1:1000; Sigma-Aldrich, St. Louis, MO, USA) for 10 min, and mounted with ProLong® Gold Antifade Mountant (Thermo Fisher Scientific; Waltham, MA, USA). To stain the cell-derived tubular networks, matrix-coated coverslips were fixed for 20 min in 4% paraformaldehyde (PFA; Santa Cruz Biotech., Santa Cruz, CA, USA) and then staining was continued as above. All steps were performed at room temperature unless otherwise indicated. For multiplexed immunohistochemistry (mIHC), the following antibodies were used: 1:50 polyclonal rabbit anti-CD31 antibody (ab28364, Abcam, Cambridge, UK); 1:100 monoclonal mouse anti-CD44 antibody (144M-95; Cell Marque, Rocklin, CA, USA); 1:100 monoclonal mouse antihuman E-cadherin antibody (M361201, Dako, Glostrup, Denmark); monoclonal mouse anti-CK c11 (ab7753, Abcam, Cambridge, UK); and 1:150 monoclonal mouse anti-CK (AE1/AE3; Dako, Glostrup, Denmark). mIHC was performed in the Digital Microscopy and Molecular Pathology Unit (FIMM Institute, University of Helsinki) as described previously [17].

2.4. Cell Line and Culture

Thirteen primary and metastatic HNSCC cell lines were used, including HSC-3 (JCRB 0623; Osaka National Institute of Health Sciences, Japan), SCC-25 (ATCC, Rockville, MD, USA) and SAS (JCRB-0260). Ten cell lines (UT-SCC, hereafter SCC) were established directly from the patient biopsy material at the Department of Otorhinolaryngology, Head and Neck Surgery Unit, Turku University Hospital (Table S1). Of these, paired primary and metastatic cell lines (SCC-24A and -24B, respectively) were obtained from the same patient. The SCC-28 cell line was derived from a primary tumour that was first treated with radiotherapy prior to surgical resection. Cancer cell lines were cultured in 1:1 DMEM-F12 medium (Gibco/Invitrogen, Tokyo, Japan) supplemented with 10% heat-inactivated fetal bovine serum (Gibco), penicillin–streptomycin (15140-122, Thermo Fisher Scientific; Waltham, MA, USA), 50 µg/mL ascorbic acid (A1052, AppliChem, Chicago, IL, USA), 250 ng/mL amphotericin B (A2942, Sigma-Aldrich, St. Louis, MO, USA) and 0.4 µg/mL hydrocortisone (H0888, Sigma-Aldrich, St. Louis, MO, USA). Cell lines were maintained in a 95% humidified incubator of 5% CO_2 at 37 °C. Human umbilical vein endothelial cells (HUVEC; Thermo Fisher Scientific; Waltham, MA, USA) were used as a positive control for the in vitro tubulogenesis. HUVECs were cultured in 200PRF medium supplemented with a low serum growth supplement (Thermo Fisher Scientific; Waltham, MA, USA).

2.5. Murine and Human-Derived 3D Matrices

We used the commercial mouse Engelbreth–Holm–Swarm (EHS) sarcoma matrix, Matrigel (Corning, NYC, NY, USA). In addition, we used our in-house gelatinous soluble matrix "Myogel" that is derived from human leiomyoma tissue [18,19]. The preparation and usage of human leiomyoma tissue have been approved by the Ethics Committee of Oulu University Hospital (no. 35/2014). Liquid handling was performed using MultiFlo™ FX automated multi-mode reagent dispenser (BioTeK, Winooski, VT, USA).

2.6. In Vitro Tube Formation Assay

The in vitro tube formation assay was performed according to a previously published protocol [20]. For the Matrigel-based assay, following a slow overnight thawing at 4 °C, 50 µL of Matrigel was dispensed into a 96-well plate and incubated for 30 min at 37 °C. Cancer cells and HUVECs were detached from 75 cm^2 flasks (Sigma-Aldrich, St. Louis, MO,

USA) with trypsin–EDTA, resuspended in serum-free DMEM or 200PRF medium, and then counted using Scepter™ 2.0 Cell Counter (Merck Millipore, Burlington, MA, USA). Cells were seeded on the top of Matrigel at a starting density of 20×10^3 in 50 µL serum-free medium and incubated at 37 °C.

For the Myogel-based assay, the optimal gel concentration (1 mg/mL) was determined using pilot experiments with HUVECs. The Myogel-fibrin matrix was prepared with serum-free medium using the following concentrations: 1 mg/mL Myogel, 1 mg/mL fibrinogen (341578, Merck, Darmstadt, Germany), 66.67 µg/mL aprotinin (A6279-10ML, Merck, Darmstadt, Germany), and 0.6 U/mL thrombin (T6884-100UN, Sigma-Aldrich, St. Louis, MO, USA). To test the potential effects of different gel constituents, Myogel was also combined with 1 mg/mL rat-tail type I collagen (354236; Corning, NYC, NY, USA) or 1–2% low-melting agarose (LMA; 50101, Lonza, Basel, Switzerland). In total, 50 µL of LMA was slowly pipetted into a 96-well plate to avoid bubbles and incubated overnight at 37 °C. The next day, Myogel was pipetted with the cells into the LMA-coated wells. The matrix-coated well plates were incubated for 12 and 24 h for endothelial- and tumour cell-derived tubulogenesis, respectively. The wells were then rinsed in phosphate-buffered solution (PBS), fixed for 20 min with 4% PFA, and stored in 4 °C.

2.7. Zebrafish Larvae Assays

In vivo zebrafish experiments were performed in the zebrafish core facility at the University of Helsinki. All procedures were approved by the ethical committee of the regional state administrative agency (license ESAVI/13139/04.10.05/2017). Two-day post-fertilization zebrafish larvae were dechorionated and anaesthetized using 0.04% Tricaine (n = 10 per matrix group). Fluorescently labelled with CellTrace™ Far Red (Thermo Fisher Scientific; Waltham, MA, USA), HSC-3 cells were washed in PBS and resuspended in 1:1 Matrigel or Myogel, and then microinjected into the perivitelline space using glass microinjection needles (about 1000 cells). Fish were maintained at 34 °C within an embryonic medium (Sigma-Aldrich, St. Louis, MO, USA) for 72 h and then collected, fixed with 10% PFA, and mounted using SlowFade Gold Antifade (Invitrogen, Carlsbad, CA, USA).

2.8. Imaging and Tube Formation Analysis

For experiments on tube formation, samples were photographed with magnifications of 4×, 10× and 20× using the reverse Nikon Digital Sight DS-U3 microscope (Nikon, Tokyo, Japan). Each experiment was repeated at least three times independently. Stained section images were acquired with magnifications of 10×, 20×, and 40× using a Leica DM6000 microscope (Leica Microsystems, Wetzlar, Germany). Imaging of zebrafish larvae was performed at the Biomedicum Imaging Unit (University of Helsinki) using a Leica TCS SP8 confocal microscope. The ImageJ software (Wayne Rasband, National Institute of Health, Bethesda, MD, USA) was used by applying the "Angiogenesis Analyzer" plugin to measure several different parameters for evaluating the tube formation as described in the Results section.

3. Results

3.1. Utility of the $CD31^{-ve}/PAS^{+ve}$ Reaction in Identifying the VM in HNSCC Patients

To identify the VM in the patient samples, we first employed the traditional staining method—a combination of the endothelial cell marker and PAS staining on FFPE sections from HNSCC patients (Figure 1A). PAS stains basement membrane components such as laminin, collagen, and glycogen, whereas CD31 was opted as a specific endothelial cell marker. Areas of PAS^{+ve} laminin and collagen-rich networks (pink) with the surrounding tumour cells were recognized in the patient samples. Additionally, $CD31^{+ve}/PAS^{+ve}$ endothelial vessels (brown/pink; Figure 1B,C) and $CD31^{-ve}/PAS^{+ve}$ areas (pink; Figure 1D) were identified. However, it was often onerous to accurately identify the $CD31^{-ve}/PAS^{+ve}$ structures due to the presence of necrotic areas or faint CD31 signals that can be easily masked by the surrounding PAS staining (Figure 1E; arrows show a faint signal of CD31).

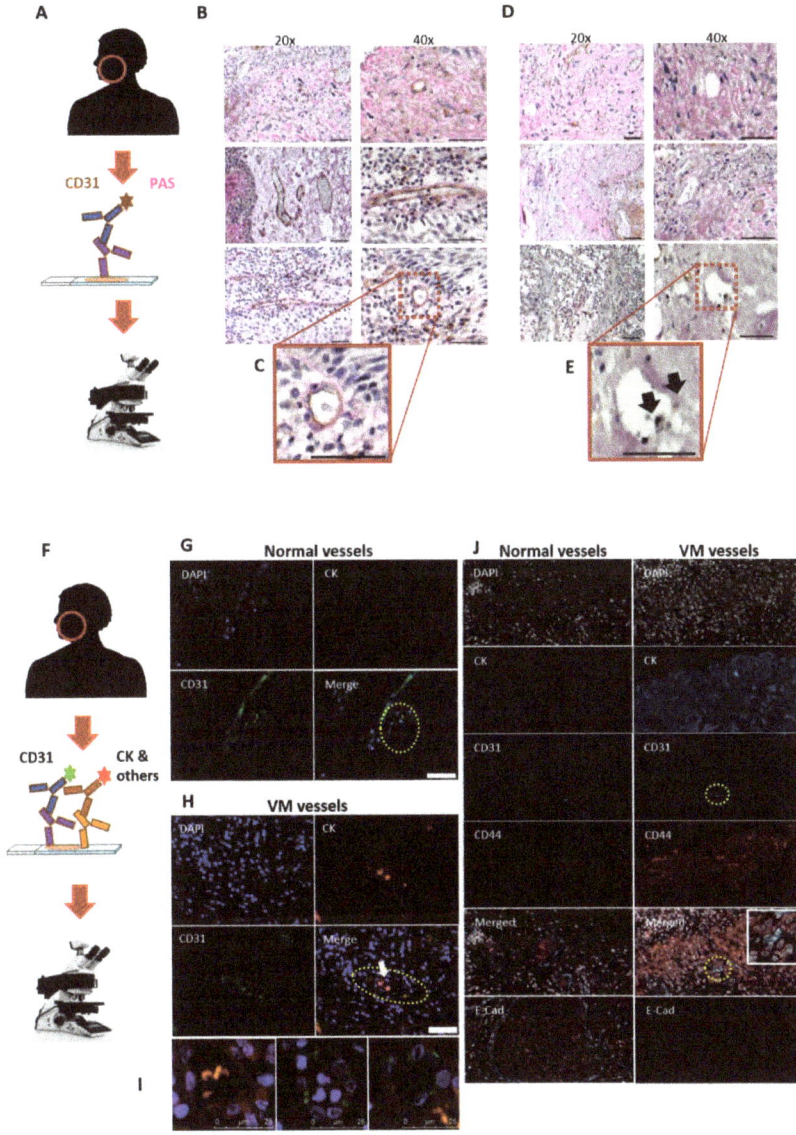

Figure 1. Identification of vascular mimicry (VM) in tumour tissues. (**A**) Representative figures from tumour sections (n = 30) obtained from patients with oral tongue squamous cell carcinoma (OTSCC) and stained using a combination of endothelial cell (EC) marker (CD31) and periodic acid–Schiff (PAS) staining. (**B,C**) Normal blood vessels express CD31^{+ve}/PAS^{+ve} (brown/pink). Scale bar: 50 μm (**D,E**) Additionally, some CD31^{-ve}/PAS^{+ve} vessel-like structures (pink) were identified. However, identifying these structures was often demanding due to the presence of necrotic areas or a faint CD31 signal (black arrows). Scale bar: 50 μm. (**F**) The double-labelled immunofluorescence assay was employed using a combination of CD31 and tumour cell marker (pan-cytokeratin, CK) to investigate the presence of mosaic vessels in HNSCC sections. (**G**) EC-lined blood vessels were easily distinguished in the peritumoral areas (dashed yellow line). Scale bar: 50 μm (**H**) The intratumoral CD31^{+ve}/CK^{+ve} mosaic vessels were also observed (dashed yellow line; white arrow). Scale bar: 50 μm.

(I) These mosaic lumens were either containing RBCs, metastasizing tumour cells or clear. Scale bar: 25 µm. (J) The multiplexed immunohistochemistry (mIHC) platform was used to identify VM (merged; inset) as well as to explore the phenotype of VM-forming tumour cells. A negative or weak staining of CD44 was observed in morphologically normal tissues (left), while a strong staining was detected in the VM-forming regions (right). By contrast, E-cadherin (E-Cad) staining was evident in normal and VM-free cancerous tissues (left, red), while it was faint around the mosaic vessels (right). The mIHC images were taken at a magnification of 63×.

3.2. The Mosaic VM Pattern Reveals Tumour Cell Plasticity

Recently, we showed that oral tongue squamous cell carcinoma (OTSCC) cells express considerable levels of the endothelial marker CD31 in vitro [21]. Due to the limited utility of the $CD31^{-ve}/PAS^{+ve}$ reaction in identifying VM in HNSCC tissues, we sought to explore the presence of intratumoral mosaic vessels using $CD31^{+ve}/CK^{+ve}$ double-labelled immunofluorescence (Figure 1F). Normal blood vessels were easily distinguished as CD31-expressing lumens mainly in the peritumoral stroma (Figure 1G). Interestingly, OTSCC patient samples revealed distinct and clear intratumoral $CD31^{+ve}/CK^{+ve}$ mosaic VM lumens, which also contain red blood cells (Figure 1H, arrow). It has been well reported that VM formation is associated with phenotype switching or "cell stemness" (i.e., tumour cell plasticity), which is mediated by certain events such as upregulation of CD44 and loss of epithelial cell markers including E-cadherin [22,23]. This observation prompted us to explore whether the mosaic vessels can also be harnessed to examine the status of these phenotype mediators. Importantly, using the mIHC platform, the mosaic $CD31^{+ve}/CK^{+ve}$ structures revealed an induced CD44-immunoreactivity, while E-cadherin staining was noticeably weaker around the mosaic vessels compared with tumoral VM-free regions (Figure 1I).

3.3. Metastatic HNSCC Cells Preferentially form VM in Matrigel

Previous pioneering studies have shown that cancer cells can form VM capillary networks similar to the endothelial tubulogenesis when cultured on a collagen-rich matrix [24]. However, there is very limited knowledge concerning the effect of the extracellular matrix (ECM) on such a phenomenon. Therefore, after identifying the VM structures in patient samples, we explored whether matrix origin and constituents can influence VM formation in vitro. To this end, 13 primary and metastatic HNSCC cell lines plus HUVEC were seeded on murine- and human-derived matrices at a density of 20×10^3 cells/well, as described previously [20]. Of note, all cell lines with high metastatic potential ($n = 3$) formed capillary networks in Matrigel but not in Myogel. By contrast, the primary cell lines showed a greater tendency to form VM in Myogel ($n = 4$) compared with Matrigel ($n = 2$; Figure 2A). Nevertheless, HUVEC formed consistent tubes in both matrices, suggesting that ECM could be an important modulator of the tumour cell-derived tubulogenesis. At this cell density, the tubes were, however, poorly networked and occupied less than half of the matrix area and were then scored (+) as illustrated in Table 1. Combining Myogel with collagen I or LMA did not noticeably alter VM formation.

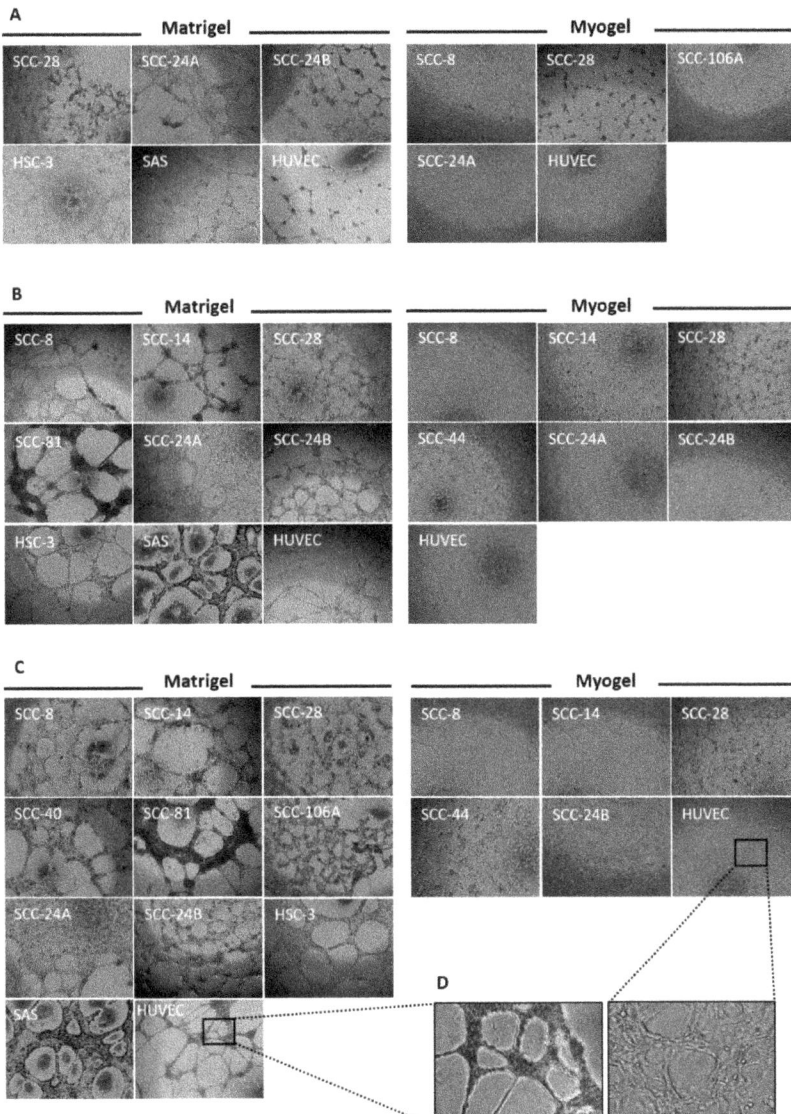

Figure 2. Assessment of tumour cell-derived tubulogenesis in vitro. (**A**) Thirteen cell lines derived from head and neck squamous cell carcinoma (HNSCC) and normal human endothelial cells (HUVEC) were seeded at a starting cell density of 20×10^3 cells on Matrigel or Myogel. All of the highly metastatic HNSCC cell lines (namely, SCC-24B, HSC-3, and SAS) formed a VM meshwork in Matrigel only, while more primary cell lines formed such tubes in Myogel ($n = 4$). HUVEC formed tubes in both matrices. (**B**) At a higher starting cell density of 40×10^3, all metastatic and some primary HNSCC cell lines ($n = 7$) developed longer and more interlaced VM meshwork in Matrigel. In Myogel, primary tumour cell lines ($n = 5$) continued to form VM structures with the most extensive meshwork attained by cells originating from the floor of the mouth and gingiva (SCC-28 and SCC-44, respectively). Additionally, the metastatic cell line (SCC-24B) started to initiate consistent tubes in Myogel that were more extensive than its primary counterpart (SCC-24A). (**C**) When the starting cell density reached 60×10^3, only metastatic and merely two primary cell lines continued to develop thicker and longer VM networks in Matrigel compared with four primary cell lines in Myogel. (**D**) The HUVEC meshwork has become shorter and more interlaced in Myogel. The images were taken at a magnification of $4\times$.

Table 1. Vascular mimicry-like network formation for head and neck squamous cell carcinoma and human endothelial cell lines in two different matrices.

	Matrigel			
Cell density [1]	SCC-8	SCC-14	SCC-28	SCC-40
A	-	-	+	-
B	++	++	++	-
C	++	+++	+++	++
	SCC-44	SCC-73	SCC-81	SCC-106A
A	-	-	-	-
B	-	-	++	-
C	-	-	++	++
	SCC-25	SCC-24A	SCC-24B	HSC-3
A	-	+	+	+
B	-	+	++	++
C	-	+	+++	+++
	SAS		HUVEC	
A	+		+	
B	++		++	
C	+++		+++	
	Myogel			
	SCC-8	SCC-14	SCC-28	SCC-40
A	+	-	+	-
B	+	+	++	-
C	+	+	+++	-
	SCC-44	SCC-73	SCC-81	SCC-106A
A	-	-	-	+
B	++	-	-	-
C	+++	-	-	-
	SCC-25	SCC-24A	SCC-24B	HSC-3
A	-	+	-	-
B	-	+	+	-
C	-	-	+	-
	SAS		HUVEC	
A	-		+	
B	-		++	
C	-		+++	

[1] Data from one representative experiment of at least three independent experiments are shown; starting cell density was as follows: **A** = 20×10^3; **B** = 40×10^3; **C** = 60×10^3 cells/well. Score description: (-) = no tube formation; (+) = poorly interconnected capillary networks that covered less than half of the matrix surface; (++) = cells formed well-defined interconnected capillary networks that covered not more than half of the matrix surface; (+++) = cells formed clear, well-defined interconnected capillary networks that covered more than half of the matrix surface. HUVEC: human umbilical vein endothelial cells.

3.4. Tumour Cell Density Influences VM Formation In Vitro

Tumour cell-derived tubulogenesis is an important assay not only for assessing VM formation but also for testing potential anti-angiogenic drugs in vitro [21]. It is therefore important to discern the optimal number of tumour cells needed to establish mature capillaries for HNSCC-related studies. For this purpose, HNSCC cell lines were seeded on Matrigel or Myogel using different starting cell densities of 20, 40, and 60×10^3 cells. Notably, all metastatic and some primary HNSCC cell lines ($n = 7$) formed longer and well-networked VM structures at 40×10^3 cells, which covered approximately half of the Matrigel (score ++; Figure 2B). Furthermore, only metastatic ($n = 3$) and merely two primary cell lines developed thicker and longer capillary networks when tumour cell density reached 60×10^3, which spread to more than half of the Matrigel (score +++; Figure 2C). In Myogel, primary tumour cell lines ($n = 5$) continued to form VM structures with the most extensive networks attained by cells originating from the floor of the mouth and gingiva (SCC-28, grade 1; SCC-44, grade 3, respectively; Figure 2B,C). Of interest, at higher cell densities, the metastatic cell line (SCC-24B) started to initiate consistent VM networks in Myogel that were more extensive than its primary counterpart (SCC-24A; Figure 2B,C). Moreover, the HUVEC meshwork has apparently become shorter and more interlaced in Myogel (Figure 2D). Two primary cell lines (SCC-73 and SCC-25) failed to form VM networks in either matrices, which remained dispersed in the matrices as round cell aggregates (Figure S1). The scores of VM formation using different cell densities and matrices are listed in Table 1.

Next, we used the Angiogenesis Analyser tool to assess the comparative capacity of various HNSCC cells in forming VM capillaries in vitro [25]. Angiogenic parameters including the number of junctions (branching capillary nodes), segments (capillaries delimited by two junctions), meshes (areas enclosed by segments), total meshes area (sum of mesh areas), total segments length (length sum of all segments), and total branching length were quantified. It is worth noting that the pre-irradiated SCC-28 cells formed unique "spiky" capillaries that spread evenly on Matrigel, regardless of their cell density (Figure 3A). Overall, starting cell densities of 40 and 60×10^3 cells were both adequate for initiating proper tubulogenesis in vitro; however, the latter density produced more looping meshwork in most cell lines (Figure 3A,B).

3.5. In Vitro VM Networks Reveal Different Morphological Patterns

Interestingly, tumour cells from different head and neck regions formed varying morphological patterns of VM networks in their respective matrix. While metastatic OTSCC cell lines (e.g., HSC-3 and SCC-24B) had the typical "honeycomb-like" pattern, the larynx-derived primary cell line (SCC-8) attained thinner and somewhat smoother capillary extensions (Figure 4A). On the other hand, cells derived from the floor of the mouth (i.e., SCC-28) formed peculiar capillary networks with thick "spike-like" projections in the two matrices (Figure 4A).

3.6. In Vitro VM Networks Express Endothelial Cell Marker

Having determined the optimal cell density to establish VM in 3D matrices, we next sought further in vitro verification that HNSCC cells, rather than endothelial cells, were responsible for the observed mosaic pattern in the clinical samples. Hence, tumour cell-derived VM networks on phenol red-free Matrigel were stained with the endothelial cell marker CD31. To unambiguously localize CD31 in relation to tumour cell junctions, VM capillaries were also labelled with Phalloidin–Alexa-594 to stain F-actin networks. Interestingly, tumour cell-derived VM capillaries clearly expressed CD31, which was mostly localized in the tubular extensions and around the capillary junctions (Figure 4B).

3.7. Larval Zebrafish as a Novel In Vivo Model for VM Formation

Testing VM formation in vivo is currently conducted in patient-derived murine xenografts [24]. However, such models can present substantial challenges, including time consumption and cost and labour intensiveness. Therefore, we assessed the utility of zebrafish larvae as a simple and yet efficient approach to optically screening the formation of VM structures in vivo. Fluorescently labelled aggressive tumour cells (HSC-3) were resuspended in their respective matrix and microinjected into the perivitelline space of anaesthetized zebrafish (Figure 5A). Using confocal microscopy at 72 h post-injection, the xenografted tumour cells displayed VM-like structures in some of the fish (n = 3) belonging to the Matrigel-injected group, which attained singular or multi-tubular pattern (Figure 5B,C). By contrast, no similar structures were observed in the Myogel-injected group (Figure 5D).

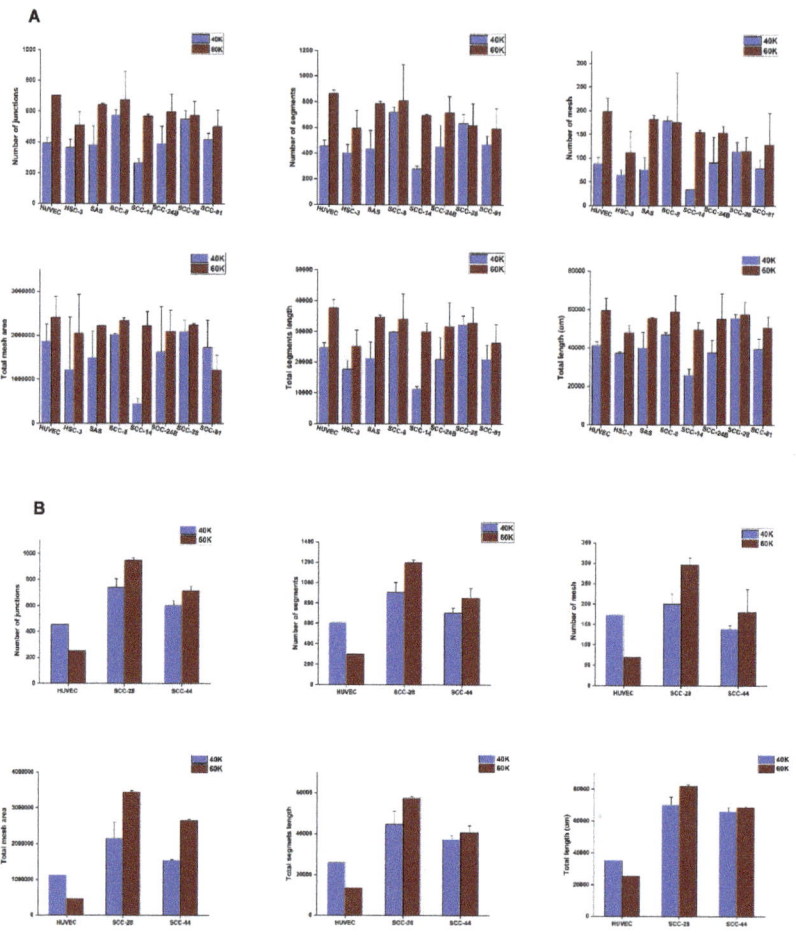

Figure 3. In vitro tube formation analysis of tumour cell-derived vascular mimicry (VM). (**A**) The Angiogenesis Analyser plugin was used to discern the optimal starting cell density needed to establish VM meshwork in vitro. Different tube formation parameters were analysed, including the number of junctions, segments, meshes, total mesh area, total segment length, and total branching lengths of the tubular networks. A starting cell density of 60×10^3 produced consistent mature looping patterns in Matrigel for almost all the included cell lines. However, overall, the analysis shows that both 40 and 60×10^3 concentrations are sufficient to initiate VM structures in vitro. (**B**) The results were comparable in Myogel, with better tubes formed with a starting cell density of 60×10^3. However, at such a higher density, HUVEC meshwork became more extensively interlaced in Myogel, which limited the analyser's capacity to recognize smaller tubular areas as shown in the figure. Data from one representative experiment, presented as mean ± SD of three technical replicates, are shown.

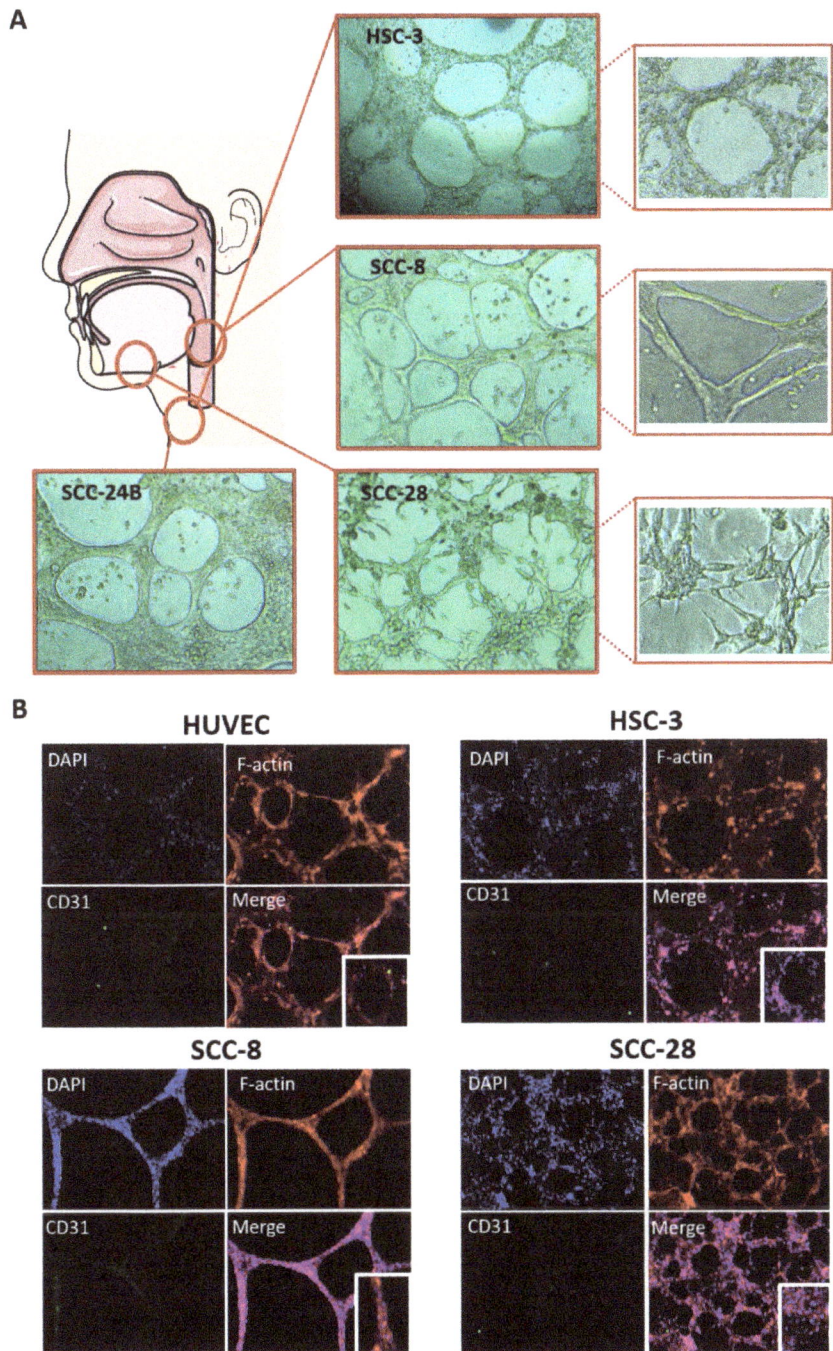

Figure 4. (**A**) Tumour cells show distinct morphological patterns of tubulogenesis in vitro. The highly metastatic tongue cancer cell lines (HSC-3 and SCC-24B) formed the classical "honeycomb-like" looping pattern, while the larynx-derived cell line (SCC-8) attained thinner branches with smoother capillaries. Evidently, cells from the floor of the mouth (SCC-28)

formed peculiar and "spike-like" networks, on both Matrigel and Myogel, that were morphologically different from any other cell line. (**B**) In vitro tumour cell-derived tubulogenesis showed substantial resemblance to the endothelial ones. These cell networks expressed the endothelial cell marker CD31, which was primarily localized in the capillary extensions and junctions. The images were taken at magnifications of 10× and 20×.

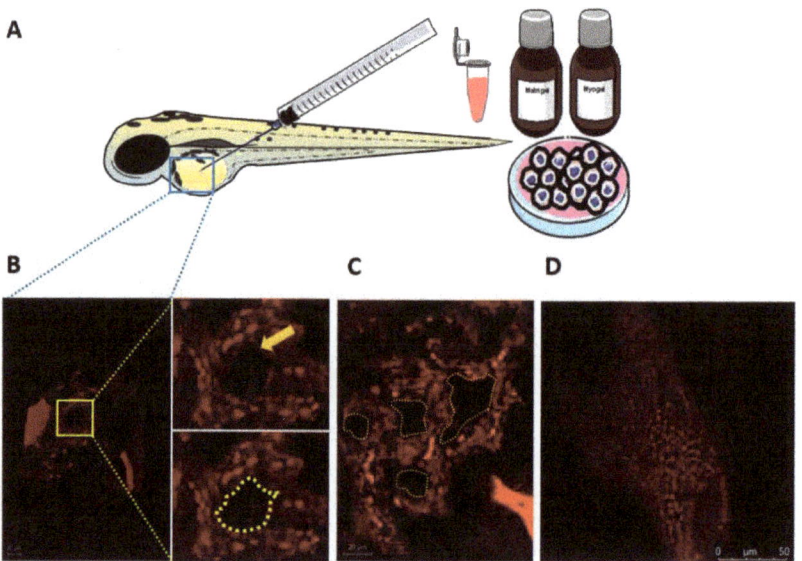

Figure 5. Larval zebrafish model to evaluate vascular mimicry (VM) formation in vitro. (**A**) Fluorescently labelled highly metastatic tumour cells (HSC-3) were resuspended in Matrigel or Myogel and microinjected into the perivitelline space of 2-day-old zebrafish larvae. Fish were screened 27 h post-injection using confocal microscopy. (**B,C**) HSC-3 cells formed seemingly VM-like structures in the Matrigel-injected fish. (**D**) No similar tube formation was detected in Myogel-containing fish, supporting a similar outcome from the in vitro assays. Scale bars: 20 and 50 µm.

4. Discussion

The VM has been well documented in a variety of cancers and is associated with a stem-like cell phenotype, aggressive disease course, and dismal survival outcomes [9,10,13,26]. However, the currently available approaches to identify VM in HNSCC are rather limited, thereby necessitating more research on this intriguing phenomenon [7,8]. In this study, we first revealed some challenges associated with identifying VM in HNSCC sections, wherein the mosaic vessels could be adopted to further assess the phenotype of VM-forming cells. Next, we reported the impact of ECM origin, tumour cell type, and density on the formation and morphology of HNSCC cell-derived tubulogenesis. We then delineated the optimal cell numbers needed to obtain such tubular meshwork in vitro, which also expressed the specific endothelial cell marker—CD31. Finally, we proposed for the first time a simple animal model, the zebrafish larvae, for assessing the development of VM in vivo.

Histologically, VM structures are often identified in cancer patients as PAS^{+ve}, RBC-containing, lumen-like structures combined with a negative staining of an endothelial cell marker [14]. However, PAS stains various ECM components including collagens, laminin, and proteoglycans and hence may not always represent the vascular mimetic structures. Using an X-ray microtomography 3D reconstruction, Racordon et al. showed that many PAS^{+ve} areas do not display actual lumens in vitro and may instead represent glycoprotein-rich regions [16]. It has therefore been recommended to be attentive when scoring PAS^{+ve} areas to differentiate VM from non-specific ECM aggregates [7,14]. Furthermore, a strong

PAS staining may conceal the expression of endothelial cell markers, making it challenging to discern CD31^{-ve}/ PAS^{+ve} patterns. In a different approach, several reports described the existence of "mosaic" vessels expressing both tumour and endothelial cell markers in cancer tissues, emphasizing the importance of tumour cell plasticity in VM formation [6,27–29]. Initially, these vessels were thought to result from endothelial and tumour cell merging in blood vessel walls. However, it was later shown that tumour cells are able to form and maintain blood vessels by expressing neuropilin-2, EphA2, and laminin-15γ2 [28]. An interesting study revealed that 20–90% of the vascular endothelium in glioblastoma was derived from VM-forming tumour cells in mice; their selective targeting resulted in tumour reduction and degeneration [26]. Supporting these findings, Kim et al. found that the intratumoral VM channels were derived from CD31^{+ve}/CD34^{+ve} gastric tumour cells [30]. Furthermore, we recently showed, by fluorescence-activated cell sorting, that 90% of the HSC-3 cells were CD31^{+ve}, compared with 96% of HUVEC [21]. In this study, we manifested this expression phenotypically by showing that tumour cell-derived tubes are CD31^{+ve} with a striking resemblance to the endothelial ones. These findings suggest that intratumoral mosaic vessels may represent an additional staining approach to identifying patterned VM structures in cancer tissues.

Using the mIHC platform, the adhesion molecule CD44—a transmembrane glycoprotein receptor known to promote tumour cell plasticity—and VM were induced around the mosaic VM-forming cells [31]. A tumour cell plasticity is best seen in crucial metastatic processes such as epithelial mesenchymal transition, wherein tumour cells lose their adhesion, polarity, and epithelial cell markers including E-cadherin [32]. It is therefore interesting that mosaic VM-forming regions revealed a faint expression of E-cadherin compared with other epithelial regions. Our results advocate the use of mIHC for the simultaneous assessment of different markers associated with the development of VM.

Previous seminal works on VM have shown that aggressive cancer cells can form tubular networks when seeded on Matrigel. However, it is worth noting that considerable variations exist among different matrices based on their origin, composition, and consistency. Our findings suggest that tumour cell-derived tubulogenesis could be influenced, in part, by the matrix type. Although it is not yet clear why tumour cells have a matrix-specific ability to form VM, variations in ECM features may underpin this interesting observation. For instance, the protein composition of Myogel is substantially different from other EHS-based matrices. Further, crucial carcinogenesis-related properties, such as tumour cell invasion and response to HNSCC-targeted therapy, were more efficiently represented in Myogel than in Matrigel [18,33]. A fascinating observation is that a primary cell line (SCC-24A) formed merely a few tubes compared with an extensively interlaced network formed by its metastatic counterpart (SCC-24B), albeit both were established from the same patient. This confirms previous studies showing that VM is associated with metastatic and highly aggressive tumours. Additionally, we infer that VM competence can differ even within the same patient, signifying the need for more precise targeting of anti-angiogenic therapies. The spike-like pattern formed by tumour cells from the floor of the mouth is another intriguing observation. Interestingly, this particular cell line (SCC-28) was established from a tumour that was treated with radiotherapy prior to surgical resection. In this context, there is abundant evidence that ionizing radiation targeting cancer cells may enhance their metastatic process [34]. Additionally, the floor of the mouth is the most high-risk site for metastasis in oral cancer patients. Thus, it has been recommended that patients with SCC in this site should be offered an elective neck dissection even at early stages of the disease [35]. We encourage further research to investigate whether this peculiar tubular morphology plays a role in the metastatic potential of HNSCC and whether radiation therapy could impact VM formation. Consistent with previous data, endothelial cells formed shorter and much interlaced networks in Myogel [18].

Cancer cell-derived tubulogenesis is a valuable assay not only to evaluate VM formation in vitro but also for testing potential anti-angiogenic therapeutic approaches in HNSCC [21]. Therefore, we presented an easy standardized protocol to establish mature capillary networks using a good number and a variety of HNSCC cell lines. Previous studies reported similar approaches to estimating such an optimal tumour cell number, for instance, in human ovarian cancer cell lines [16]. In this study, authors provided solid evidence that VM tubes in vitro represent in most cases functional hollow channels. Additionally, 15 and 75×10^3 starting numbers of the ovarian cancer cells produced clear tubular formation on day 4 of the experiment. In another protocol, Francescone et al. suggested a starting density of $10 - 20 \times 10^3$ cells using melanoma, glioblastoma, and breast cancer cell lines [20]. In the present HNSCC cell lines, comparable starting cell densities (20, 40, and 60×10^3 cells) were used to obtain VM channels within 24 h in culture, confirming that this phenomenon could vary based on the tumour cell type.

Zebrafish larvae have recently emerged as a popular in vivo model of HNSCC to mimic key tumorigenic events such as metastasis [36]. Indeed, zebrafish provides many advantages over other animal models considering its efficiency, feasibility, and cost- and labour-effectiveness [37]. Currently, most in vivo model systems of VM are conducted in murine xenografts. However, in addition to cost and labour challenges, screening of VM in these models can be made only post-mortem, restricting further follow-up studies [24]. Thus, we proposed the use of zebrafish larvae as a simple and cost-effective in vivo model of VM. Although VM-like structures were observed in some xenografts, their formation should be interpreted with caution as there is no evidence indicating that they represent actual lumens. In addition, it is not clear why these structures were not formed in all xenografts. Such disparity in the formation of in vivo mimetic vessels has been nonetheless observed in murine xenografts [36]. However, several technical limitations may arise when using the larval zebrafish model. Firstly, there is a possibility of tumour cell leakage out of the fish due to poor resealing of the yolk sac membrane. Secondly, their smaller body size restricts the number of microinjected cells and the resulting tumour size compared with larger animal models. Finally, larval assays are performed at 34 °C, which may not be suitable for some cell lines and hence fail to form proper tumour colonies [38]. Further studies would be paramount to optimizing this model and testing its feasibility for real-time imaging as well as for therapeutic and functional assays.

5. Conclusions

In conclusion, our study provides a comprehensive comparative analysis of VM in HNSCC using a variety of experimental approaches. We, however, acknowledge some limitations, including the lack of perfusion assays to assess the functionality of the tubular networks, which has already been revealed in previous reports. Overall, our findings could offer a valuable resource for designing future studies that may facilitate the therapeutic exploitation of VM in HNSCC as well as in other recalcitrant tumours.

Supplementary Materials: The following are available online at https://www.mdpi.com/article/10.3390/cancers13194747/s1: Figure S1: Two primary cell lines (SCC-73 and SCC-25) were not able to initiate own tubulogenesis in either Matrigel or Myogel, where they remained dispersed as round cell aggregates (A, 40×10^3 cells; B, 60×10^3 cells); Table S1: Patient-derived cell lines and their corresponding data.

Author Contributions: Conceptualization, T.S. and A.S.; methodology, R.H., R.A. and A.S.; software, R.H. and R.A.; validation, R.H., R.A., T.S. and A.S.; formal analysis, R.H., R.A., T.S. and A.S.; investigation, R.H., R.A. and A.S.; resources, T.S. and A.S.; data curation, R.H. and R.A.; writing—original draft preparation, R.H.; writing—review and editing, A.S.; visualization, R.H. and A.S.; supervision, T.S. and A.S.; project administration, T.S. and A.S.; funding acquisition, T.S. and A.S. All authors have read and agreed to the published version of the manuscript.

Funding: This research was funded by the Jane and Aatos Erkko Foundation; the Minerva Foundation Institute for Medical Research; Cancer Society of Finland; Sigrid Jusélius Foundation; Helsinki University Central Hospital research funds; and an Oulu University Hospital MRC grant.

Institutional Review Board Statement: The study was conducted according to the guidelines of the Declaration of Helsinki and approved by the Ethics Committee of the National Supervisory

Authority for Welfare and Health (VALVIRA) and the Northern Ostrobothnia Hospital District. The preparation and usage of human leiomyoma tissue has been approved by the Ethics Committee of Oulu University Hospital (no. 35/2014; 28.4.2014). Zebrafish procedures were approved by the ethical committee of the regional state administrative agency (license ESAVI/13139/04.10.05/2017).

Informed Consent Statement: The patient sections in this study were obtained a long time ago (1990–2010), and no consent forms were possible to obtain in this case. Therefore, the Finnish National Supervisory Authority for Welfare and Health (VALVIRA) has approved the use and publishing these patient materials. In addition, we confirm that there is NO use of any "identifying" personal information or images of the patients in our article.

Data Availability Statement: The datasets used in this study are available from the corresponding author upon a reasonable request.

Acknowledgments: The authors would like to thank Antti Isomäki (Biomedicum Imaging Unit, University of Helsinki) for his kind assistance with confocal microscopy imaging and Wafa Wahbi for helpful discussions on the zebrafish assays. Multiplexed immunohistochemistry was performed in the Digital Microscopy and Molecular Pathology Unit (FIMM Institute, University of Helsinki). Zebrafish experiments were performed in the zebrafish core facility at the University of Helsinki. Open access funding provided by University of Helsinki.

Conflicts of Interest: The authors declare no conflict of interest.

References

1. Marur, S.; Forastiere, A.A. Head and Neck Squamous Cell Carcinoma: Update on Epidemiology, Diagnosis, and Treatment. *Mayo Clin. Proc.* **2016**, *91*, 386–396. [CrossRef]
2. Sung, H.; Ferlay, J.; Siegel, R.L.; Laversanne, M.; Soerjomataram, I.; Jemal, A.; Bray, F. Global cancer statistics 2020: GLOBOCAN estimates of incidence and mortality worldwide for 36 cancers in 185 countries. *CA Cancer, J. Clin.* **2021**, *71*, 209–249. [CrossRef]
3. Pisani, P.; Airoldi, M.; Allais, A.; Aluffi Valletti, P.; Battista, M.; Benazzo, M.; Briatore, R.; Cacciola, S.; Cocuzza, S.; Colombo, A.; et al. Metastatic disease in head & neck oncology. *Acta Otorhinolaryngol. Ital.* **2020**, *40*, S1–S86. [CrossRef]
4. Ferlito, A.; Shaha, A.R.; Silver, C.E.; Rinaldo, A.; Mondin, V. Incidence and sites of distant metastases from head and neck cancer. *ORL J. Otorhinolaryngol. Relat. Spec.* **2001**, *63*, 202–207. [CrossRef] [PubMed]
5. Maniotis, A.J.; Folberg, R.; Hess, A.; Seftor, E.A.; Gardner, L.M.; Pe'er, J.; Trent, J.M.; Meltzer, P.S.; Hendrix, M.J. Vascular channel formation by human melanoma cells in vivo and in vitro: Vasculogenic mimicry. *Am. J. Pathol.* **1999**, *155*, 739–752. [CrossRef]
6. Hendrix, M.J.C.; Seftor, E.A.; Hess, A.R.; Seftor, R.E.B. Vasculogenic mimicry and tumour-cell plasticity: Lessons from melanoma. *Nat. Rev. Cancer* **2003**, *3*, 411–421. [CrossRef]
7. Salem, A.; Salo, T. Vasculogenic Mimicry in Head and Neck Squamous Cell Carcinoma—Time to Take Notice. *Front. Oral. Health* **2021**, *2*, 666895. [CrossRef]
8. Hujanen, R.; Almahmoudi, R.; Karinen, S.; Nwaru, B.I.; Salo, T.; Salem, A. Vasculogenic Mimicry: A Promising Prognosticator in Head and Neck Squamous Cell Carcinoma and Esophageal Cancer? A Systematic Review and Meta-Analysis. *Cells* **2020**, *9*, 507. [CrossRef] [PubMed]
9. Hendrix, M.J.; Seftor, E.A.; Seftor, R.E.; Chao, J.T.; Chien, D.S.; Chu, Y.W. Tumor cell vascular mimicry: Novel targeting opportunity in melanoma. *Pharmacol. Ther.* **2016**, *159*, 83–92. [CrossRef] [PubMed]
10. Wagenblast, E.; Soto, M.; Gutiérrez-Ángel, S.; Hartl, C.A.; Gable, A.L.; Maceli, A.R.; Erard, N.; Williams, A.M.; Kim, S.Y.; Dickopf, S.; et al. A model of breast cancer heterogeneity reveals vascular mimicry as a driver of metastasis. *Nature* **2015**, *520*, 358–362. [CrossRef]
11. Ren, H.Y.; Shen, J.X.; Mao, X.M.; Zhang, X.Y.; Zhou, P.; Li, S.Y.; Zheng, Z.W.; Shen, D.Y.; Meng, J.R. Correlation Between Tumor Vasculogenic Mimicry and Poor Prognosis of Human Digestive Cancer Patients: A Systematic Review and Meta-Analysis. *Pathol. Oncol. Res.* **2019**, *25*, 849–858. [CrossRef] [PubMed]
12. Zhang, X.; Zhang, J.; Zhou, H.; Fan, G.; Li, Q. Molecular Mechanisms and Anticancer Therapeutic Strategies in Vasculogenic Mimicry. *J. Cancer* **2019**, *18*, 6327–6340. [CrossRef] [PubMed]
13. Yang, J.P.; Liao, Y.D.; Mai, D.M.; Xie, P.; Qiang, Y.Y.; Zheng, L.S.; Wang, M.Y.; Mei, Y.; Meng, D.F.; Xu, L.; et al. Tumor vasculogenic mimicry predicts poor prognosis in cancer patients: A meta-analysis. *Angiogenesis* **2016**, *19*, 191–200. [CrossRef] [PubMed]
14. Valdivia, A.; Mingo, G.; Aldana, V.; Pinto, M.P.; Ramirez, M.; Retamal, C.; Gonzalez, A.; Nualart, F.; Corvalan, A.H.; Owen, G.I. Fact or Fiction, It Is Time for a Verdict on Vasculogenic Mimicry? *Front. Oncol.* **2019**, *2*, 680. [CrossRef]
15. Ayala-Domínguez, L.; Olmedo-Nieva, L.; Muñoz-Bello, J.O.; Contreras-Paredes, A.; Manzo-Merino, J.; Martínez-Ramírez, I.; Lizano, M. Mechanisms of Vasculogenic Mimicry in Ovarian Cancer. *Front. Oncol.* **2019**, *27*, 998. [CrossRef]
16. Racordon, D.; Valdivia, A.; Mingo, G.; Erices, R.; Aravena, R.; Santoro, F. Structural and functional identification of vasculogenic mimicry in vitro. *Sci. Rep.* **2017**, *7*, 6985. [CrossRef]

17. Blom, S.; Paavolainen, L.; Bychkov, D.; Turkki, R.; Mäki-Teeri, P.; Hemmes, A.; Välimäki, K.; Lundin, J.; Kallioniemi, O.; Pellinen, T. Systems pathology by multiplexed immunohistochemistry and whole-slide digital image analysis. *Sci. Rep.* **2017**, *14*, 15580. [CrossRef]
18. Salo, T.; Sutinen, M.; Hoque Apu, E.; Sundquist, E.; Cervigne, N.K.; de Oliveira, C.E. A novel human leiomyoma tissue derived matrix for cell culture studies. *BMC Cancer* **2015**, *16*, 981. [CrossRef]
19. Salo, T.; Dourado, M.R.; Sundquist, E.; Apu, E.H.; Alahuhta, I.; Tuomainen, K.; Vasara, J.; Al-Samadi, A. Organotypic three-dimensional assays based on human leiomyoma-derived matrices. *Philos. Trans. R. Soc. Lond. B Biol. Sci.* **2018**, *5*, 20160482. [CrossRef]
20. Francescone, R.A.3rd; Faibish, M.; Shao, R. A Matrigel-based tube formation assay to assess the vasculogenic activity of tumor cells. *J. Vis. Exp.* **2011**, *7*, 3040. [CrossRef]
21. Almahmoudi, R.; Salem, A.; Hadler-Olsen, E.; Svineng, G.; Salo, T.; Al-Samadi, A. The effect of interleukin-17F on vasculogenic mimicry in oral tongue squamous cell carcinoma. *Cancer Sci.* **2021**, *112*, 2223–2232. [CrossRef] [PubMed]
22. Chen, L.; Fu, C.; Zhang, Q.; He, C.; Zhang, F.; Wei, Q. The role of CD44 in pathological angiogenesis. *FASEB J.* **2020**, *34*, 13125–13139. [CrossRef]
23. Luo, Q.; Wang, J.; Zhao, W.; Peng, Z.; Liu, X.; Li, B.; Zhang, H.; Shan, B.; Zhang, C.; Duan, C. Vasculogenic mimicry in carcinogenesis and clinical applications. *J. Hematol. Oncol.* **2020**, *14*, 19. [CrossRef] [PubMed]
24. Wechman, S.L.; Emdad, L.; Sarkar, D.; Das, S.K.; Fisher, P.B. Vascular mimicry: Triggers, molecular interactions and in vivo models. *Adv. Cancer Res.* **2020**, *148*, 27–67. [CrossRef] [PubMed]
25. Carpentier, G.; Berndt, S.; Ferratge, S.; Rasband, W.; Cuendet, M.; Uzan, G.; Albanese, P. Angiogenesis Analyzer for ImageJ —A comparative morphometric analysis of "Endothelial Tube Formation Assay" and "Fibrin Bead Assay". *Sci. Rep.* **2020**, *14*, 11568. [CrossRef]
26. Ricci-Vitiani, L.; Pallini, R.; Biffoni, M.; Todaro, M.; Invernici, G.; Cenci, T.; Maira, G.; Parati, E.A.; Stassi, G.; Larocca, L.M.; et al. Tumour vascularization via endothelial differentiation of glioblastoma stem-like cells. *Nature* **2010**, *9*, 468, 824–828. [CrossRef]
27. Chang, Y.S.; di Tomaso, E.; McDonald, D.M.; Jones, R.; Jain, R.K.; Munn, L.L. Mosaic blood vessels in tumors: Frequency of cancer cells in contact with flowing blood. *Proc. Natl. Acad. Sci. USA* **2000**, *19*, 14608–14613. [CrossRef]
28. El Hallani, S.; Boisselier, B.; Peglion, F.; Rousseau, A.; Colin, C.; Idbaih, A. A new alternative mechanism in glioblastoma vascularization: Tubular vasculogenic mimicry. *Brain* **2010**, *133*, 973–982. [CrossRef]
29. Tong, M.; Han, B.B.; Holpuch, A.S.; Pei, P.; He, L.; Mallery, S.R. Inherent phenotypic plasticity facilitates progression of head and neck cancer: Endotheliod characteristics enable angiogenesis and invasion. *Exp. Cell Res.* **2013**, *319*, 1028–1042. [CrossRef]
30. Kim, H.S.; Won, Y.J.; Shim, J.H.; Kim, H.J.; Kim, J.; Hong, H.N.; Kim, B.S. Morphological characteristics of vasculogenic mimicry and its correlation with EphA2 expression in gastric adenocarcinoma. *Sci. Rep.* **2019**, *49*, 3414. [CrossRef]
31. Paulis, Y.W.; Huijbers, E.J.; van der Schaft, D.W.; Soetekouw, P.M.; Pauwels, P.; Tjan-Heijnen, V.C.; Griffioen, A.W. CD44 enhances tumor aggressiveness by promoting tumor cell plasticity. *Oncotarget* **2015**, *14*, 19634–19646. [CrossRef]
32. Chin, V.L.; Lim, C.L. Epithelial-mesenchymal plasticity-engaging stemness in an interplay of phenotypes. *Stem. Cell Investig.* **2019**, *6*, 25. [CrossRef] [PubMed]
33. Tuomainen, K.; Al-Samadi, A.; Potdar, S.; Turunen, L.; Turunen, M.; Karhemo, P.R. Human Tumor-Derived Matrix Improves the Predictability of Head and Neck Cancer Drug Testing. *Cancers* **2019**, *12*, 92. [CrossRef] [PubMed]
34. Sundahl, N.; Duprez, F.; Ost, P.; De Neve, W.; Mareel, M. Effects of radiation on the metastatic process. *Mol. Med.* **2018**, *24*, 16. [CrossRef]
35. Montero, P.H.; Patel, S.G. Cancer of the oral cavity. *Surg. Oncol. Clin. N. Am.* **2015**, *24*, 491–508. [CrossRef]
36. Karinen, S.; Juurikka, K.; Hujanen, R.; Wahbi, W.; Hadler-Olsen, E.; Svineng, G.; Eklund, K.K.; Salo, T.; Åström, P.; Salem, A. Tumour cells express functional lymphatic endothelium-specific hyaluronan receptor in vitro and in vivo: Lymphatic mimicry promotes oral oncogenesis? *Oncogenesis* **2021**, *10*, 23. [CrossRef] [PubMed]
37. Zhao, S.; Huang, J.; Ye, J. A fresh look at zebrafish from the perspective of cancer research. *J. Exp. Clin. Cancer Res.* **2015**, *34*, 80. [CrossRef] [PubMed]
38. Fazio, M.; Ablain, J.; Chuan, Y.; Langenau, D.M.; Zon, L.I. Zebrafish patient avatars in cancer biology and precision cancer therapy. *Nat. Rev. Cancer* **2020**, *20*, 263–273. [CrossRef]

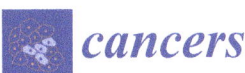

Article

Sleep Disorders and Psychological Profile in Oral Cancer Survivors: A Case-Control Clinical Study

Roberta Gasparro [1], Elena Calabria [1,*], Noemi Coppola [1], Gaetano Marenzi [1], Gilberto Sammartino [1], Massimo Aria [2], Michele Davide Mignogna [1,†] and Daniela Adamo [1,†]

[1] Department of Neurosciences, Reproductive Science and Dentistry, Federico II University of Naples, Via Pansini 5, 80138 Naples, Italy; roberta.gasparro@unina.it (R.G.); noemi.coppola@unina.it (N.C.); gaetano.marenzi@unina.it (G.M.); gilberto.sammartino@unina.it (G.S.); mignogna@unina.it (M.D.M.); danielaadamo.it@gmail.com (D.A.)
[2] Department of Economics and Statistics, Federico II University of Naples, Via Cinthia, Monte Sant'Angelo, 80126 Naples, Italy; aria@unina.it
* Correspondence: calabriaelena92@gmail.com
† These two authors equally contributed to the manuscript and need to be considered as last authors.

Simple Summary: Sleep disorders have been increasingly investigated in several medical illnesses as their presence may affect patients' quality of life. However, the research examining sleep disorders in oral cancer is relatively weak. Indeed, the majority of the available studies present a cross-sectional or retrospective designs. Moreover, very few of them have evaluated quality of sleep in oral cancer survivors (OC survivors). We aimed to carry out a case-control study with the purpose to investigate sleep disorders and mood impairment in 50 OC survivors. Our research has shown that quality of sleep is significantly affected in OC survivors compared to a healthy population and that OC survivors suffers from higher levels of anxiety and depression. Our results may suggest that an appropriate assessment of quality of sleep and psychological profile should be performed in OC survivors as a prompt treatment for both sleep and mood disorders is crucial for the overall improvement of patients' quality of life.

Abstract: Quality of sleep (QoS) and mood may impair oral cancer survivors' wellbeing, however few evidences are currently available. Therefore, we aimed to assess the prevalence of sleep disorders, anxiety and depression among five-year oral cancer survivors (OC survivors). 50 OC survivors were compared with 50 healthy subjects matched for age and sex. The Pittsburgh Sleep Quality Index (PSQI), the Epworth Sleepiness Scale (ESS), the Hamilton Rating Scales for Depression and Anxiety (HAM-D, HAM-A), the Numeric Rating Scale (NRS), the Total Pain Rating Index (T-PRI) were administered. The global score of the PSQI, ESS, HAM-A, HAM-D, NRS, T-PRI, was statistically higher in the OC survivors than the controls (p-value: <0.001). QoS of OC survivors was significantly impaired, especially with regard to some PSQI sub-items as the subjective sleep quality, sleep latency and daytime dysfunction (p-value: 0.001, 0.029, 0.004). Moreover, poor QoS was negatively correlated with years of education (p-value: 0.042 *) and positively correlated with alcohol consumption (p-value: 0.049 *) and with the use of systemic medications (p-value: 0.044 *). Sleep disorders and mood disorders are common comorbidities in OC survivors; therefore, early assessment and management before, during and after treatment should be performed in order to improve the quality of life of OC survivors.

Keywords: oral cancer; sleep disturbance; depression; anxiety; insomnia; oral cancer survivors; psychiatric profile

Citation: Gasparro, R.; Calabria, E.; Coppola, N.; Marenzi, G.; Sammartino, G.; Aria, M.; Mignogna, M.D.; Adamo, D. Sleep Disorders and Psychological Profile in Oral Cancer Survivors: A Case-Control Clinical Study. *Cancers* **2021**, *13*, 1855. https://doi.org/10.3390/cancers13081855

Academic Editors: Carlo Lajolo, Gaetano Paludetti and Romeo Patini

Received: 8 March 2021
Accepted: 8 April 2021
Published: 13 April 2021

Publisher's Note: MDPI stays neutral with regard to jurisdictional claims in published maps and institutional affiliations.

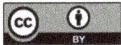

Copyright: © 2021 by the authors. Licensee MDPI, Basel, Switzerland. This article is an open access article distributed under the terms and conditions of the Creative Commons Attribution (CC BY) license (https://creativecommons.org/licenses/by/4.0/).

1. Introduction

Oral cancer is a life-threatening disease and a burden for health care systems worldwide. According to Global Cancer Statistics, GLOBOCAN, there were 354,864 new cases of oral cavity cancer causing 177,384 deaths during 2018 [1]. Despite the improvement in diagnosis and treatment by health care providers with a subsequent decrease in mortality, the quality of life of oral cancer survivors (OC survivors) remains poor on account of the impact of this disease on mental and emotional well-being. Indeed, oral cancer patients often suffer from emotional distress, fatigue, sleep disturbance, anxiety and depression that can arise during treatment and persist long-term, aggravating the burden of the disease [2,3].

Recently, a growing interest has been focused on the evaluation of sleep disorders in relation to several medical illnesses as their presence may worsen the underlying disease and increase the rate of mortality [4]. Furthermore, sleep disorders are considered to be an extremely sensitive marker for psychiatric comorbidities which may also precede mood disorders, especially depression or anxiety, and its early detection and treatment is crucial to improve the prognosis and quality of life of patients.

Insomnia is the most frequent sleep disorder; generally, patients report a difficulty in falling asleep, and often experience restless sleep and excessive daytime sleepiness (hypersomnolence) [5].

The overall incidence of insomnia in cancer patients has been found to be three times higher than that reported in the general population and ranges from 30.0% to 93.1%, depending on the type of cancer [6,7].

This high incidence is probably related to a post-diagnosis experience marked by a series of stressors that can act as a trigger for insomnia and, if they persist, may contribute to a chronic development causing long-lasting sleep disturbance even after the cancer treatment ends.

In a recent systematic review, the prevalence of insomnia in oral cancer patients was 29.0% before, 45% during and 40% after the treatment while hypersomnolence was reported by 16% and 32% of patients before and after the treatment, respectively [8].

The persistence of sleep disorders such as insomnia and hypersomnolence may negatively affect the quality of life of OC survivors and has a powerful influence on the increased risk of infectious disease, and on the occurrence and progression of several major medical illnesses including cardiovascular diseases and mood disorders [9]. Sleep disorders activate biological mechanisms, such as inflammation which are increasingly thought to contribute to depression, and potentially increase the risk of cancer morbidity and related mortality [10]. Indeed, sleep duration has been closely related to a poor overall survival and cancer-specific death over a ten-year follow-up period [11].

In contrast to the substantial literature on depression, research examining sleep disorders in oral cancer is relatively weak, with the majority of studies using a cross-sectional or retrospective analysis. In addition, most of the studies have evaluated the prevalence of sleep disorders before the start or during the treatment while very few studies have included OC survivors in follow-up. Moreover, the role of predictors in sleep disorders remains unclear.

Therefore, we have designed a case-control study to better evaluate the difference in the prevalence of sleep disorders between OC survivors and healthy subjects. The purposes of this study were: (1) to investigate the prevalence of sleep disorders (insomnia and daytime sleepiness), pain, anxiety and depression among OC survivor patients, (2) and to evaluate the potential predictors of sleep disorders such as socio-demographic data, habits, body mass index (BMI), pain, anxiety, depression, medical comorbidities and drug intake and the staging and grading of the oral cancer.

2. Material and Methods

2.1. Study Design and Participants

A case-control study was carried out at the Oral Medicine Department of Federico II University of Naples in accordance with the ethical principles of the World Medical Association Declaration of Helsinki. The study was approved by the Research Ethics Committee (protocol number 188: 2014). The methods adopted conformed with the Strengthening the

Reporting of Observational Studies in Epidemiology (STROBE) guidelines for observational studies (Figure S1) [12].

The recruitment of OC survivors and healthy subjects was conducted between January and September 2018 and was based upon convenience sampling. All potentially eligible individuals were invited to participate in the present study and provided their written informed consent.

The case and the control groups were matched by age and gender. Specifically, first we recruited the patients and then calculated the gender distribution and the average age; secondly, we recruited the controls to obtain a matched sample.

Participants of either gender and aged 18 or older were included. The inclusion criteria for the OC survivors' group were: (i) clinical and histopathological findings of oral squamous cell carcinoma (OSCC) or tobacco-related verrucous cell carcinoma (VCC) (ii) patients with a follow-up of at least five years after the diagnosis of OSCC or VCC and being free from malignancy for at least one year, (iii) all stages based on the American Joint Committee on Cancer Staging Manual 8th edition and (iv) patients managed by surgery, radiotherapy and/or chemotherapy.

On the contrary, the exclusion criteria for the case group were: (i) patients affected by human papillomavirus (HPV)-related OSCC, (ii) patients affected by another type of tumor localized at the head and neck region, (iii) patients who had concomitant tumors in another organ, and (iv) patients who had experienced severe and irreversible side effects from OSCC treatment such as fibrosis, a mouth opening restriction of less than 30 mm, trismus, hyposalivation or osteoradionecrosis of the jaw.

The inclusion criteria for the control group were: (i) patients treated at the University Dental Clinic only for routine dental care during the study period; and (ii) the absence of any oral mucosal lesions or any previous history of OSCC/VCC.

For both groups the exclusion criteria were (i) breastfeeding or pregnant participants, (ii) patients affected by autoimmune disease or another debilitating condition or unstable disease (such as osteonecrosis of the jaw or dementia), (iii) participants with a medical history of a psychiatric disorder as defined by the DSM-5 or regularly treated with a psychotropic drug, (iv) drug-addicted or alcoholic participants and (v) individuals unable or not willing to give their consent or to understand and complete the questionnaires.

2.2. Procedure

A comprehensive intra- and extra-oral examination was carried out by two oral medicine experts (RG and AD). Upon admission, demographic data such as gender, age, educational level (in years), marital status, employment status, risk factors (smoking and alcohol consumption) body mass index (BMI), comorbidities and associated drug use were recorded for both groups.

Details of clinical oral cancer related characteristics were also noted for the case-group, such as the clinical stage and grading at the time of diagnosis, the location of the tumor, any clinical nodal involvement, any metastasis, the type of treatment, and any need for further treatment during the 5-year follow-up. The performance status was assessed using the Eastern Cooperative Oncology Group (ECOG) scale in OC survivors whose scores range from 0 (fully active) to 5 (death), with higher values indicating a poorer performance status [13].

A predefined set of questionnaires was given to the participants of both groups in order to assess their quality of sleep (QoS), their psychological status (level of anxiety and depression) and the intensity and quality of any pain. The questionnaires comprised:

- the Pittsburgh Sleep Quality Index (PSQI) [14] for the evaluation of insomnia;
- the Epworth Sleepiness Scale (ESS) [15] for the assessment of hypersomnolence;
- the Hamilton Rating Scale for Depression (HAM-D) [16] and the Hamilton rating scale for Anxiety (HAM-A) [17] to evaluate depression and anxiety, respectively;
- the Numeric Rating Scale (NRS) [18] and the short form of the McGill Pain Questionnaire (SF-MPQ) [19] for the evaluation of the intensity and quality of any pain. All

the questionnaires were administered in their Italian version and were reviewed for completeness before collection.

2.3. Outcome Measures

2.3.1. Measures of the Quality of Sleep

The Pittsburgh Sleep Quality Index (PSQI) is a standardized questionnaire used for the assessment of the QoS and the incidence of sleep disturbances. This tool consists of 19 items which generate 7 'component' scores: subjective sleep quality, sleep latency, sleep duration, habitual sleep efficiency, sleep disturbances, use of sleep medication and daytime dysfunction. The scores for each item range from 0 to 3, with higher scores indicating a poorer QoS. The items are combined to yield the seven components, each component having a score ranging from 0 to 3, and the sum of the scores for these seven components yields a global score ranging from 0 to 21. Global scores above five distinguish poor sleepers from good sleepers with a high sensitivity (90–99%) and specificity (84–87%) [14].

The Epworth Sleepiness Scale (ESS) is used to measure an individual's general level of daytime sleepiness. The tool consists of 8 items assessing the propensity for sleep in eight common situations. Subjects rate their likelihood of dozing in each situation on a scale of 0 (would never doze) to 3 (would have a high chance of dozing). The ESS score is the sum of the eight items, ranging from 0 to 24, with a cut-off value of >10 indicating excessive daytime sleepiness [15].

2.3.2. Measures of Psychological Factors

The Hamilton Rating Scale for Anxiety (HAM-A) is a measure of symptoms of anxiety and it consists of 14 items. Scores can range from 0 to 56, with scores from 7 to 17 indicating mild symptoms, between 18 and 24 indicating mild-to-moderate severity, and >25 indicating moderate-to-severe anxiety [16].

The Hamilton Rating Scale for Depression (HAM-D) is a measure of symptoms of depression that is comprised of 21 items pertaining to the affective field. Scores can range from 0 to 54. Scores between 7 and 17 indicate mild depression, between 18 and 24 moderate depression, and over 24 severe depression [17].

2.3.3. Measures of Pain

The Numeric Rating Scale (NRS-11) is a well-validated instrument for the evaluation of pain intensity. whose scale ranges from 0 to 10 (0 = no oral symptoms and 10 = the worst imaginable discomfort). Respondents are asked to report pain intensity in the last 24 h [18].

The Total Pain Rating Index (T-PRI) from the short form of the McGill Pain Questionnaire (SF-MPQ) is a measure of the quality of pain and it is a multidimensional pain questionnaire which measures the sensory, affective and evaluative aspects of the perceived pain. It comprises 15 items from the original MPQ, each scored from 0 (none) to 3 (severe). The T-PRI score is obtained by summing the item scores (range 0–45). There are no established critical cut-off points for the interpretation of the scores and, as for the MPQ, a higher score indicates worse pain [19].

2.4. Statistical Analysis

Descriptive statistics, including means, standard deviations, medians and the interquartile range (IQR) were used to analyse all the socio-demographic and clinical characteristics of the two groups. For the qualitative variables, the significance was calculated by the Exact Chi Square Test. For the demographic numerical variables the significance difference between means was calculated by the parametric two-samples t-test procedure. The significance difference between the recorded medians of the PSQI, ESS, HAM-D, HAM-A, NRS and T-PRI, was measured by the Mann-Whitney Test.

The addition of the clinical characteristics predictors of a poor QoS in OC survivors, hierarchical multiple regression analyses were performed and unadjusted coefficient estimations were obtained for each predictor. A total of six models was computed. The coefficient estimated for binary variables, such as smoking and alcohol consumption, measures the effect of the Yes response on the outcome estimation. For each model, we reported the adjusted R2 which measures the overall goodness of fit adjusted for the number of variables included into the model. The demographic model (model 1) was performed to test the contribution of the demographic variables to a poor QoS. Next, the clinical model (model 2), the psychological model (model 3), the daytime sleepiness model (model 4) and the pain model (model 5) were each performed after controlling for demographic variables to test the contribution of the clinical variables of the OSCC, anxiety and depression (HAM-A; HAM-D), daytime sleepiness (ESS), intensity and quality of pain (NRS, T-PRI) to a poor QoS. Finally, a standard regression analysis (model 6) was computed by entering all the variables simultaneously into the model in order to determine the relative contributions of all the variables to a poor QoS. In all the steps, standard errors of the model coefficients, which measure the statistical precision of the inference estimation of the model parameters, were provided. The IBM SPSS version 22.0 was used to conduct all the statistical analyses in this study, and p-value < 0.05 (two-tails) was considered as statistically significant.

3. Results

The demographic characteristics, BMI and habits of the case and control groups are summarized in Table 1. A total of 100 participants were included in this study, 50 OC survivors and 50 healthy participants and no missing data were recorded.

Table 1. Socio-demographic profile, body mass index, disease onset, and risk factors in the 50 OC survivors and 50 controls.

	OC Survivors	Controls	
	Mean ± SD	Mean ± SD	p-Value
Age	59.5 ± 10.1	65.1 ± 14.4	0.051
Years of education	8.5 ± 3.0	10.3 ± 5.0	0.054
	N° (%)	N° (%)	
Gender M:F	26:24 (52%, 48%)	26:24 (52%, 48%)	1.00
Marital status (married)	33 (66%)	40 (80%)	0.115
Full-time employment			
Employed	14 (28.0%)	36 (72.0%)	<0.001 **
Not employed	12 (24.0%)	8 (16.0%)	
Retired	24 (48.0%)	3 (12.0%)	
BMI			
<16.5	1 (2.0%)	0 (0.0%)	
16.5–18.4	1 (2.0%)	0 (0.0%)	
18.5–24.9	19 (38.0%)	29 (58.0%)	
25.0–29.9	21 (42.0%)	21 (42.0%)	0.068
30.0–34.9	5 (10.0%)	0 (0.0%)	
35.0–39.9	3 (6.0%)	0 (0.0%)	
≥40.0	0 (0.0%)	0 (0.0%)	
Mean ± SD	26.1 ± 4.6	27.4 ± 1.8	
Smoking	9 (18.0%)	23 (46%)	0.005 **
Alcohol consumption	21 (42.0%)	18 (36.0%)	0.619

The significance difference between means was measured by the t-student test. The significance difference between the percentages was measured by the Pearson Chi Square test. * Significant $0.01 < p \leq 0.05$, ** Significant $p \leq 0.01$. Legend: BMI = body mass index; OSCC = oral squamous cell carcinoma.

Of these participants, 54% (n = 26) and 46% (n = 24) were male and female for each group, respectively, with a mean age of 59.5 ± 10.1 years for the cases and 65.1 ± 14.4 years for the controls (p-value: 0.051). No statistically significant difference was found in terms of marital status, years of education, BMI or alcohol consumption (p-values: 0.115, 0.054, 0.068, 0.619, respectively). However, the number of healthy participants in full-time employment and with a current smoking habit was significantly higher (*p*-value: <0.001 ** and 0.005 *** respectively) in comparison to the case group.

Table 2 shows the prevalence of systemic diseases and drug intake in the study sample. The OC survivors presented with a statistically higher number of systemic comorbidities in comparison to the control group (*p*-value: 0.012 *), especially with respect to hypertension, hypercholesterolemia, prostatic hypertrophy and gastrointestinal diseases (*p*-values: <0.001 **, 0.001 **, 0.16 * and <0.001 *** respectively). Consequently, the number of OC survivors taking medications, such as angiotensin II receptor antagonists, beta blockers, proton pump inhibitors and statin agents was significantly higher compared to the controls (*p*-value: <0.001 **).

Table 2. Frequency of systemic diseases and drug consumption in the 50 OSCC patients and 50 controls.

	OC Survivors	Controls	*p*-Value
	N° (%)	N° (%)	
SYSTEMIC DISEASES	37 (74.0)	24 (48.0)	0.012 *
Hypothyroidism	5 (10.0)	14 (7.0)	0.244
Hyperthyroidism	3 (6.0)	8 (16.0)	0.084
Hypertension	26 (52.0)	9 (18.0)	0.001 **
Hypercholesterolemia	22 (44.0)	3 (6.0)	<0.001 **
Previous Heart Attack	2 (4.0)	2 (4.0)	0.457
Arrhythmia	7 (14.0)	2 (4.0)	0.074
HCV +	2 (4.0)	0 (0.0)	0.437
Other hepatitis	0 (0.0)	0 (0.0)	1.000
Type 2 diabetes	3 (6.0)	0 (0.0)	0.189
Type 1 diabetes	3 (6.0)	0 (0.0)	0.189
Other cancer	3 (6.0)	0 (0.0)	0.189
Prostatic hypertrophy	5 (10.0)	0 (0.0)	0.016 *
Gastro-intestinal disease	9 (8.0)	0 (0.0)	<0.001 **
Respiratory illness	2 (4.0)	0 (0.0)	0.189
Other	2 (4.0)	0 (0.0)	0.189
DRUG CONSUMPTION			
ACE inhibitors	8 (16.0)	0 (0.0)	<0.001 **
Antiplatelets	12 (24.0)	5 (10.0)	0.010 **
Anticoagulants	3 (6.0)	0 (0.0)	0.189
Beta adrenergic blocking agents	14 (28.0)	3 (6.0)	<0.001 **
Biphosphonates	2 (4.0)	0 (0.0)	0.438
CCB (calcium channel antagonists)	5 (10.0)	0 (0.0)	0.034 *
Diuretics	9 (18.0)	4 (8.0)	0.026 *
Proton pump inhibitors	14 (28.0)	0 (0.0)	<0.01 **
Insulin	3 (6.0)	0 (0.0)	0.189
Hypoglycemic agents	3 (6.0)	0 (0.0)	0.189
Levothyroxine	4 (8.0)	12 (24.0)	0.017 *
ARB (angiotensin II receptor antagonists)	14 (28.0)	4 (8.0)	0.004 **
Statins	18 (36.0)	3 (6.0)	<0.001 **
Other drugs	0 (0.0)	1 (2.0)	0.478

The significance difference between percentages was measured by the Pearson Chi Square test. * Significant $0.01 < p \leq 0.05$, ** Significant $p \leq 0.01$.

Table 3 summarizes the clinical characteristics of the OC survivors. The majority of the patients were diagnosed with stages 0–1 (52%) while 48% were diagnosed with stages 3–4 and with differentiated OSCC (G1-2 88% of the patients). Most of the tumors were localized at the tongue (52%) and alveolar ridges (22%), while 16% and 10% at the buccal mucosa and hard/soft palate, respectively. All the patients with OSCC were managed with surgical treatments ranging from local conservative tumor excision (66.0%) to more invasive surgical treatments. such as hemiglossectomy (20%), maxillary osteotomy (8.0%), hemimandibulectomy (6%) and cervical neck dissection (42%). Only a few patients received, in addition, radiotherapy (16%) or chemotherapy (2%). Tracheostomy was not performed in respect of any OC survivors. Overall, the OSCC patients were further treated with incisional or excisional biopsies over the five-year follow-up period (a mean of 4.8 +/− 2.9) due to local relapses, especially in respect of the 29 (58%) OC survivors with associated potentially malignant disorders such as lichenoid lesions 8 (16%), leukoplakia 7 (14%) erythroleukoplakia 14 (28%).

Table 3. Medical characteristics of the OC survivors.

OC Survivors	N° (%)
TUMOR TYPE	
Squamous cell carcinoma	47 (94.0)
Verrucous cell carcinoma	3 (6.0)
TUMOR LOCALIZATION	
Tongue and mouth floor	26 52.0)
Alveolar ridge and gingiva	11 (22.0)
Buccal mucosa	8 (16.0)
Soft and hard palate	5 (10.0)
STAGING	
TISN0M0 (stage 0)	25 (50.0)
T1N0M0 (stage 1)	1 (2.0)
T2N0M0 (stage 2)	0 (0.0)
T3N0M0 (stage 3)	1 (2.0)
T3N1M0 (stage 3)	3 (6.0)
T4N0M0 (stage 4)	1 (2.0)
T4N1M0 (stage 4)	19 (38.0)
GRADING	
G1	13 (26.0)
G2	31 (62.0)
G3	5 (10.0)
G4	1 (2.0)
ORAL POTENTIALLY MALIGNANT DISORDERS	29 (58.0)
SURGICAL TREATMENT OF PRIMARY OSCC	
Local tumor resection	33 (66.0)
Hemiglossectomy	10 (20.0)
Maxillary Osteotomy	4 (8.0)
Hemimandibulectomy	3 (6.0)
Cervical neck dissection	21 (42.0)
CHEMOTHERAPY	1 (2.0)
RADIOTHERAPY	8 (16.0)
N° OF PATIENTS WITH LOCAL RECURRENCES	30 (60.0)
N° OF SECONDARY SURGICAL LOCAL RESECTIONS	Mean ± SD (Range) 1.74 ± 2.18 (1−9)
ECOG	
Status 0	33 (66.0)
Status 1	17 (34.0)

At the time of the assessment, 66% of the OSCC patients presented with an ECOG performance status of 0 ("fully active") and 34% with an ECOG performance status of 1 ("restricted in physically strenuous activity").

Among the OC survivors, 52% were poor sleepers (PSQI > 5), whereas only 12% of the controls reported a poor QoS. Moreover, mild to severe anxiety was reported in 84% of the OC survivors (48% mild, 12% moderate and 24% severe anxiety) along with mild to severe depression in 74% of cases (40% mild, 16% moderate and 18% severe depression). On the contrary, only 20% and 18% of the healthy participants showed mild anxiety and depression symptoms, respectively, and no cases of moderate to severe anxiety or depression were recorded in the control group.

Table 4 shows the differences in all the psychological factors between the case and control group. A Cronbach alpha value of 0.76 and 0.91 was indicative of a good reliability of the PSQI scale in both groups. The OC survivors presented a mean of hours of sleep of 6.94 ± 1.024, while the controls slept a mean of 7.16 ± 0.681 h. A statistically significant difference was found between the medians of all the psychological variables assessed in terms of QoS, anxiety and depression and intensity and quality of pain. The OC survivors showed statistically significant higher scores in the global PSQI (p-value: 0.017 *), especially for the items "subjective sleep quality", "sleep latency" and daytime dysfunction" (p-values: <0.001 **, 0.029 * and 0.004 ** respectively), and in the total ESS score (p-value: 0.001 **) in comparison with the controls. Furthermore, statistically significant higher levels of anxiety and depression, as reflected by the total scores of the HAM-A and HAM-D, were also recorded among the OC survivors (p-value: <0.001 **), together with higher levels of oral discomfort and pain according to the NRS and T-PRI total scores (p-value: 0.001). Taken together, these findings suggest that QoS and psychological status may be severely impaired in OC survivors.

Table 4. Differences in sleep quality, anxiety, depression and pain in 50 OSCC patients and 50 controls.

	OC Survivors	Controls	
PSQI Cronbach Alpha	0.76	0.91	p-Value
	Median-IQR	Median-IQR	
PSQI			
Subjective sleep quality	6; [3–9]	4; [3–5]	0.017 *
Sleep latency	1; [1–2]	1; [0–1]	<0.001 **
Sleep duration	1; [0–2]	0; [0–1]	0.029 *
Habitual sleep efficiency	1; [0–2]	1; [0–1]	0.512
Sleep disturbances	0; [0–2]	0; [0–1]	0.400
Use of sleep medications	1; [1–2]	1; [1–1]	0.740
Daytime dysfunction	0; [0–1]	0; [0–0]	0.004 **
HAM-A	12; [9–24]	5; [3–6]	<0.001 **
HAM-D	10; [6–24]	4; [3–6]	<0.001 **
ESS	5; [2–9]	3; [3–4]	0.001 **
NRS	2; [0–5]	0; [0–0]	<0.001 **
T-PRI	2; [0–9]	0; [0–0]	<0.001 **

Legend: ESS = Epworth Sleepiness Scale; HAM-A = Hamilton Anxiety Scale; HAM-D = Hamilton Depression Scale; IQR = interquartile range. NRS = Numeric Rating Scale; McGill: PSQI = Pittsburgh Sleep Quality Index; T-PRI: Total Pain Rating Index. The significance difference between medians was measured by the Mann–Whitney test. * Significant $0.01 \leq p \leq 0.05$ ** Significant $p \leq 0.01$.

Furthermore, in the case group, a statistically significant positive correlation was found between the global PSQI score and the HAM-A, HAM-D and T-PRI scores (p-values: <0.001 **, <0.001 ** and 0.019 * respectively) but not with the ESS and the NRS. Specifically, the majority of the PSQI sub-items (except for "use of sleep medication" and "sleep latency") were positively correlated with the HAM-A and HAM-D (except for "use of sleep medication"), whereas the T-PRI was correlated only with "sleep disturbances and daytime dysfunction" which also correlated, as expected, with the ESS. Overall, patients with a poorer QoS presented with higher levels of anxiety and depression and a worse quality of pain but not with increasing daytime sleepiness or pain intensity (Table 5).

Table 5. Correlation analysis between the PSQI items and anxiety, depression and pain in 50 OSCC patients and 50 controls.

	HAM-A		HAM-D		ESS		NRS		T-PRI	
	Rho	p-Value	Rho	p-Value	Rho	p-Value	Rho	p-Value	Rho	p-Value
PSQI	,671	<0.001 **	,735	<0.001 **	,242	0.138	,250	0.125	,374	0.019 *
Subjective sleep quality	,423	0.007 **	,528	0.001 **	,078	0.636	-,023	0.891	,251	0.124
Sleep latency	,305	0.059	,470	0.003 **	,285	0.079	,172	0.295	,181	0.271
Sleep duration	,488	0.002 **	,572	<0.001 **	,139	0.398	,206	0.209	,216	0.187
Habitual sleep efficiency	,542	<0.001 **	,573	<0.001 **	-,004	0.981	,194	0.237	,232	0.155
Sleep disturbances	,480	0.002 **	,599	<0.001 **	,102	0.535	,189	0.249	,395	0.013 *
Use of sleep medications	,298	0.066	,149	0.364	,003	0.984	,167	0.309	,051	0.760
Daytime dysfunction	,561	<0.001 **	,506	0.001 **	,461	0.003 **	,118	0.473	,389	0.014 *

Legend: ESS = Epworth Sleepiness Scale; HAM-A = Hamilton Anxiety Scale; HAM-D = Hamilton Depression Scale; NRS = Numeric Rating Scale; McGill: PSQI = Pittsburgh Sleep Quality Index; T-PRI: Total Pain Rating Index. Correlation between PSQI items and other variables was measured with the Spearman correlation analysis. * Moderately significant $0.01 < p \leq 0.05$; ** strongly significant $p \leq 0.01$.

The hierarchical multiple regression analyses predicting QoS are shown in Table 6. The first model (the demographic model), testing the contribution of demographic variables and risk factors (alcohol and smoking) to QoS, showed that the PSQI was negatively correlated with years of education (p-value: 0.042 *) and resulted in a strongly significant increase in the coefficient of determination (R2) ($\Delta R2 = 31.7\%$, p-value: 0.009). The addition of the clinical characteristics showed that the PSQI was positively correlated with alcohol consumption (p-value: 0.018 *) and with the use of systemic medications (p-value: 0.045 *). When entering all the variables simultaneously in the second model, we found an increase in the R2 value with a $\Delta R2$ of 6.2%, possibly due to both the parameters, namely alcohol consumption and medications, although it was not statistically significant (p-value: 0.222). The third model (the psychological model), testing the contribution of anxiety and depression to QoS, showed that the PSQI was positively correlated with the HAM-A and HAM-D (p-value: 0.001 **) and resulted in a strongly significant increase in the R2 ($\Delta R2 = 20.4\%$, p-value: <0.001 **). The daytime sleepiness and pain models (models 4 and 5) did not result in a significant increase in the R2 value ($\Delta R2 = -2.1\%$, 0.0%; p-value: 0.749 and 0.377 respectively). The final full model (model 6, the standard multiple regression analysis) in which all of the variables were entered simultaneously (including demographic variable, risk factors, clinical characteristics, medications, anxiety, depression, daytime sleepiness, pain) resulted in a moderate increase in the R2 value ($\Delta R2 = 12.6\%$; p-value: 0.043 *) and could explain the 44.3% of variance of poor QoS. In this last model, depression has shown a strong correlation to sleep disorders (p-value: 0.001 **) contributing significantly to a poor QoS.

Table 6. Multiple linear regression analysis predicting poor QoS (PSQI > 5) in 50 OC survivors.

Parameter	Model 1 Beta (SE)	Model 1 p-Value	Model 2 Beta (SE)	Model 2 p-Value	Model 3 Beta (SE)	Model 3 p-Value	Model 4 Beta (SE)	Model 4 p-Value	Model 5 Beta (SE)	Model 5 p-Value	Model 6 Beta (SE)	Model 6 p-Value
Gender Male vs. Female	−2.93 (1.70)	0.094	−4.12 (1.78)	0.029	−1.44 (1.53)	0.354	−2.85 (1.74)	0.113	−2.46 (1.74)	0.168	−2.55 (1.04)	0.226
Age	0.04 (0.06)	0.583	−0.03 (0.08)	0.739	0.02 (0.05)	0.618	0.04 (0.07)	0.546	0.04 (0.06)	0.522	0.07 (0.07)	0.399
Education	−0.29 (0.14)	0.042 *	−0.24 (0.18)	0.207	−0.11 (0.12)	0.364	−0.30 (0.14)	0.045 *	−0.21 (0.14)	0.155	−0.09 (0.17)	0.579
Employment Yes vs. No	1.41 (2.12)	0.511	1.94 (2.15)	0.376	0.53 (1.79)	0.788	1.61 (2.25)	0.477	0.97 (2.17)	0.659	2.57 (2.30)	0.277
Married Yes vs. No	−2.51 (1.52)	0.110	−1.42 (1.75)	0.425	−1.30 (1.31)	0.327	−2.70 (1.66)	0.114	−2.83 (1.62)	0.092	−2.58 (1.88)	0.186
BMI	0.10 (0.13)	0.442	−0.02 (0.16)	0.871	0.11 (0.11)	0.311	0.11 (0.13)	0.419	0.12 (0.14)	0.429	−0.09 (0.19)	0.634
Smoking Yes vs. No	0.71 (1.94)	0.715	3.89 (1.52)	0.098	1.25 (1.65)	0.455	0.60 (1.99)	0.765	0.94 (1.94)	0.631	2.82 (2.05)	0.184
Alcohol consumption Yes vs. NO	2.54 (1.40)	0.079	3.90 (1.52)	0.018 *	1.95 (1.27)	0.135	2.54 (1.42)	0.084	2.63 (1.40)	0.071	3.32 (1.78)	0.077
Potentially malignant disorders Yes vs. No			2.66 (1.54)	0.097							1.63 (1.63)	0.330
Number of operations			0.16 (0.32)	0.613							0.20 (0.29)	0.497
Radiotherapy Yes vs. NO			1.52 (2.40)	0.534							−0.56 (3.01)	0.852
T3N0M0 vs. TISN0M0			1.71 (2.41)	0.486							2.61 (2.59)	0.327
T4N0M0 vs. TISN0M0			1.13 (1.64)	0.497							0.67 (2.29)	0.773

Table 6. *Cont.*

Parameter	Model 1 Beta (SE)	Model 1 p-Value	Model 2 Beta (SE)	Model 2 p-Value	Model 3 Beta (SE)	Model 3 p-Value	Model 4 Beta (SE)	Model 4 p-Value	Model 5 Beta (SE)	Model 5 p-Value	Model 6 Beta (SE)	Model 6 p-Value
Medications Yes vs. NO			−10.2 (4.98)	0.045 *							−7.32 (5.42)	0.193
HAM-A					0.08 (0.08)	0.352					0.09 (0.13)	0.499
HAM-D					0.15 (0.06)	0.001 **					0.16 (0.07)	0.001 **
ESS							−0.04 (0.14)	0.749			−0.13 (0.15)	0.378
NRS									0.06 (0.33)	0.853	0.30 (0.33)	0.374
T-PRI									0.09 (0.11)	0.423	−0.11 (0.13)	0.431
R2 Adjusted	31.7%		37.9%		52.1%		29.6%		31.7%		44.3%	
ΔR2 Adjusted	31.7% ($p = 0.009$ **)		6.2% ($p = 0.222$)		20.4% ($p < 0.001$ **)		−2.1% ($p = 0.749$)		0.0% ($p = 0.377$)		12.6% ($p = 0.043$ *)	

SE are the standard errors of the beta estimates. The *p*-values were obtained from the hypothesis test on the regression coefficients. * Moderately significant $0.01 < p\text{-value} \leq 0.05$ ** Strongly significant $p\text{-value} \leq 0.01$. Legend: ESS = Epworth Sleepiness Scale; HAM-A = Hamilton Anxiety Scale; HAM-D = Hamilton Depression Scale; NRS = Numeric Rating Scale; McGill: PSQI = Pittsburgh Sleep Quality Index; T-PRI: Total Pain Rating Index.

4. Discussion

The aim of this study has been to investigate the prevalence of sleep disorders (insomnia and hypersomnolence), anxiety and depression in OC survivors with a 5-year follow-up and to analyze potential predictors in the development of sleep disorders. The detection and treatment of factors which could influence the well-being of OC survivors are becoming increasingly important for healthcare systems in order to improve the follow-up care of these patients.

Among this population, insomnia, poor QoS, short sleep duration, excessive daytime sleepiness and sleep-related breathing are commonly reported and tend to become often chronic and pervasive in patients during and after treatment for OSCC [3].

In a recent systematic review, the prevalence of self-reported insomnia (defined with a PSQI cut-off of 5) in patients with head and neck cancer was 29% before treatment, 45% during treatment and 40% after treatment, while the prevalence rate of hypersomnolence (ESS cut-off > 10) was 16% before and 32% after treatment [8].

In this study, a higher prevalence of insomnia among the OC survivors within the 5-year follow-up was found, in comparison with the study of Santoso et al. [8] as 52% of the patients were poor sleepers (median PSQI score 6), while hypersomnolence was found in 24 % of OC survivors, in line with previous research [20,21].

With regard to the PSQI components a higher percentage of OC survivors reported an impaired subjective sleep quality, sleep latency, and daytime dysfunction.

Pain, fatigue, medical treatment, psychological profile (anxiety and depression) and comorbidities [22] may cause poor sleep in cancer patients. In this study, the full model of the multiple regression analysis, where all the variables were entered simultaneously, could explain only 44.3% of the variance of the PSQI in OC survivors, suggesting that the occurrence of insomnia could be independent of the cancer characteristics, staging of the malignancy, type of treatment (surgery, or radiotherapy), pain and presence of potentially malignant disorders. Instead, poor sleep was negatively correlated with years of education and positively correlated with mood disorders (anxiety and depression), the use of systemic medications and the consumption of alcohol. Therefore, a lower education level, the use of systemic drugs, the consumption of alcohol and the presence of anxiety and depression were predictors for poor sleep in OC survivors.

In a previous study, a lower education level, the presence of systemic comorbidities and the use of systemic drugs, adversely affected quality of life outcomes in survivors of cancer [23]. Moreover, there is evidence that sleep disorders may be associated with cardiovascular diseases and cardiovascular risk factors, such as hypertension and elevated resting heart rate in the general population [24], and that cardiovascular medications such as beta adrenergic blocking agents, ACE inhibitors, calcium channel antagonists may negatively affect sleep quality in individuals with other comorbidities, especially those with sleep disorders breathing [25].

Our results are in line with these studies, suggesting that the use of medications for systemic comorbidities could have a detrimental effect on the life of patients that over time could also influence QoS. However, medications with alcohol consumption contributed to sleep disorders on the account of 6.2% of the variance of poor QoS based on the second model of the regression analysis which suggests that medications may not have a pivotal role in explaining the higher prevalence of sleep disorders in this group of OC survivors, possibly for the absence of sleep disorder breathing and obstructive sleep apnea in our sample.

In addition, the low intensity of pain (NRS: 2) reported by OC survivors is considered as a predictor of poor sleep, as suggested by the regression analysis. Although xerostomia was not detected in our sample of patients probably because radiotherapy was prescribed in only 16% (8) of patients, Shuman et al [26] similarly reported that pain in the mouth and xerostomia (dry mouth) were strong predictors of poor sleep.

Regarding habits, alcohol abuse and tobacco smoking might play a role in the development of sleep disorders. Indeed, heavy alcohol users often experience insomnia even after they stop their alcohol consumption, while smokers suffer more frequently from poor sleep, compared with non-smokers [27,28]. In this study, at the time of evaluation, only 16% (8) were current smokers, as the majority had stopped their smoking habit after their OSCC diagnosis. Conversely, 42% (21) continued to consume alcohol (<14 units per week), although no one was a heavy drinker. Therefore, the positive correlation between poor sleep and alcohol consumption could be related to a previous higher alcohol consumption.

While in a recent study insomnia and hypersomnolence were found to be associated with chemotherapy and radiotherapy, [23] in the present study we could not find this correlation, presumably because the majority of the patients were in stage 0/1 (52%, 26 individuals) and only 2% (1) and 16% (8) of patients, respectively, had received these protocols. A recent review article suggested that surgery may have a positive effect on sleep quality; indeed, patients with oral cancer treated with surgery were less prone to develop insomnia, probably because they considered the operation as a resolution of the disease. The authors found a prevalence of insomnia of 31.9% in oral cancer patients who had undergone surgery and of 44.9% in those who were not receiving surgery, especially females. An explanation of these results could be that women are more vulnerable to the stress related to a cancer diagnosis and subsequently to mood disorders on account of their hormonal status [29]. In the current study we did not find any differences between male and female OC survivors, all the patients having been treated with surgical procedures.

Previous studies have suggested that obesity (BMI > 30) is considered a significant predictor of sleep disorders [30]. In our study, only 16% (8) of OC survivors were overweight, however, based on the result of the regression analyses, BMI may not have contributed to sleep disorders, similarly to the findings from the study of Bardewell et al [31].

Regarding the psychological profile, the current literature has reported a prevalence of anxiety and depression, ranging from 19 to 50%, in cancer survivors, suggesting that the burden of cancer diagnosis and its treatment could have a strong impact on the psychological profile, persisting over time despite a successful operation and subsequently decreasing the quality of life of the affected patients. Moreover, Espie et al. reported that from 22% to 32% of OC survivors were anxious or depressed even ten years after the diagnosis and treatment [32]. Factors identified as contributing to an increased risk of psychological distress among oral cancer patients include persistent pain, age (generally, younger patients more seriously affected than older patients), gender (females more seriously affected than males), stage of cancer, type of treatment, and fear of cancer recurrence. Moreover, anxiety and oral dysfunction, including trismus, xerostomia, sticky saliva and problems with eating and social contacts, are also considered a barrier to any return to work after treatment among head and neck cancer survivors [33]. As a consequence, a lack of full-time employment can exacerbate the depressive symptoms.

In this study, a higher prevalence of mood disorders has been found in comparison with the current literature; indeed, anxiety and depression were identified in 84% (42%) and 74% (37) of OC survivors, respectively. In addition, in the final full model, depression was found to be the most contributive factor to poor QoS. The higher level of depression may be related to the stress associated with a fear of cancer recurrence, since almost 40% [3] of patients presented a local cancer recurrence and, therefore, underwent a subsequent operation during the five years of follow-up.

Mood disorders and poor sleep were closely interconnected, as shown by the correlation analysis. In addition, anxiety and depression were predictors of poor sleep, as confirmed by the regression analysis. No differences between male and female patients were detected, and neither the stage and treatment nor the number of operations for cancer recurrence affected the incidence of sleep disorders. In line with previous studies, an impaired mood and sleep affected the functional recovery of patients and their return to work because, despite their age, the majority of OC survivors (48%) had retired.

The results of this study suggest that the high prevalence of insomnia may be related not only to psychiatric symptoms or to a fear of cancer recurrence but could also be considered in some cases an independent variable (as shown by the regression analysis) which needs to be addressed regardless of all the other factors. It is possible to consider that cancer itself can lead to the development of sleep disorders through inflammation. Inflammation has emerged as a crucial pathway which may be especially relevant with respect to cancer survivors. The sleep-wake cycle has emerged as a homeostatic regulator of inflammatory biology in which sleep loss induces an activation of nuclear factor KB (NF-kb) [34] and circulating levels of IL-6 [35], which coordinate the production of inflammatory mediators and systemic inflammation. In turn, pro-inflammatory cytokines are thought to contribute in part to the onset of depressive symptoms, which can amplify sleep disorders [36,37]. Moreover, chronic inflammation may predispose to a second primary recurrence [38].

Adequate sleep is a biological requirement for healthy physical, cognitive and psychological functioning so the management of sleep disturbance should be targeted by clinicians with appropriate interventions. In particular, the prominent role of cognitive behavior therapy has been studied [39]. * Additionally, the administration of melatonin in relation to the management of the sleep-wake cycle and mood disturbance as well as with respect to the quality of life of cancer patients has been proposed [40].

The findings of the current study should be understood in the light of some limitations. First, the sample is small and all the patients were recruited at a single hospital, thus preventing the possibility of any geographical generalizability and slightly affecting the power of the regression analyses. Secondly, the exclusion of patients who had developed severe and permanent side effects due to the radiotherapy, may have produced a potential underestimation of the prevalence of sleep disorders in OC survivors. Moreover, the study design does not allow the drawing of any conclusive inferences about the temporality and causality of the relationships between the variables explored. Finally, only subjective sleep quality was investigated in this study, with objective sleep quality not being considered, and therefore additional measurement systems should be incorporated to verify our findings.

5. Conclusions

Sleep disorders (including insomnia and hypersomnolence) continue to be prevalent both during and after treatment for OSCC. A lower level of education, the use of systemic drugs, the consumption of alcohol and the presence of anxiety and especially depression are predictors of poor sleep in OC survivors.

The treatment of oral cancer must clearly remain the major goal, but the treatment of any psychological comorbidities is also important in order to improve the quality of life in these patients. Therefore, healthcare professionals should be encouraged to include sleep disorders assessment at the time of diagnosis, during treatment and in follow-up consultations. Further clinical and prospective studies should be conducted not only to evaluate the real prevalence of sleep disorders but also to plan an adequate treatment over time with respect to all OC survivors.

Supplementary Materials: The following are available online at https://www.mdpi.com/article/10.3390/cancers13081855/s1, Figure S1: Flow chart.

Author Contributions: D.A. and M.D.M. equally contributed for the conceptualization of the study, the methodology, the data collection and curation and drafted the paper; R.G., E.C. and N.C. contributed to the data curation and collection and drafted the paper; G.M. and G.S. drafted and reviewed the paper; M.A. analyzed the data and contributed to writing the manuscript. All authors have read and agreed to the published version of the manuscript.

Funding: The authors have not been supported by any private or corporate financial institutions, nor have they received any grant for this study.

Institutional Review Board Statement: The study was conducted according to the guidelines of the Declaration of Helsinki, and approved by the Institutional Review Board (or Ethics Committee) of University of Naples Federico II (protocol number 188: 2014).

Informed Consent Statement: Informed consent was obtained from all subjects involved in the study.

Data Availability Statement: The data presented in this study are available on request from the corresponding author. The data are not publicly available due to patient sensitive data.

Conflicts of Interest: The authors declare no conflict of interest.

References

1. Bray, F.; Ferlay, J.; Soerjomataram, I.; Siegel, R.L.; Torre, L.A.; Jemal, A. Global cancer statistics 2018: GLOBOCAN estimates of incidence and mortality worldwide for 36 cancers in 185 countries. *CA Cancer J. Clin.* **2018**, *68*, 394–424. [CrossRef]
2. Irwin, M.R. Depression and Insomnia in Cancer: Prevalence, Risk Factors, and Effects on Cancer Outcomes. *Curr. Psychiatry Rep.* **2013**, *15*, 1–9. [CrossRef] [PubMed]
3. Roscoe, J.A.; Kaufman, M.E.; Matteson-Rusby, S.E.; Palesh, O.G.; Ryan, J.L.; Kohli, S.; Perlis, M.L.; Morrow, G.R. Cancer-Related Fatigue and Sleep Disorders. *Oncologist* **2007**, *12* (Suppl. 1), 35–42. [CrossRef]
4. Ferrie, J.E.; Shipley, M.J.; Cappuccio, F.P.; Brunner, E.; Miller, M.A.; Kumari, M.; Marmot, M.G. A Prospective Study of Change in Sleep Duration: Associations with Mortality in the Whitehall II Cohort. *Sleep* **2007**, *30*, 1659–1666. [CrossRef] [PubMed]
5. Davidson, J.R.; MacLean, A.W.; Brundage, M.D.; Schulze, K. Sleep disturbance in cancer patients. *Soc. Sci. Med.* **2002**, *54*, 1309–1321. [CrossRef]
6. Grandner, M.A. Sleep, Health, and Society. *Sleep Med. Clin.* **2020**, *15*, 319–340. [CrossRef] [PubMed]
7. Slade, A.N.; Waters, M.R.; Serrano, N.A. Long-term sleep disturbance and prescription sleep aid use among cancer survivors in the United States. *Support Care Cancer* **2020**, *28*, 551–560. [CrossRef]
8. Santoso, A.M.M.; Jansen, F.; de Vries, R.; Leemans, C.R.; van Straten, A.; Verdonck-de Leeuw, I.M. Prevalence of sleep disturbances among head and neck cancer patients: A systematic review and meta-analysis. *Sleep Med. Rev.* **2019**, *47*, 62–73. [CrossRef]
9. Dickerson, S.S.; Connors, L.M.; Fayad, A.; Dean, G.E. Sleep-wake disturbances in cancer patients: Narrative review of literature focusing on improving quality of life outcomes. *Nat. Sci. Sleep* **2014**, *6*, 85–100. [CrossRef]
10. Mantovani, A.; Allavena, P.; Sica, A.; Balkwill, F.R. Cancer-related inflammation. *Nat. Cell Biol.* **2008**, *454*, 436–444. [CrossRef]
11. Palesh, O.; Aldridge-Gerry, A.; Zeitzer, J.; Koopman, C.; Neri, E.; Giese-Davis, J.; Jo, B.; Kraemer, H.; Nouriani, B.; Spiegel, D. Actigraphy-Measured Sleep Disruption as a Predictor of Survival among Women with Advanced Breast Cancer. *Sleep* **2014**, *37*, 837–842. [CrossRef]
12. Von Elm, E.; Altman, D.G.; Egger, M.; Pocock, S.J.; Gøtzsche, P.C.; Vandenbroucke, J.P. The Strengthening the Reporting of Observational Studies in Epidemiology (STROBE) Statement: Guidelines for reporting observational studies. *Int. J. Surg.* **2014**, *12*, 1495–1499. [CrossRef]
13. Oken, M.M.; Creech, R.H.; Tormey, D.C.; Horton, J.; Davis, T.E.; McFadden, E.T.; Carbone, P.P. Toxicity and response criteria of the Eastern Cooperative Oncology Group. *Am. J. Clin. Oncol.* **1982**, *5*, 649–655. [CrossRef] [PubMed]
14. Curcio, G.; Tempesta, D.; Scarlata, S.; Marzano, C.; Moroni, F.; Rossini, P.M.; Ferrara, M.; De Gennaro, L. Validity of the Italian version of the Pittsburgh Sleep Quality Index (PSQI). *Neurol. Sci.* **2013**, *34*, 511–519. [CrossRef] [PubMed]
15. Vignatelli, L.; Plazzi, G.; Barbato, A.; Ferini-Strambi, L.; Manni, M.; Pompei, F.; D'Alessandro, R. Italian version of the Epworth sleepiness scale: External validity. *Neurol. Sci.* **2003**, *23*, 295–300. [CrossRef]
16. Hamilton, M. A rating scale for depression. *J. Neurol. Neurosurg. Psychiatry* **1960**, *23*, 56–62. [CrossRef] [PubMed]
17. Hamilton, M. The assessment of anxiety states by rating. *Br. J. Med. Psychol.* **1959**, *32*, 50–55. [CrossRef] [PubMed]
18. Hjermstad, M.J.; Fayers, P.M.; Haugen, D.F.; Caraceni, A.; Hanks, G.W.; Loge, J.H.; Fainsinger, R.; Aass, N.; Kaasa, S. Studies Comparing Numerical Rating Scales, Verbal Rating Scales, and Visual Analogue Scales for Assessment of Pain Intensity in Adults: A Systematic Literature Review. *J. Pain Symptom Manag.* **2011**, *41*, 1073–1093. [CrossRef]
19. Melzack, R. The short-form McGill pain questionnaire. *Pain* **1987**, *30*, 191–197. [CrossRef]
20. Ritterband, L.M.; Bailey, E.T.; Thorndike, F.P.; Lord, H.R.; Farrell-Carnahan, L.; Baum, L.D. Initial evaluation of an Internet intervention to improve the sleep of cancer survivors with insomnia. *Psycho-Oncology* **2012**, *21*, 695–705. [CrossRef]
21. Yilmaz, M. Evaluation of sleep disorders in nonmetastatic breast cancer patients based on pittsburgh sleep quality index. *J. Cancer Res. Ther.* **2020**, *16*, 1274–1278. [PubMed]
22. Dahiya, S.; Ahluwalia, M.S.; Walia, H.K. Sleep disturbances in cancer patients: Under recognized and undertreated. *Clevel. Clin. J. Med.* **2013**, *80*, 722–732. [CrossRef] [PubMed]
23. Palesh, O.G.; Roscoe, J.A.; Mustian, K.M.; Roth, T.; Savard, J.; Ancoli-Israel, S.; Heckler, C.; Purnell, J.Q.; Janelsins, M.C.; Morrow, G.R. Prevalence, demographics, and psychological associations of sleep disruption in patients with cancer: University of Rochester Cancer Center-Community Clinical Oncology Program. *J. Clin. Oncol.* **2010**, *28*, 292–298. [CrossRef] [PubMed]
24. Spiegelhalder, K.; Scholtes, C.; Riemann, D. The association between insomnia and cardiovascular diseases. *Nat. Sci. Sleep* **2010**, *2*, 71–78. [CrossRef] [PubMed]
25. Fender, A.D. CV Drugs That Negatively Affect Sleep Quality. American College of Cardiology. Available online: https://www.acc.org/latest-in-cardiology/articles/2014/07/18/15/46/cv-drugs-that-negatively-affect-sleepquality#:~{}:text=ACE%20inhibitors%20are%20thought%20to,bradykinin%20may%20worsen%20the%20AHI (accessed on 3 April 2021).
26. Shuman, A.G.; Duffy, S.A.; Ronis, D.L.; Garetz, S.L.; McLean, S.A.; Fowler, K.E.; Terrell, J.E. Predictors of poor sleep quality among head and neck cancer patients. *Laryngoscope* **2010**, *120*, 1166–1172. [CrossRef] [PubMed]
27. Brower, K.J. Alcohol's effects on sleep in alcoholics. *Alcohol Res. Health* **2001**, *25*, 110–125.

28. Sabanayagam, C.; Shankar, A. The association between active smoking, smokeless tobacco, second-hand smoke exposure and insufficient sleep. *Sleep Med.* **2011**, *12*, 7–11. [CrossRef]
29. Del Pup, L. Is there any evidence of the belief that stress could increase the risk of female cancers? *World Cancer Res.* **2017**, *4*, e976.
30. Polesel, D.N.; Nozoe, K.T.; Tufik, S.; Andersen, M.L. Considering the effect of sleep disorders on the relation between obesity and cardiometabolic risk. *Am. J. Clin. Nutr.* **2013**, *98*, 1592. [CrossRef]
31. Bardwell, W.A.; Profant, J.; Casden, D.R.; Dimsdale, J.E.; Ancoli-Israel, S.; Natarajan, L.; Rock, C.L.; Pierce, J.P.; Women's Healthy Eating & Living (WHEL) Study Group. The relative importance of specificriskfactors for insomnia in womentreated for early-stage breastcancer. *Psychooncology* **2008**, *17*, 9–18. [CrossRef]
32. Espie, C.A.; Freedlander, E.; Campsie, L.M.; Soutar, D.S.; Robertson, A.G. Psychological distress at follow-up after major sur-gery for intra-oral cancer. *J. Psychosom. Res.* **1989**, *33*, 441–448. [CrossRef]
33. Verdonck-de Leeuw, I.M.; van Bleek, W.J.; Leemans, C.R.; de Bree, R. Employment and return to work in head and neck can-cer survivors. *Oral Oncol.* **2010**, *46*, 56–60. [CrossRef] [PubMed]
34. Irwin, M.R.; Wang, M.; Ribeiro, D.; Cho, H.J.; Olmstead, R.; Breen, E.C.; Martinez-Maza, O.; Cole, S. Sleep loss activates cellular inflammatory signaling. *Biol. Psychiatry* **2008**, *64*, 538–540. [CrossRef] [PubMed]
35. Meier-Ewert, H.K.; Ridker, P.M.; Rifai, N.; Regan, M.M.; Price, N.J.; Dinges, D.F.; Mullington, J.M. Effect of sleep loss on C-Reactive protein, an inflammatory marker of cardiovascular risk. *J. Am. Coll. Cardiol.* **2004**, *43*, 678–683. [CrossRef]
36. Irwin, M.R.; Olmstead, R.E.; Ganz, P.A.; Haque, R. Sleep disturbance, inflammation and depression risk in cancer survivors. *Brain Behav. Immun.* **2013**, *30*, S58–S67. [CrossRef]
37. Eisenberger, N.I.; Inagaki, T.K.; Mashal, N.M.; Irwin, M.R. Inflammation and social experience: An inflammatory challenge induces feelings of social disconnection in addition to depressed mood. *Brain Behav. Immun.* **2010**, *24*, 558–563. [CrossRef]
38. Silverman, S. Demographics and occurrence of oral and pharyngeal cancers. *J. Am. Dent. Assoc.* **2001**, *132*, 7S–11S. [CrossRef]
39. Howell, D.; Oliver, T.K.; Keller-Olaman, S.; Davidson, J.R.; Garland, S.; Samuels, C.; Savard, J.; Harris, C.; Aubin, M.; Olson, K.; et al. Sleep disturbance in adults with cancer: A systematic review of evidence for best practices in assessment and management for clinical practice. *Ann. Oncol.* **2014**, *25*, 791–800. [CrossRef]
40. Rondanelli, M.; Faliva, M.A.; Perna, S.; Antoniello, N. Update on the role of melatonin in the prevention of cancer tumor-igenesis and in the management of cancer correlates, such as sleep-wake and mood disturbances: Review and remarks. *Aging Clin. Exp. Res.* **2013**, *25*, 499–510. [CrossRef] [PubMed]

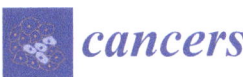

Systematic Review

Is Systemic Immunosuppression a Risk Factor for Oral Cancer? A Systematic Review and Meta-Analysis

Romeo Patini [1], Massimo Cordaro [1], Denise Marchesini [1], Francesco Scilla [1], Gioele Gioco [1,*], Cosimo Rupe [1], Maria Antonietta D'Agostino [2] and Carlo Lajolo [1]

[1] Department of Head, Neck and Sense Organs, School of Dentistry, Catholic University of Sacred Heart, Fondazione Policlinico Universitario "A. Gemelli"—IRCCS Rome, 00135 Rome, Italy; romeo.patini@unicatt.it (R.P.); massimo.cordaro@unicatt.it (M.C.); denise.marchesini01@icatt.it (D.M.); francesco.scilla01@icatt.it (F.S.); cosimorupe@gmail.com (C.R.); carlo.lajolo@unicatt.it (C.L.)

[2] Department of Geriatric and Orthopedic Sciences, Catholic University of Sacred Heart, Fondazione Policlinico Universitario "A. Gemelli"—IRCCS Rome, 00135 Rome, Italy; mariaantonietta.dagostino@unicatt.it

* Correspondence: gioele.gioco@guest.policlinicogemelli.it

Simple Summary: Immunosuppression is a medical condition in which a person's immune system is unable to function properly, or it does not function at all. It is a well-known fact that an ill-functioning immune system can favor the generation and development of potentially malignant lesions, autoimmune and allergic diseases, and even neoplasms. At present, the amount of risk for the development of oral cancer in immunosuppressed patients has not been quantitatively reported. Such a topic has been investigated, revealing that immunosuppression increases the risk of developing cancer from 0.2% to 1% (95% CI: 0.2% to 1.4%), giving further importance to the accurate follow-up of this category of patients.

Abstract: Even if the relationship between immunosuppression and increased incidence of systemic cancers is well known, there is less awareness about the risk of developing oral cancer in immunosuppressed patients. The aim of this review was to evaluate the association between immunosuppression and the development of oral cancer. Two authors independently and, in duplicate, conducted a systematic literature review of international journals and electronic databases (MEDLINE via OVID, Scopus, and Web of Science) from their inception to 28 April 2023. The assessment of risk of bias and overall quality of evidence was performed using the Newcastle–Ottawa Scale and GRADE system. A total of 2843 articles was identified, of which 44 met the inclusion criteria and were included in either the qualitative or quantitative analysis. The methodological quality of the included studies was generally high or moderate. The quantitative analysis of the studies revealed that immunosuppression should be considered a risk factor for the development of oral cancer, with a percentage of increased risk ranging from 0.2% to 1% (95% CI: 0.2% to 1.4%). In conclusion, the results suggest that a constant and accurate follow-up should be reserved for all immunosuppressed patients as a crucial strategy to intercept lesions that have an increased potential to evolve into oral cancer.

Keywords: immunosuppression; oral cancer; systematic review; meta-analysis

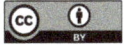

1. Introduction

According to official data from the World Health Organization (WHO, Geneva, Switzerland), 377,713 new cases of oral and lip cancer were diagnosed in 2020, making it the 16th most common cancer in the world. It still has a severe prognosis today, as approximately 50% of oral and lip cancer patients will die in the 5 years following diagnosis, while the remaining 50% have aesthetic and functional relics that make their quality of life rather low. Historically, the main risk factors for this neoplasm are being male, having a diet low in vitamins, having MPDs, past/present viral infections, radiation exposure, having genetic predispositions and immunodeficiencies, and engaging in luxuriant habits such as smoking and alcohol and betel consumption [1].

Oral cancer treatment is challenging and requires a multidisciplinary approach with a team of specialists, which includes head and neck surgeons, radiation oncologists, medical oncologists, and oral oncologists [2].

Although surgery is the most common initial definitive treatment for the majority of oral cancers, adjunctive radiotherapy (RT), with or without chemotherapy (CT) may be performed [3].

The immune system performs numerous functions, among which its primary functions are defense against infections, self-control and immunosurveillance at the onset and during the proliferation of solid and liquid cancers, identifying and suppressing genetically modified cells that have already passed the normal checkpoints, and the intracellular control of proliferation. The possible role of the immune system in the development of cancers has been defined in the theory of "immune surveillance", which configures the active role of the immune system in preventing the onset of cancers [4].

Immune surveillance against cancer is the process in which the immune system identifies cancerous and/or precancerous cells and eliminates them.

According to the most recent findings, the immune system can play a role in preventing tumors, throughout different mechanisms. First, the virus-induced tumors can be prevented when a functioning immune system can eliminate or suppress viral infections. Second, this action against pathogens may cause a prompt resolution of inflammation, preventing the establishment of an inflammatory environment, which is a risk factor for carcinogenesis [5]. Third, the immune system can identify and eliminate tumor cells on the basis of their expression of tumor-specific antigens. Therefore, the theory of immunosurveillance is essentially based on two generally accepted claims: (I) most cancers are antigenic (an obvious requirement for immunological recognition) and (II) such antigenic differences can, "under appropriate conditions", elicit an immune response [4].

Despite immune surveillance, cancers develop even in the presence of a functioning immune system, and therefore, currently, we speak of "cancer immunoediting", a term which is used to describe the evolution of tumors, wherein tumor cells become less effectively recognized and killed by the immune system [6,7].

A first consideration concerns the definition that is used for patients with disorders of the immune system. The terms immunosuppression and immunodeficiency are often used interchangeably. This confusion is related to the subtle nuance that separates them. It could be specified that immunosuppression identifies a medical condition of a general malfunction of the immune system. Immunodeficiency, on the other hand, classifies the severity of this physical deficit according to two categories: primary and secondary.

Immunosuppression is a pathological condition characterized by the inhibition of one or more components of the immune system, whether natural or acquired, resulting in the impossibility of a person's immune system to function properly. However, currently, there is no description illustrating the relationship between immunoediting and immunosuppression. The incorrect functioning of the immune system can favor the development of autoimmune and allergic diseases or neoplasms. Immunodeficiencies are divided into primary (if they are derived from congenital defects) and secondary (if they are derived from infections or pharmacological treatments) classifications. This condition involves the onset of infections that develop and recur very often, manifesting themselves in a more serious and longer-lasting form.

Among the many alterations of the immune system, immunodeficiency can be caused by numerous and different causes, and it can involve acquired or innate immunity, both in the humoral and cellular components, as follows: innate pathologies (e.g., agammaglobulinemia linked to the X sex chromosome, one common variable immunodeficiency, severe combined immunodeficiency, DiGeorge syndrome, and congenital hypogammaglobulinemia), systemic diseases (e.g., autoimmune diseases, diabetes, chronic infections, and solid and liquid malignancies, such as leukemia, lymphoma, and multiple myeloma), and pharmacological therapies (e.g., chemotherapy, antirheumatics, immunosuppressants, and glucocorticoids), which are the main causes of immunodeficiency [8,9].

By definition, immunodeficiency is characterized by a functional deficit of the immune system (either congenital or acquired). Immunosuppression is a pathological condition characterized by the inhibition of one or more components of the immune system (natural or acquired), and it occurs following an intercurrent disease or autoimmune pathologies [10]. Immunosuppression also refers to pharmacological treatment with immunosuppressive drugs capable of inhibiting an immune system response [11]. Therefore, immunocompromised patients have a reduced ability to fight infections and other diseases.

Numerous studies have shown that in immunosuppressed subjects, there is a higher incidence of cancers than in a population with normal immunity [12]. The increased susceptibility to infections (i.e., HPV, candida, Helicobacter pylori, etc.) and the reduced immune response to infections in immunosuppressed subjects could represent a further mechanism that favors the onset of neoplasms. Furthermore, immunosuppression is, at the same time, one of the risk factors for the onset of oncological pathologies, but it is also a condition that could favor the loco-regional and distant growth and spread of cancers. In fact, the literature shows that immunosuppression is not only a risk factor for the genesis of a cancer but also a factor for the prognosis of its course [13].

Although the relationship between immunosuppression and the increased incidence of systemic cancers is now well documented, currently, it is not clear how much the risk of developing oral cancer increases in immunosuppressed subjects and what effect immunosuppression has on prognosis in terms of survival. The purpose of this systematic review was, therefore, to evaluate the association and the possible correlation between the state of depression of the immune system and the development of oral cancer through the evaluation of the incidence of oral cancer in patients with systemic immunosuppression and to compare that to data from official databases (Globocan, WHO), which lacked precise data on non-immunosuppressed subjects.

2. Materials and Methods

In the present systematic review, the adopted protocol followed the Preferred Reporting Items for Systematic Reviews and Meta-Analyses (PRISMA) statement. The review protocol was registered in PROSPERO database (CRD42021243898).

2.1. PICOS Question

The following question was developed according to the population, intervention, comparison, outcome, and study design (PICOS).

Population: immunosuppressed patients who later developed oral cancer were included in this systematic review.

Intervention: patients with systemic immunodepression due to various factors (immunodepression, malnutrition, infections, autoimmune diseases, genetic immunosuppression, immunosuppression as a consequence of immunosuppressive therapy or radiotherapy, and oncologic immunosuppression) who subsequently developed oral cancer were considered.

Comparison: the rates of development of oral cancer in non-immunosuppressed patients and the rates of development of oral cancer in immunosuppressed patients were compared.

Outcome: the primary outcome was to evaluate the incidence of oral carcinoma in immunosuppressed patients.

Study design: cohorts, case controls, cross-sectional studies, and randomized clinical trials (RCTs) with no fewer than 10 patients were included. All case reports, case series with less than 10 patients, in vitro or in vivo studies based on animals, systematic reviews, letters to the editor, cases of oral cancer related to human papilloma virus (HPV), and articles published in languages other than Italian, English, and Spanish were excluded.

2.2. Focused Question

The question on which attention was focused was formulated on the basis of the PICOS criteria: "Do immunosuppressed patients have a higher rate of development of oral cancer than healthy patients?".

2.3. Research

The research was conducted on three databases (MEDLINE via OVID, Scopus, and Web of Science) from the start of their activity in May 2022, using a combination of key words and MeSH terms as follows: ((immunosuppression OR malnutrition OR infections OR autoimmune disease OR X-linked agammaglobulinemia OR common variable immunodeficiency OR selective immunoglobulin A deficiency OR hyper IgM syndrome OR DiGeorge syndrome OR severe combined immunodeficiency OR Wiskott–Aldrich syndrome OR acquired immunodeficiency syndrome OR AIDS OR immunosuppressive therapy OR radiotherapy OR "other systemic cancers" OR leukaemia OR lymphoma) AND "Oral Cancer"), ("Oral Carcinoma" AND (immunosuppression OR malnutrition OR infections OR autoimmune disease OR X-linked agammaglobulinemia OR common variable immunodeficiency OR selective immunoglobulin A deficiency OR hyper IgM syndrome OR DiGeorge syndrome OR severe combined immunodeficiency OR Wiskott–Aldrich syndrome OR acquired immunodeficiency syndrome OR AIDS OR immunosuppressive therapy OR radiotherapy OR "other systemic cancers" OR leukaemia OR lymphoma)), and ("Oral Neoplasms" AND (immunosuppression OR malnutrition OR infections OR autoimmune disease OR X-linked agammaglobulinemia OR common variable immunodeficiency OR selective immunoglobulin A deficiency OR hyper IgM syndrome OR DiGeorge syndrome OR severe combined immunodeficiency OR Wiskott–Aldrich syndrome OR acquired immunodeficiency syndrome OR AIDS OR immunosuppressive therapy OR radiotherapy OR "other systemic cancers" OR leukaemia OR lymphoma)). The date of the last search was 28 April 2023.

2.4. Manual Search

A manual search of articles published between 2002 and 2022 in the following peer-reviewed journals was performed: *Oral Oncology, Oral Diseases, Lancet Oncology,* and *Journal of Hematology and Oncology.*

2.5. Search of Unpublished Articles

Unpublished literature was searched in the U.S. National Institutes of Health clinical trials registry and the European Multidisciplinary Database to identify incumbent studies and grey literature. In addition, bibliographic references of all included articles and reviews were similarly checked to identify additional potentially relevant studies and increase the sensitivity of the search.

2.6. Study Selection

Based on the inclusion criteria, two authors independently and in duplicate (D.M. and F.S.) analyzed the titles and abstracts of the articles found. The authors retrieved the full versions of articles whose titles and abstracts appeared to meet the inclusion criteria or those, which reported insufficient data to make a clear decision. Next, the two authors independently read the full texts to determine whether the articles met these criteria. In cases where the two authors disagreed, agreement was sought through a comparison between the two, and when a solution could not be reached, a third senior author (R.P.) stepped in.

To calculate the agreement between the reviewers, Cohen's kappa coefficient was used. The level of agreement was considered excellent when k was greater than 0.75, fair to good when it was between 0.40 and 0.74, and poor when it was less than 0.4 [14].

All articles that met the inclusion criteria were subjected to data extraction and quality assessments. All irrelevant articles were excluded, and the reasons for exclusion were as described.

2.7. Extraction Data

The data were collected using a purpose-built data extraction form. In cases where the publication did not provide all the necessary data, the corresponding author was contacted by e-mail to obtain the missing data. In the event that the two authors disagreed about one of the publications, a discussion was opened, which, in cases of disagreement, required the intervention of the third author.

In cases of redundant publications, the most recent article and the one with the largest follow-up were included.

2.8. Quality Assessment

The risk of bias in the included studies was independently assessed in duplicate by two authors as part of the data extraction process.

An assessment of risk of bias was undertaken using the Newcastle–Ottawa Scale (NOS) [15]. The presence of each parameter was recorded with a green mark, while absence was recorded with a red mark (0). Papers with 1–3 green marks were classified as high risk of bias, those with 4–6 green marks were classified as medium risk, and those with 7–9 green marks were classified as low risk. A supplemental analysis was performed independently by the two examiners regarding the overall quality of the evidence for any performed meta-analysis using the Grading of Recommendations, Assessment, Development, and Evaluations (GRADE) system [16]. Any disagreement between the two reviewers (D.M. and F.S.) was solved by discussion with the author supervisor (R.P.).

Publication bias was assessed through a funnel plot, which was made using Excel software (Microsoft Excel®).

2.9. Heterogeneity Assessment

The OpenMeta software was used for assessing the heterogeneity of the studies included in any conducted meta-analysis (OpenMeta, Inc.©, Zug, Zug, Switzerland). The authors calculated the comparability of the observed proportions across the results with chance alone using the I2 test. In cases where the p-value was <0.1, the heterogeneity was considered significant. Moreover, the same test was considered as a measure of heterogeneity across studies, following the subsequent scheme [17]: 0–40%, negligible; 30–60%, moderate; 50–90%, substantial; and 75–100%, considerable.

2.10. Data Analysis

Descriptive characteristics of the studies are expressed as means/medians and/or frequencies, as appropriate, depending on the variables.

Meta-analyses were performed only when there were studies comparing similar groups and reporting the same outcomes. In such cases, the meta-analyses were performed with a fixed-effect model. A random-effect model was used only in the case of not-negligible heterogeneity across the included studies (>50%).

A forest plot was created to illustrate the effects on the meta-analysis of individual studies and the overall estimate. OpenMeta-analyst [18] was used to perform all analyses. The cut-off value of significance was set at $p < 0.05$.

3. Results

3.1. Study Selection

A flowchart of the search strategy and study selection is shown in Figure 1.

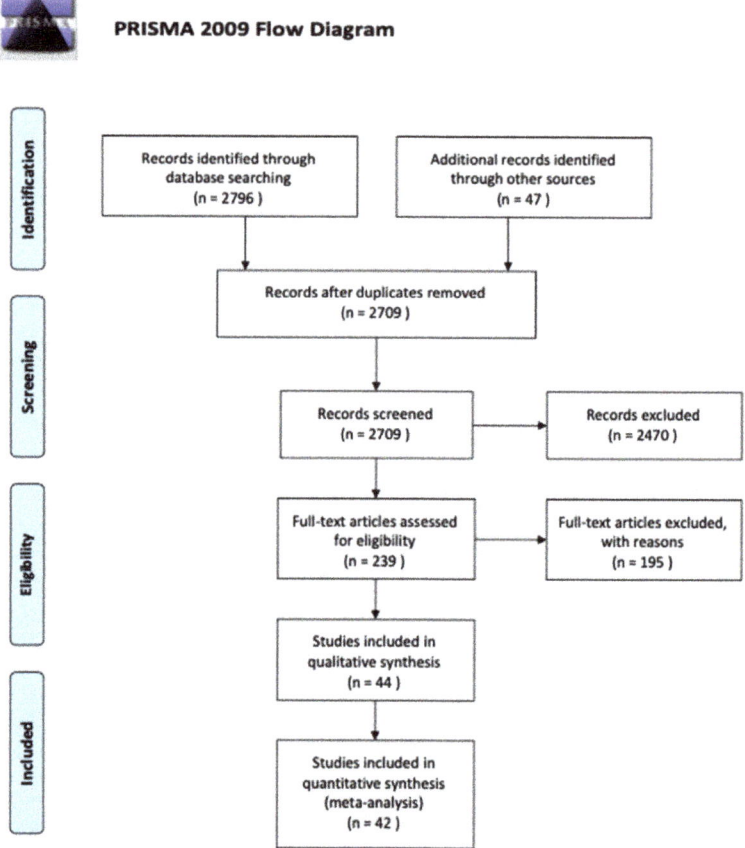

Figure 1. Flowchart of the selection of the studies for the review.

A total of 2843 articles was identified, with 2796 found through electronic searches and 47 found through other sources. Out of the 2709 studies that resulted after removal of the duplicates, 2470 were excluded as a result of title and abstract reading (inter-reader agreement, k = 0.78). Eventually, out of the 239 articles that remained to be evaluated in the full-text, 44 met the inclusion criteria and were included in either the qualitative or quantitative analyses (meta-analysis); in contrast, 195 were excluded. All information about full-text articles excluded, with reasons are included in the Supplementary Materials File (Table S1).

3.2. Study Characteristics

The characteristics of the included studies are summarized in Table 1.

Both prospective (five studies) and retrospective (nine studies) cohort studies were included in the review. Twenty-four studies presented data from national registries, and therefore, they were analyzed separately. In addition, six studies presented results related to a single immunosuppression condition, namely, graft-versus-host disease, and for this reason, they were analyzed separately, as this condition is, itself, a potentially malignant disorder of the oral cavity. All studies were conducted in an institutional environment.

Table 1. Characteristics of the included studies.

Authors-Year	Study Setting	Study Design	No. Patients (Gender)	Cause of Immunodepression	No. Patients Who Developed Oral Cancer	% of Oral Cancer (Cancer/Tot)	Age (Mean)	Gender	Aim	Oral Cancer Site	Follow Up (Years)
Spolidorio, 2006 [19]	São Paulo Hospital	P	155 (120 M, 35 F)	Organ Transplant Cyclosporin A or tacrolimus	3	1.93%	Unknown	NR	To determine the oral status of renal transplant recipients receiving cyclosporin A or tacrolimus as immunosuppressant	Lip	unknown
Jiang, 2010 [20]	Canadian Organ Replacement Register	R	1703 (1405 M, 298 F)	Heart transplantation	10	0.58%	54.4	NR	To assess the long-term risk of developing cancer among heart transplant recipients compared to the Canadian general population	NR	6.08 years
López-Pintor, 2010 [21]	Hospital Universitario 12 de Octubre, Madrid, Spain	R	500 (193 F, 307 M)	Renal transplantation	6	1.2%	57.33	M	To establish the incidence of lip cancer (LC) in a population of renal transplant patients (RTPs)	lip	18
Ferreira da Silva, 2012 [22]	Department of the federal university of Sergipe, Brazil	R	21 (7 F, 14 M)	Kidney transplantation	1	4.76%	42	M	To investigate oral lesions in kidney transplant patients	lip	2.5 (mean)
Ohman, 2014 [23]	Sahlgrenska University Hospital Register	R	4590 (2839 M, 1751 F)	Transplantation	51	1.11%	62	NR	To verify an increased risk of oral and lip cancer in solid organ transplantation patients	4 tongue, 5 salivary glands, 3 floor of mouth, 3 gingiva, palate, bucca, 34 lip	Median 6.3 years
Narayan, 2018 [24]	Medwin Hospitals, Telangana, India	P	332	Renal transplantation	5	1.50%	NR	NR	To identify the number of patients with renal transplant who developed second cancer	tongue	26
Jaamaa-Holmberg, 2019 [25]	NA	R	479 (381 M, 98 F)	Heart transplantation	13	2.71%	Unknown	NR	To demonstrate that cancer incidence in Finnish HTx-recipients is six times higher than in general Finnish population	7 lip, 4 tongue, 1 salivary glands, 1 non specified	Median 7.8 years
Laprise, 2019 [26]	The scientific Registry of transplant recipients	R	261,500 (174,475 M, 109,357 F)	Transplantation	231	0.09%	50	NR	To evaluate the incidence of lip cancer after solid organ transplantation	231 lip	Median 3.96 years

167

Table 1. Cont.

Authors-Year	Study Setting	Study Design	No. Patients (Gender)	Cause of Immunode-pression	No. Patients Who Deleveped Oral Cancer	% of Oral Cancer (Cancer/Tot)	Age (Mean)	Gender	Aim	Oral Cancer Site	Follow Up (Years)
Lin, 2019 [27]	Changhua Christian Hospital	R	455-2 (453)	Liver transplantation	5	1.10%	56	1 F, 4 M	To identify the number of head and neck cancer in liver transplant recipients	3 tongue, 1 retromolar trigone, 1 buccal mucosa, 1 parotid gland	NR
				Other Cancers							
Johns, 1986 [28]	Johns Hopkins Medical Istitutions, Baltimore	R	384 (206 F, 178 M)	Salivary gland or thyroid gland malignancies	3	0.78%	NR	1 F, 2 M	To determine the exact risk of multiple primary neoplasms in patients with salivary gland or thyroid gland malignancies	3 salivary glands	10
Guttman, 1991 [29]	Tel Aviv Medical Center	P	370 (133 M, 237 F)	Melanoma	3	0.81%	60.5	F	To identify the number of patients with GVHD who developed second cancer	NR	Different based on stages
Lishner, 1991 [30]	Princess Margaret Hospital, Toronto	R	321	Non-Hodgkin's lymphoma	4	1.24%	48	3 M, 1 unknown	To evaluate the incidence of second malignant tumors in patients with Non-Hodgkin's lymphoma	3 tongue, 1 gingiva	At least 6 months
Hiyama, 1991 [31]	Department of field research, Osaka	R	61,168 (22,391 F; 38,777 M)	Stomach cancer	51	0.08%	NR	NR	To determine the risk of second primary cancer after diagnosis of stomach cancer in Osaka	NR	30
Spitz, 1992 [32]	National Cancer Institute	R	48,940 (F)	Cervix cancer	34	0.07%	NR	F	To evaluate the association between malignancies of the upper aerodigestive tract and uterine cervix	NR	11 years
Rabkin, 1992 [33]	National cancer institute, Belthesda	R	28,160 (25,295 F; 2865 M)	Anal and cervical carcinoma	51	0.18%	NR	NR	To determine the risk of second primary cancer following anal and cervical carcinoma	NR	NR
Levi, 1997 [34]	The Cancer Registries, Switzerland	R	4639	Skin Cancer	16	0.34%	74	NR	To evaluate the incidence of second primary cancers in patients with skin cancer	5 lip, 3 salivary gland, 8 mouth	23 years

Table 1. *Cont.*

Authors-Year	Study Setting	Study Design	No. Patients (Gender)	Cause of Immunode-pression	No. Patients Who Deleveped Oral Cancer	% of Oral Cancer (Cancer/Tot)	Age (Mean)	Gender	Aim	Oral Cancer Site	Follow Up (Years)
Levi, 1999 [35]	University of Milan, Italy	R	5794	Lung carcinoma	15	0.26%	NR	NR	To determine the risk of second primary cancer in patients with lung carcinoma	NR	22
Levi, 2007 [36]	Université de Lausanne	R	1672 (424 F, 1248 M)	Esophageal cancer	67	4.00%	55	NR	To determine the risk of second neoplasms after esophageal cancer	NR	30
Chuang, 2008 [37]	Lyon, France	R	52,589 (19,110 F, 33,479 M)	Esophageal cancer	92	0.18%	NR	NR	To assess the risk of second primary cancers following a first primary esophageal cancer	NR	10
Brown, 2010 [38]	The National Cancer Institute's Survival	R	69,620 (F)	Endometrial cancer	143	0.20%	62	F	To examine the risk of subsequent primary malignancies (SPMs) in women diagnosed with endometrial cancer.	NR	11.2 years
Zhu, 2011 [39]	Academy of Medical Sciences, Gansu, China	R	24,557 (6253 F, 18,304 M)	Treatment of esophageal cancer	162	0.66%	NR	NR	To determine the risk of second primary cancer after treatment for esophageal cancer	NR	34
Hsu, 2014 [40]	Taiwan's National Health Insurance	R	9423 (1940 M, 7483 F)	Thyroid cancer	53	0.56%	NR	NR	To determine the association of thyroid cancer with other malignancies in Taiwan.	40 mouth, 13 salivary glands	NR
Robsahm, 2014 [41]	Cancer Registry of Norway	R	52,689 (28,069 CMM, 24,620 SCC)	Squamous cell carcinoma and melanomas	47 (CMM), 152 (SCC)	0.37%	NR	33 M, 14 F (CMM)/ 114 M, 38 F (SCC)	To examine the risk of a new primary cancer following an initial skin cancer	NR	10.1
Davis, 2014 [42]	University of Michigan Medical school	R	441,504 (M)	Prostate cancer	1251	0.28%	NR	NR	To determine the risk of second primary tumors in men with prostate cancer	NR	10
Hyeon Bae, 2015 [43]	Chonnam National University Hospital, Hwasun, Korea	R	452 (208 M, 244 F)	Melanoma	1	0.22%	Unknown	NR	To assess the presence of other primary cancer in patients with acral and non-acral melanomas	NR	No
Krilaviciute, 2016 [44]	National cancer institute, Vilnius, Lithuania	R	12,584 (8074 F, 4510 M)	Basal cell carcinoma	39	0.31%	NR	NR	To determine the risk of second primary cancer in basal cell carcinoma patients in Lithuania	14 lip, 25 other in oral cavity	14

Table 1. Cont.

Authors-Year	Study Setting	Study Design	No. Patients (Gender)	Cause of Immunodepression	No. Patients Who Developed Oral Cancer	% of Oral Cancer (Cancer/Tot)	Age (Mean)	Gender	Aim	Oral Cancer Site	Follow Up (Years)
Schlieve, 2016 [45]	University of Tennessee	R	19,406/849	Primary Non-head-neck cancer	32	80%/	67	NR	To determine the rate of second primary head and neck cancer development among patients with a primary cancer diagnosed outside of the head and neck region, to present the clinical characteristics of this population, and to determine if any variables are associated with survival.	11 gingiva, 7 tongue, 4 base of tongue, 4 buccal, 3 floor of mouth, 2 palate, 1 parotid	10 years
Boakye, 2020 [46]	National Cancer Institute's Surveillance	R	2,903,241	First primary cancers	1877	0.064	63.1	1303 M, 574 F	To describe the risk of developing a second primary cancer among survivors of 10 cancer sites with the highest survival rates in the United States	1462 tongue, 343 floor, 72 salivary glands	3.8 years
Wu, 2020 [47]	People's hospital of Nanjing, China	R	1161 (542 F, 619 M)	Pulmonary high-grade neuroendocrine carcinoma	13	1.12%	NR	NR	To determine the risk of second primary cancer in patients with pulmonary high-grade neuroendocrine carcinoma	floor of mouth, and gum and other mouth	16
				Infectious Diseases							
Song, 2019 [48]	The China Kadoorie Biobank	R	(a) 496,732 (203,660 M, 294,072 F) (b)37,336 (c) 97 (73 M, 24 F)	HBV	(a) 415 (b) no cases c) NR	(a) 1.98%/ 0.08% (b) no c) NR	(a) 51.5 (b)	NR	To assess the association between chronic HBV infection and risk of all cancer types	NR	(a) 8.85 (b)
Su, 2020 [49]	National Health insurance Research Database	P	100,058 (50,029 HCV-50,029 NO HCV) + 47,904 (23 952 therapy-23,952 no therapy)	HCV and anti-HCV therapy	229 (NO-HCV) 265 (HCV) + 146 (no therapy) 58 (therapy)	0.47%	59 (1 group)- 51 (2 group)	NR	To investigate the association between chronic hepatitis C and oral cancer, and the development of oral cancer after anti-hepatitis C virus (HCV) therapy	NR	7.9 years non-HCV/5.1 years HCV + 4.9 years no therapy/ 3.4 years therapy

Table 1. Cont.

Authors-Year	Study Setting	Study Design	No. Patients (Gender)	Cause of Immunode-pression	No. Patients Who Developed Oral Cancer	% of Oral Cancer (Cancer/Tot)	Age (Mean)	Gender	Aim	Oral Cancer Site	Follow Up (Years)
Mahale, 2020 [50]	Surveillance, Epidemiology, and End Results (SEER)	R	531,460 (384,777 M, 146,683 F)	HIV+/lymphoid malignancies	511	0.01%	NR	NR	To describe the risk of cancers following lymphoid malignancies among HIV-infected people.	NR	NR
				HSC							
Yokota, 2010 [51]	Kanto Study Group for Cell Therapy	R	2062 (1225 M, 837 F)	Allogeneic hematopoietic SCT	10	35.7%/0.48%	42	5 M, 4 F, 1 Unknown	To evaluate the incidence and risk factors for secondary solid tumors in Japan after hematopoietic SCT	5 tongue, 3 gingiva, 2 oral mucosa	Median 5.7 years
Curtis, 2016 [52]	Center for International Blood and Marrow Transplant Research	P	24011	GVHD	24	13.11%/0.1%	NR	NR	To identify the number of patients with GVHD who developed second cancer	NR	30
Majhail, 2016 [53]	Center for International Blood and Marrow Transplant Research	R	4318 (2415 M, 1903 F)	Hematopoietic cell transplant	11	16.6%/0.25%	44	NR	To evaluate the risk of secondary solid cancers among allogeneic hematopoietic cell transplant recipients	NR	NR
Dyer, 2018 [54]	Blood and Marrow Transplant Network, Australia.	P	441 (191 F, 250 M)	Blood and marrow transplant	4	1.5%	NR	NR	To investigate oral health in blood and marrow transplant recipients	NR	12
Anak, 2018 [55]	Istanbul University Faculty of Medicine, Our Istanbul Children Leukemia Foundation BMT Center	P	24 (12 M, 12 F)	Hematopoietic cell transplantation in Fanconi Anemia patients	4	21	NR	To investigate SCC development after HSCT and examine features of the follow-up patients	4 retromolar trigone	NR	NR

Table 1. Cont.

Authors-Year	Study Setting	Study Design	No. Patients (Gender)	Cause of Immunode-pression	No. Patients Who Deleveped Oral Cancer	% of Oral Cancer (Cancer/Tot)	Age (Mean)	Gender	Aim	Oral Cancer Site	Follow Up (Years)
Santarone, 2020 [56]	Bone marrow transplant center, Ospedale civile, Pescara, Italy	R	908 (498 M, 410 F)	Hematopoietic cell transplantation	12	100%/1.32%	47	8 M, 4 F	To demonstrate that oral cGVHD and a diagnosis of non-malignant hematologic disease are strong risk factors in the SOC development	6 tongue, 1 lower lip, 3 cheek mucosa, 1 gingival fornix, 1 hard palate	Unknown
				Inflammatory Diseases							
Bensing, 2008 [57]	National Death Register/Swedish Cancer Register	R	3299 (1359 M, 1940 F)	Autoimmune primary adrenocortical insufficiency	10	0.30%	NR	NR	To assess the increased death risk and altered cancer incidence in patients with autoimmune primary adrenocortical insufficiency	NR	29 years
Zhang, 2009 [58]	Peking Union Medical College Hospital	R	1320 (1201 F, 119 M)	Sjögren's syndrome	3	10%	50.7	NR	To identify the incidence of malignancy in primary Sjögren's syndrome	2 tongue, 1 parotid gland	4.4 (mean)
Katsanos KH, 2015 [59]	Clinical Gastroenterology and Hepatology, NT; USA	R	7294 (3785 F, 3509 M)	Inflammatory bowel disease (IBD)	11	0.15%	44.6	4 F, 7 M	To identify the number of patients with IBD that developed oral cancer	6 tongue, 2 hard palate, 3 buccal	NR
Rautemaa, 2016 [60]	Helsinki Hospital, Finland	R	92 (47 F, 45 M)	APECED	6	6.52%	37	2 F, 4 M	To study the possible association of APECED with oral and esophageal carcinoma.	buccal mucosa	NR
Derk, 2019 [21]	Thomas Jefferson University Philadelphia, Pennsylvania, USA	P	769	Systemic sclerosis	9	1.17%	49.2	NR	To describe the incidence of carcinoma of the tongue in a cohort of patients with systemic sclerosis	tongue	16
				NR							
Atsuta, 2014 [61]	Transplant Registry Unified Management Program	R	17545 (10,386 M, 7149 F)	NR	64	23.80%	NR	NR	To determine the incidence and the risk factors for secondary solid tumors after allogenic stem cell transplantation	NR	NR

NR: Not reported, P: Prospective, R: Retrospective.

3.3. Assessment of the Risk of Bias

The risk of bias is summarized in Figures 2 and 3. The methodological quality of the included studies was high for 12 studies [19,22,24,25,28,31–33,36,51,53,58], moderate for 26 studies [20,21,23,25,26,29,30,32,34,37–50,52,54–57,60–62], and low for six studies [23,26,27,35,48,59].

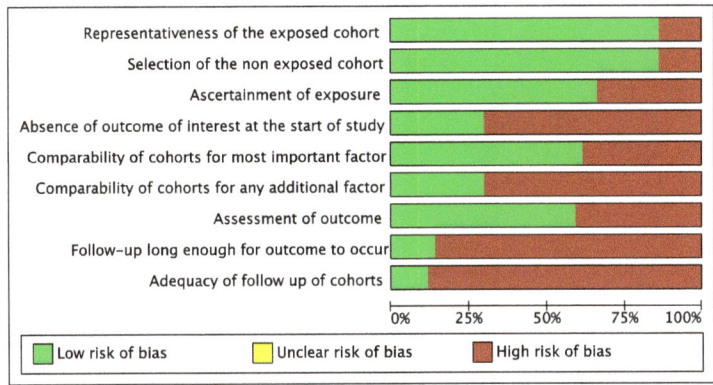

Figure 2. Risk of bias graph.

The results regarding publication bias are presented in Figures 4–6. Significant publication bias was found in the studies that presented results related to Graft Versus Host Disease (GVHD) and the national registries. The Grading of Recommendations, Assessment, Development, and Evaluations (GRADE) system provided information on the certainty of the conclusions and the strength of the evidence (Table 2). Although the meta-analyses drew conclusions from cohort studies, which are considered to be among the best-available evidence, they were considered to have only moderate strength of evidence because of the presence of at least one study with a high risk of bias and very wide confidence intervals.

Table 2. GRADE summary of findings for meta-analysis on immunosuppression and oral cancer incidence.

Quality Assessment, Outcome: Oral Cancer Incidence in Patients with Immunosuppression						
Question: Does the Immunosuppression Condition Have Influence on Oral Cancer Incidence?						
Number of Studies according to meta-analysis	Study design	Risk of Bias	Inconsistency	Indirectness	Imprecision	Publication bias
Meta-analysis on data from national registers (Figure 7): 23 studies	Cohort studies	Serious	Serious [a]	Not Serious	Serious [b]	Detected (1 study)
Meta-analysis on data not from national registers (Figure 8): 14 studies	Cohort studies	Serious	Not Serious	Not Serious	Serious [b]	Undetected
Meta-analysis on GVHD patients (Figure 9): 5 studies	Cohort studies	Serious	Serious [a]	Not Serious	Serious [b]	Detected (1 study)

[a]. Due to high heterogeneity across studies. [b]. Due to wide confidence intervals.

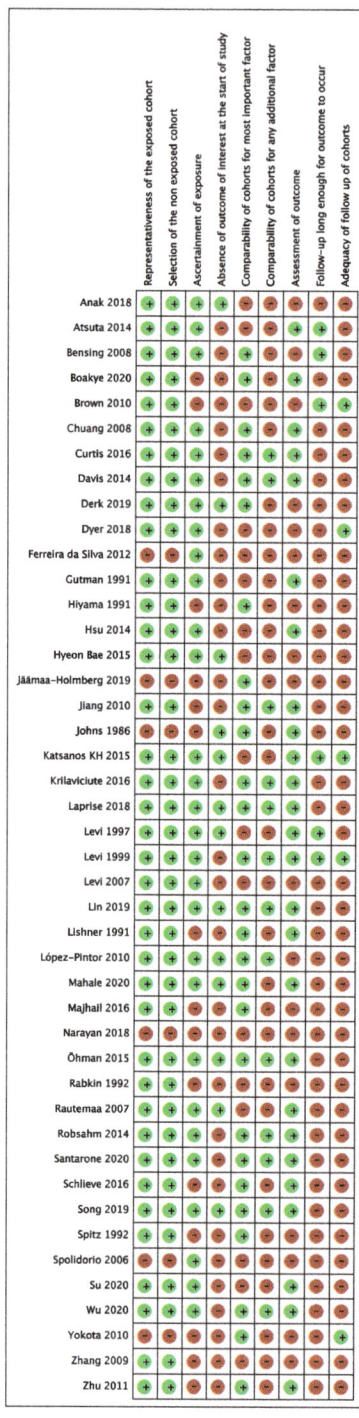

Figure 3. Risk of bias summary [19–62].

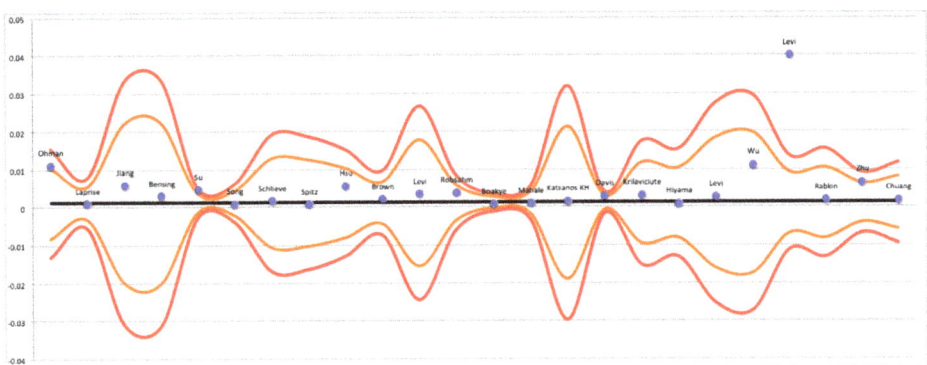

Figure 4. Funnel plot of studies with data from national registries [20,23,26,31–42,44–50,57,59].

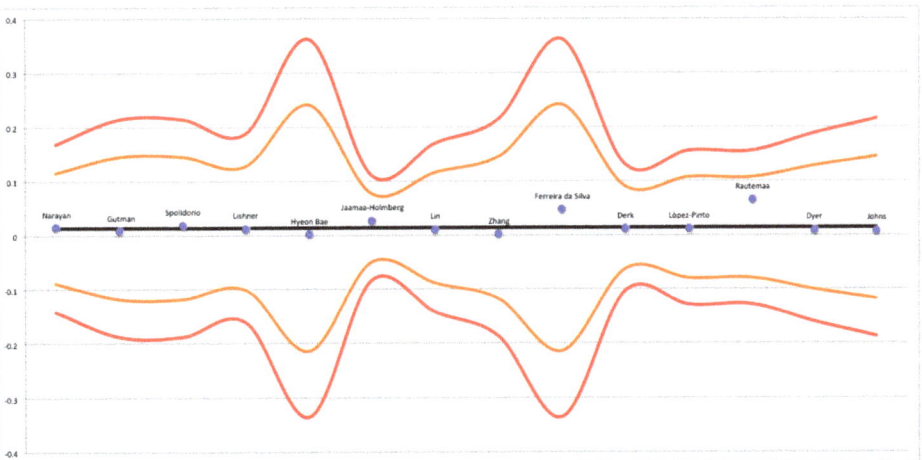

Figure 5. Funnel plot of studies with data not from national registries [19,21,22,24,25,27–30,43,54,58,60].

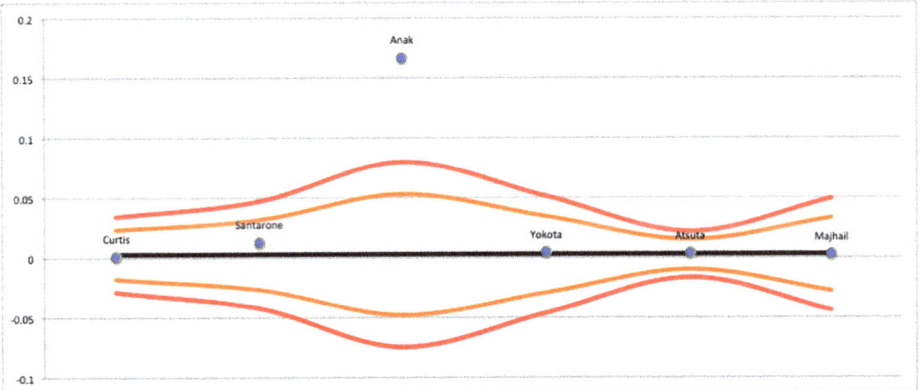

Figure 6. Funnel plot of studies with data about GVHD [51–53,55,56,61].

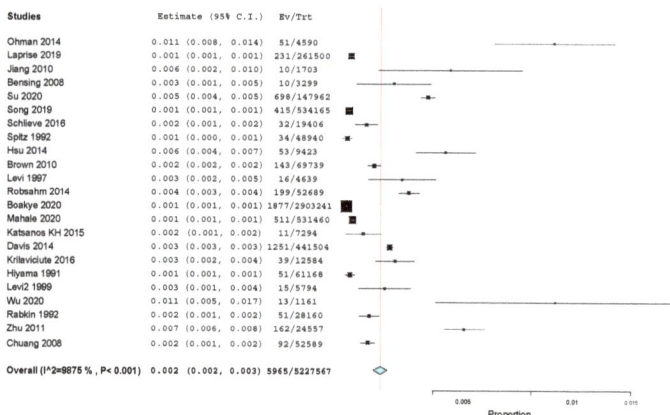

Figure 7. Meta-analysis related to data coming from national registries [20,23,26,31–35,37–42,44–50,57,59].

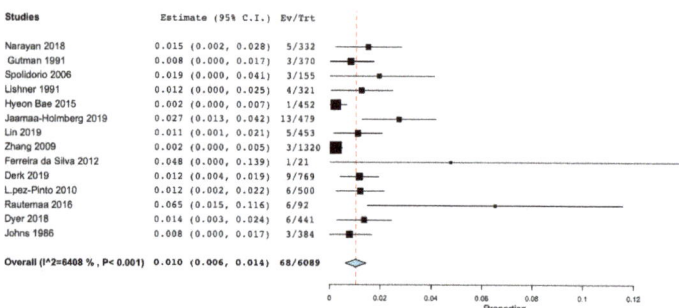

Figure 8. Meta-analysis related to data not coming from national registries [19,21,22,24,25,27–30,43,54,58,60,62].

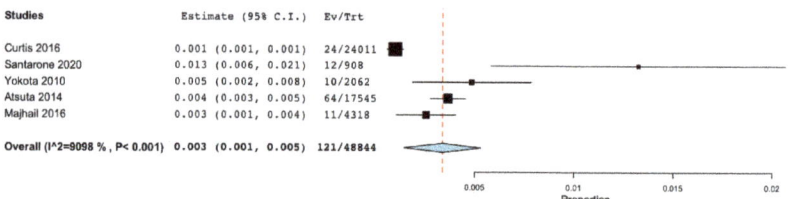

Figure 9. Meta-analysis regarding data about GVHD [51–53,56,61].

3.4. Results of the Meta-Analyses

As reported earlier, three separate meta-analyses were conducted. The meta-analysis related to the national registries (Figure 7) was conducted on 23 studies with a total of 5,227,567 patients and found an "untransformed proportion" (PR) of 0.2% (95% CI: 0.002–0.003) (p-value of <0.001).

The meta-analysis concerning data not derived from the national registries (Figure 8) was conducted on 15 studies with a total of 6997 patients and found an "untransformed proportion" (PR) of 1% (95% CI: 0.006–0.014) (p-value of <0.001).

The meta-analysis regarding data about GVHD (Figure 9) was conducted on six studies with a total of 49,285 patients and found an "untransformed proportion" (PR) of 0.3% (95% CI: 0.001–0.005) (p-value of < 0.001).

The meta-analyses conducted on the three groups of patients revealed a general increased risk of developing an oral cancer in immunosuppressed populations. Such risk ranges from 0.2% to 1% depending on whether data from national registries are considered. In immunosuppressed patients, this evidence emphasizes the need to provide for a careful follow-up of suspicious lesions and potentially malignant disorders of the oral cavity.

4. Discussion

4.1. Summary of the Main Findings

The close relationship between the immune system and cancer immunoediting has been documented for many years for numerous cancers, including oral carcinoma, and this systematic review highlighted an incidence of oral carcinoma in immunosuppressed patients of 200 new cases per 100,000. If this is compared to data from registries on the incidence of oral cancer in the general population, which is approximately 4.1 per 100,000 subjects (ASR incidence = 4.1 per 100,000), immunosuppressed subjects have a risk of developing oral cancer that is 50 times higher than the general population. These raw data emphasize the need to establish clinical protocols for primary prevention and screening in all immunosuppressed subjects, likely with tailor-made protocols that depend on the cause of immunosuppression and the severity of the immunosuppression.

Some considerations of a methodological nature that emerged from this systematic review should be made in light of the literature. A first consideration concerns the definition that is used for patients with disorders of the immune system. The terms immunosuppression and immunodeficiency are often used interchangeably. This confusion is related to the subtle nuance that separates them. It could be specified that immunosuppression identifies a medical condition involving a general malfunction of the immune system, whereas immunodeficiency classifies the severity of this deficit into primary and secondary in relation to the cause. Furthermore, an aspect still unresolved concerns the identification of clinical and/or instrumental parameters that can identify the state of immunosuppression (considering both innate and acquired immunity, both cellular and humoral) and classify it in relation to the severity of the immunosuppression.

The present systematic review demonstrated that immunosuppression should be considered a risk factor for the development of oral cancer, with a percentage of increased risk ranging from 0.2% to 1% (95% CI: 0.2% to 1.4%). Considering the main causes of immunosuppression reported in the selected articles, there are some interesting considerations. In fact, in this systematic review, the authors decided to divide the results from the included papers into three main groups: the results derived from the literature analysis of the main reasons for immunosuppression (not from national registries), those from articles related to GVHD, and those from the registry analysis, which depict an increased risk of 1% (95% CI: 0.6% to 1.4%), of 0.3% (95% CI: 0.1% to 0.5%), and of 0.2% (95% CI: 0.2% to 0.3%), respectively. Articles referring to states of malnutrition were not included in this review, as they did not report adequate information regarding immune status.

4.2. Organ Transplantation

Organ transplantation, in particular, kidney transplantation, represents one of the main causes of immunosuppression most frequently associated with the onset of oral cavity neoplasms. The increased life expectancy of transplant recipients exposes them to prolonged immunosuppressive therapy (mainly cyclosporine), which is necessary to avoid the phenomenon of transplant rejection. In the study conducted by López-Pintor [62], 500 kidney transplant patients were recruited, and during follow-up, six cases of oral cancer were reported out of 500 patients (incidence of 1 patient per 100 subjects).

The same trend was seen for patients undergoing heart transplantation (HTx). Due to new techniques introduced in transplant surgery, survival after heart transplantation has improved significantly in recent decades. In the study conducted by Jäämä-Holmberg (2019) [25], the risk of oral cancer after organ transplantation was two to four times higher than that of the general population, becoming one of the main long-term complications in this group of patients. Furthermore, it would appear that oral cancer occurs with a higher frequency in subjects who have undergone thoracic organ transplantation rather than those who have undergone abdominal organ transplants (i.e., liver and kidney). This different risk of oral cancer in relation to the type of organ transplanted could be partly related to the different pharmacological regimens adopted and partly linked to the underlying pathologies that lead to the need for transplants. Further studies should stratify the risk of oral cancer in relation to the type of organ transplanted.

4.3. Other Cancers

Another cause of immunosuppression associated with a greater risk of developing oral cavity cancer is represented by the treatment of thyroid neoplasms. The number of newly diagnosed cases of thyroid cancer has increased in recent years due to technological advances and the spread of cytological tests for early diagnosis. Patients who underwent partial or total thyroidectomy and those who received radio-iodine treatment for the treatment of thyroid cancer reported an increased risk of developing oral cancer. The study by Hsu et al. (2014) [40] showed an increased association between thyroid cancer and subsequent head and neck cancer. This association found that its biochemical-molecular explanation was related to the intrinsic carcinogenic action of radio-iodine, which can possibly be enhanced by pre-existing molecular genetic mutations in a framework of immunological impairment linked to the partial or total removal of the thyroid.

4.4. Infectious Agents

Other known causes of immunosuppressive states are infectious agents (i.e., HCV, HIV, and HPV). This literature review reported only one study, which was conducted by Su et al. [49] that highlighted an incidence of 698 cases of carcinoma out of 147,962 patients. The risk of oral cancer appears to be lower in HCV patients receiving pegylated interferon (PEG-IFN) therapy than that of untreated HCV patients. Further studies should investigate the role of HCV infection in oral cancer oncogenesis, with particular attention paid to the type of therapy administered to patients.

Studies investigating the role of HIV as a cause of immunosuppression were not included in this review. In fact, it is known that HIV infection causes a depletion of CD4+ T lymphocytes, with consequent impairment of the immune system. Acquired immunodeficiency could, therefore, lead to an increased risk of oral cancer. The study conducted by Precious K. Motlokwa et al. (2022) on an oral cancer population in sub-Saharan Africa did not show an increased risk of carcinogenicity in a group of HIV-infected patients [63]. This could be partly explained by new antiretroviral therapies, which allow clinicians to gain control of HIV infections and, therefore, reduce the impairment of patients' immune systems. Further studies are needed to evaluate whether there is a real risk in HIV-positive patients and whether there are associated risk factors (CD4 T lymphocyte count or traditional antiretroviral therapies vs HAART).

4.5. Hematopoietic Stem Cell Transplantation (HSC)

Within the selected articles, it was possible to identify a group of articles conducted on patients undergoing hematopoietic stem cell transplantation (HSC), which now represents an essential therapy for the treatment of various haemato-lymphoproliferative diseases and other benign conditions (multiple myeloma, lymphomas, autoimmune disorders, etc.). In the study conducted by Santarone et al. (2020) [56], patients undergoing HSC transplantation reported the incidence of developing a malignancy at double the rate of the general population. In support of this, Dyer and colleagues [54] also found a similar incidence rate in patients undergoing HSC transplantation, underlining the importance of regular follow-ups with patients.

Furthermore, GVHD is among the adverse events associated with HSC transplantation. This clinical condition represents an adverse immunological phenomenon following HSC transplantation. GVHD oral lesions are among the so-called potentially malignant disorders, as they have a greater risk of neoplastic degeneration than healthy mucosa. Furthermore, the most frequently used therapy in the treatment of GVHD involves the use of immunosuppressive agents (e.g., both topical and high potency systemic corticosteroids and calcineurin inhibitors), which, although they reduce the inflammatory component of GVHD lesions, could increase the risk of developing a secondary malignancy. The risk of developing malignancy in patients with chronic GVHD was significantly increased compared with the general population, with a standard incidence ratio (SIR) of 1.8 and a 95% confidence interval (95% CI) of 1.5–2.0. The risk is much higher for cancer of the oral cavity (SIR = 15.7, 95% CI, 12.1–20.1), cancer of the esophagus (SIR = 8.5, 95% CI, 6.1–11.5), colon cancer (SIR = 1.9, 95% CI, 1.2–2.7), skin cancer (SIR = 7.2, 95% CI, 3.9–12.4), and cancers of the nervous system (SIR = 4.1, 95% CI, 1.2–8.4). The risk of developing oral, esophageal, or skin cancer appears to have a maximum incidence 1 year after transplantation [61].

4.6. Strengths and Limitations of the Present Systematic Review

Finally, the data obtained from this systematic review were partly extrapolated from the analysis of national registers from China, Japan, Republic of Korea, India, Taiwan, and Nordic Scandinavian countries. As these databases have a large amount of data, they can lead to significant statistical variations capable of creating very significant discrepancies in the results. In light of this, a meta-analysis dedicated solely to the analysis of the data obtained from these registries was conducted in this systematic review. It is also known that cancer of the oral cavity has a notably high incidence in the aforementioned countries (e.g., China and India) due to the different cultural and social habits. The funnel plot shown in Figure 4 revealed the presence of some studies with particularly discrepant data with respect to the confidence interval of the meta-analysis. Specifically, the study conducted by Levi et al. was discrepant to the funnel plot, and for this reason, it was removed from the statistical analysis and presented only in a qualitative form.

From a methodological point of view, all the studies included in this review had the main objective of investigating the incidence of cancer in other sites. Therefore, further prospective observational studies evaluating the occurrence of oral cancers in immunosuppressed patients as the main outcome while also taking into account the main risk factors of oral cancer that may influence this association (e.g., smoking, candida, HPV, and alcohol) are required. Moreover, it is essential to consider adequate follow-ups to avoid an underestimation of the real incidence of oral carcinomas. The time factor certainly plays an important role in the carcinogenic process, considering that a prolonged state of immunosuppression can increase the risk of the onset of neoplasms.

5. Conclusions

The results obtained from the systematic review indicated that immunosuppression is to be considered a risk factor for the development of oral cancer.

Particular attention and accurate follow-ups with all immunosuppressed patients are, therefore, essential in order to intercept clinical situations at an early stage that could evolve into oral cancer.

Further studies are needed to investigate the effective role of immunosuppression in carcinogenesis and to identify any risk factors.

Supplementary Materials: The following supporting information can be downloaded at: https://www.mdpi.com/article/10.3390/cancers15123077/s1, Table S1. Full-text articles excluded, with reason [64–218].

Author Contributions: Conceptualization, C.L.; methodology, R.P.; validation, C.L., M.A.D. and R.P.; formal analysis, G.G.; data curation, F.S. and D.M.; writing—original draft preparation, R.P., F.S. and D.M.; writing—review and editing, C.L. and R.P.; visualization, C.R. and M.A.D.; supervision, M.C. All authors have read and agreed to the published version of the manuscript.

Funding: This research received no external funding.

Institutional Review Board Statement: Not applicable.

Informed Consent Statement: Not applicable.

Data Availability Statement: Data are available upon request to the corresponding author.

Conflicts of Interest: The authors declare no conflict of interest.

References

1. Rivera, C. Essentials of oral cancer. *Int. J. Clin. Exp. Pathol.* **2015**, *8*, 11884–11894. [PubMed]
2. Liu, J.; Kaplon, A.; Blackman, E.; Miyamoto, C.; Savior, D.; Ragin, C. The Impact of the Multidisciplinary Tumor Board on Head and Neck Cancer Outcomes. *Laryngoscope* **2020**, *130*, 946–950. [CrossRef] [PubMed]
3. Shanti, R.M.; O'Malley, B.W. Surgical Management of Oral Cancer. *Dent. Clin. N. Am.* **2018**, *86*, 77–86. [CrossRef] [PubMed]
4. Burnet, M. Immunological factors in the process of carcinogenesis. *Br. Med. Bull.* **1964**, *20*, 154–158. [CrossRef] [PubMed]
5. Swann, J.B.; Smyth, M.J. Immune surveillance of tumors. *J. Clin. Investig.* **2007**, *117*, 1137–1146. [CrossRef] [PubMed]
6. Bird, L. Innate surveillance. *Nat. Rev. Immunol.* **2016**, *16*, 132–133. [CrossRef] [PubMed]
7. Lodish, H. *Molecular Biology of the Cell*, 5th ed.; Macmillan: New York, NY, USA, 2004.
8. Chinen, J.; Shearer, W.T. Secondary immunodeficiencies, including HIV infection. *J. Allergy Clin. Immunol.* **2010**, *125*, S195–S203. [CrossRef] [PubMed]
9. Notarangelo, L.D.; Bacchetta, R.; Casanova, J.L.; Su, H.C. Human inborn errors of immunity: An expanding universe. *Sci. Immunol.* **2020**, *5*, eabb1662. [CrossRef] [PubMed]
10. Rice, J.M. Immunosuppression. In *Tumour Site Concordance and Mechanisms of Carcinogenesis*; IARC Scientific Publications (No. 165); Baan, R.A., Stewart, B.W., Straif, K., Eds.; International Agency for Research on Cancer: Lyon, France, 2019; Chapter 16.
11. Geisser, E.K. Immunosuppression. *Cancer Treat. Res.* **2009**, *146*, 23–43.
12. Kumar, M. Oral cancer: Etiology and risk factors: A review. *J. Cancer Res. Ther.* **2016**, *12*, 458–463. [CrossRef] [PubMed]
13. Vial, T.; Descotes, J. Immunosuppressive drugs and cancer. *Toxicology* **2003**, *185*, 229–240. [CrossRef] [PubMed]
14. Landis, J.R.; Koch, G.G. The measurement of observer agreement for categorical data. *Biometrics* **1977**, *33*, 159–174. [CrossRef] [PubMed]
15. Wells, G.A. The Newcastle-Ottawa Scale (NOS) for Assessing the Quality of Nonrandomised studies in Meta-Analyses. *Eur. J. Epidemiol.* **2014**, *25*, 603–605.
16. Guyatt, G.H. GRADE: An emerging consensus on rating quality of evidence and strength of recommendations. *BMJ* **2008**, *336*, 924. [CrossRef] [PubMed]
17. Higgins, J.P.T. Measuring in consistency in meta-analyses. *BMJ* **2003**, *327*, 557–560. [CrossRef] [PubMed]
18. Wallace, B.C. Closing the Gap between Methodologists and End-Users: R as a Computational Back-End. *J. Stat. Softw.* **2012**, *49*, 1–15. [CrossRef]
19. Spolidorio, L.C. Oral health in renal transplant recipients administered cyclosporin A or tacrolimus. *Oral Dis.* **2006**, *12*, 309–314. [CrossRef] [PubMed]
20. Jiang, Y.; Villeneuve, P.J.; Wielgosz, A.; Schaubel, D.E.; Fenton, S.S.; Mao, Y. The incidence of cancer in a population-based cohort of Canadian heart transplant recipients. *Am. J. Transpl.* **2010**, *10*, 637–645. [CrossRef] [PubMed]
21. Derk, C.T.; Rasheed, M.; Spiegel, J.R.; Jimenez, S.A. Increased incidence of carcinoma of the tongue in patients with systemic sclerosis. *J. Rheumatol.* **2005**, *32*, 637–641.
22. Da Silva, L.C.; de Almeida Freitas, R.; de Andrade, M.P., Jr.; Piva, M.R.; Martins-Filho, P.R.; de Santana Santos, T. Oral lesions in renal transplant. *J. Craniofac. Surg.* **2012**, *23*, e214–e218. [CrossRef] [PubMed]
23. Öhman, J.; Rexius, H.; Mjörnstedt, L.; Gonzalez, H.; Holmberg, E.; Dellgren, G.; Hasséus, B. Oral and lip cancer in solid organ transplant patients—A cohort study from a Swedish Transplant Centre. *Oral. Oncol.* **2015**, *51*, 146–150. [CrossRef] [PubMed]
24. Narayan, G. Carcinoma of the Tongue in Renal Transplant Recipients: An Unusual Spectrum of De Novo Malignancy at a Tertiary Care Center in India over a Period of 26 Years. *Indian J. Nephrol.* **2018**, *28*, 119–126. [PubMed]
25. Jäämaa-Holmberg, S.; Salmela, B.; Lemström, K.; Pukkala, E.; Lommi, J. Cancer incidence and mortality after heart transplantation—A population-based national cohort study. *Acta. Oncol.* **2019**, *58*, 859–863. [CrossRef] [PubMed]
26. Laprise, C.; Cahoon, E.K.; Lynch, C.F.; Kahn, A.R.; Copeland, G.; Gonsalves, L.; Madeleine, M.M.; Pfeiffer, R.M.; Engels, E.A. Risk of lip cancer after solid organ transplantation in the United States. *Am. J. Transpl.* **2019**, *19*, 227–237. [CrossRef] [PubMed]
27. Lin, N.C.; Chen, Y.L.; Tsai, K.Y. Head and neck cancer in living donor liver transplant recipients: Single center retrospective study. *Medicine* **2019**, *98*, PMC6709202. [CrossRef]
28. Johns, M.E.; Shikhani, A.H.; Kashima, H.K.; Matanoski, G.M. Multiple primary neoplasms in patients with salivary gland or thyroid gland tumors. *Laryngoscope* **1986**, *96*, 718–721. [CrossRef]
29. Gutman, M. Are malignant melanoma patients at higher risk for a second cancer? *Cancer* **1991**, *68*, 660–665. [CrossRef] [PubMed]
30. Lishner, M. Second malignant neoplasms in patients with non Hodgkin's lymphoma. *Hematol. Oncol.* **1991**, *9*, 169–179. [CrossRef] [PubMed]
31. Hiyama, T.; Hanai, A.; Fujimoto, I. Second primary cancer after diagnosis of stomach cancer in Osaka, Japan. *Jpn. J. Cancer Res.* **1991**, *82*, 762–770. [CrossRef] [PubMed]
32. Spitz, M.R.; Sider, J.G.; Schantz, S.P.; Newell, G.R. Association between malignancies of the upper aerodigestive tract and uterine cervix. *Head Neck* **1992**, *14*, 347–351. [CrossRef] [PubMed]

33. Rabkin, C.S.; Biggar, R.J.; Melbye, M.; Curtis, R.E. Second primary cancers following anal and cervical carcinoma: Evidence of shared etiologic factors. *Am. J. Epidemiol.* **1992**, *136*, 54–58. [CrossRef] [PubMed]
34. Levi, F.; Randimbison, L.; La Vecchia, C.; Erler, G.; Te, V.C. Incidence of invasive cancers following squamous cell skin cancer. *Am. J. Epidemiol.* **1997**, *146*, 734–739. [CrossRef] [PubMed]
35. Levi, F.; Randimbison, L.; Te, V.C.; La Vecchia, C. Second primary cancers in patients with lung carcinoma. *Cancer* **1999**, *86*, 186–190. [CrossRef]
36. Levi, F.; Randimbison, L.; Maspoli, M.; Te, V.C.; La Vecchia, C. Second neoplasms after oesophageal cancer. *Int. J. Cancer* **2007**, *121*, 694–697. [CrossRef] [PubMed]
37. Chuang, S.C.; Hashibe, M.; Scelo, G.; Brewster, D.H.; Pukkala, E.; Friis, S.; Tracey, E.; Weiderpass, E.; Hemminki, K.; Tamaro, S.; et al. Risk of second primary cancer among esophageal cancer patients: A pooled analysis of 13 cancer registries. *Cancer Epidemiol. Biomark. Prev.* **2008**, *17*, 1543–1549. [CrossRef] [PubMed]
38. Brown, A.P.; Neeley, E.S.; Werner, T.; Soisson, A.P.; Burt, R.W.; Gaffney, D.K. A population-based study of subsequent primary malignancies after endometrial cancer: Genetic, environmental, and treatment-related associations. *Int. J. Radiat. Oncol. Biol. Phys.* **2010**, *78*, 127–135. [CrossRef] [PubMed]
39. Zhu, G.; Chen, Y.; Zhu, Z.; Lu, L.; Bi, X.; Deng, Q.; Chen, X.; Su, H.; Liu, Y.; Guo, H.; et al. Risk of second primary cancer after treatment for esophageal cancer: A pooled analysis of nine cancer registries. *Dis. Esophagus* **2012**, *25*, 505–511. [CrossRef] [PubMed]
40. Hsu, C.H.; Huang, C.L.; Hsu, Y.H.; Iqbal, U.; Nguyen, P.A.; Jian, W.S. Co-occurrence of second primary malignancy in patients with thyroid cancer. *QJM* **2014**, *107*, 643–648. [CrossRef] [PubMed]
41. Robsahm, T.E.; Karagas, M.R.; Rees, J.R.; Syse, A. New malignancies after squamous cell carcinoma and melanomas: A population-based study from Norway. *BMC Cancer* **2014**, *19*, 210. [CrossRef] [PubMed]
42. Davis, E.J.; Beebe-Dimmer, J.L.; Yee, C.L.; Cooney, K.A. Risk of second primary tumors in men diagnosed with prostate cancer: A population-based cohort study. *Cancer* **2014**, *120*, 2735–2741. [CrossRef] [PubMed]
43. Bae, S.H. Other primary systemic cancers in patients with melanoma: Analysis of balanced acral and nonacral melanomas. *J. Am. Acad. Dermatol.* **2016**, *72*, 333–340. [CrossRef]
44. Krilaviciute, A.; Vincerzevskiene, I.; Smailyte, G. Basal cell skin cancer and the risk of second primary cancers: A cancer registry-based study in Lithuania. *Ann. Epidemiol.* **2016**, *26*, 511–514. [CrossRef]
45. Schlieve, T.; Heidel, R.E.; Carlson, E.R. Second Primary Head and Neck Cancers after Non-Head and Neck Primary Cancers. *J. Oral. Maxillofac. Surg.* **2016**, *74*, 2515–2520. [CrossRef] [PubMed]
46. Adjei Boakye, E.; Wang, M.; Sharma, A.; Jenkins, W.D.; Osazuwa-Peters, N.; Chen, B.; Lee, M.; Schootman, M. Risk of second primary cancers in individuals diagnosed with index smoking- and non-smoking- related cancers. *J. Cancer Res. Clin. Oncol.* **2020**, *146*, 1765–1779. [CrossRef] [PubMed]
47. Wu, X.; Zhang, X.; Tao, L.; Chen, P. Risk of second primary malignancy in adults with pulmonary high-grade neuroendocrine carcinoma (HGNEC). *BMC Cancer* **2020**, *20*, 719. [CrossRef] [PubMed]
48. Song, C.; Lv, J.; Liu, Y.; Chen, J.G.; Ge, Z.; Zhu, J.; Dai, J.; Du, L.B.; Yu, C.; Guo, Y.; et al. Virus Infection and Risk of All Cancer Types. *JAMA Netw. Open.* **2019**, *2*, 6. [CrossRef]
49. Su, T.H.; Tseng, T.C.; Liu, C.J.; Chou, S.W.; Liu, C.H.; Yang, H.C.; Chen, P.J.; Chen, D.S.; Chen, C.L.; Kao, J.H. Antiviral therapy against chronic hepatitis C is associated with a reduced risk of oral cancer. *Int. J. Cancer* **2020**, *147*, 901–908. [CrossRef] [PubMed]
50. Mahale, P.; Ugoji, C.; Engels, E.A.; Shiels, M.S.; Peprah, S.; Morton, L.M. Cancer risk following lymphoid malignancies among HIV-infected people. *AIDS* **2020**, *34*, 1237–1245. [CrossRef] [PubMed]
51. Yokota, A.; Ozawa, S.; Masanori, T.; Akiyama, H.; Ohshima, K.; Kanda, Y.; Takahashi, S.; Mori, T.; Nakaseko, C.; Onoda, M.; et al. Secondary solid tumors after allogeneic hematopoietic SCT in Japan. *Bone Marrow Transpl.* **2012**, *47*, 95–100. [CrossRef] [PubMed]
52. Curtis, R.E.; Metayer, C.; Rizzo, J.D.; Socié, G.; Sobocinski, K.A.; Flowers, M.E.; Travis, W.D.; Travis, L.B.; Horowitz, M.M.; Deeg, H.J. Impact of chronic GVHD therapy on the development of squamous-cell cancers after hematopoietic stem-cell transplantation: An international case-control study. *Blood* **2005**, *105*, 3802–3811. [CrossRef] [PubMed]
53. Majhail, N.S.; Brazauskas, R.; Rizzo, J.D.; Sobecks, R.M.; Wang, Z.; Horowitz, M.M.; Bolwell, B.; Wingard, J.R.; Socie, G. Secondary solid cancers after allogeneic hematopoietic cell transplantation using busulfan-cyclophosphamide conditioning. *Blood* **2011**, *117*, 316–322. [CrossRef] [PubMed]
54. Dyer, G.; Brice, L.; Schifter, M.; Gilroy, N.; Kabir, M.; Hertzberg, M.; Greenwood, M.; Larsen, S.R.; Moore, J.; Gottlieb, D.; et al. Oral health and dental morbidity in long-term allogeneic blood and marrow transplant survivors in Australia. *Aust. Dent. J.* **2018**, *63*, 312–319. [CrossRef] [PubMed]
55. Anak, S.; Yalman, N.; Bilgen, H.; Sepet, E.; Deviren, A.; Gürtekin, B.; Tunca, F.; Başaran, B. Squamous cell carcinoma development in Fanconi anemia patients who underwent hematopoietic stem cell transplantation. *Pediatr. Transpl.* **2020**, *24*, e13706. [CrossRef]
56. Santarone, S.; Natale, A.; Angelini, S.; Papalinetti, G.; Vaddinelli, D.; Di Bartolomeo, A.; Di Bartolomeo, P. Secondary oral cancer following hematopoietic cell transplantation. *Bone Marrow Transpl.* **2021**, *56*, 1038–1046. [CrossRef] [PubMed]
57. Bensing, S.; Brandt, L.; Tabaroj, F.; Sjöberg, O.; Nilsson, B.; Ekbom, A.; Blomqvist, P.; Kämpe, O. Increased death risk and altered cancer incidence pattern in patients with isolated or combined autoimmune primary adrenocortical insufficiency. *Clin. Endocrinol.* **2008**, *69*, 697–704. [CrossRef] [PubMed]

58. Zhang, W.; Feng, S.; Yan, S.; Zhao, Y.; Li, M.; Sun, J.; Zhang, F.C.; Cui, Q.; Dong, Y. Incidence of malignancy in primary Sjogren's syndrome in a Chinese cohort. *Rheumatology* **2010**, *49*, 571–577. [CrossRef] [PubMed]
59. Katsanos, K.H.; Roda, G.; McBride, R.B.; Cohen, B.; Colombel, J.F. Increased Risk of Oral Cancer in Patients with Inflammatory Bowel Diseases. *Clin. Gastroenterol. Hepatol.* **2016**, *14*, 413–420. [CrossRef]
60. Rautemaa, R.; Hietanen, J.; Niissalo, S.; Pirinen, S.; Perheentupa, J. Oral and oesophageal squamous cell carcinoma—A complication or component of autoimmune polyendocrinopathy-candidiasis-ectodermal dystrophy (APECED, APS-I). *Oral Oncol.* **2007**, *43*, 607–613. [CrossRef] [PubMed]
61. Atsuta, Y.; Suzuki, R.; Yamashita, T.; Fukuda, T.; Miyamura, K.; Taniguchi, S.; Iida, H.; Uchida, T.; Ikegame, K.; Takahashi, S.; et al. Continuing increased risk of oral/esophageal cancer after allogeneic hematopoietic stem cell transplantation in adults in association with chronic graft-versus-host disease. *Ann. Oncol.* **2014**, *25*, 435–441. [CrossRef] [PubMed]
62. López-Pintor, R.M.; Hernández, G.; de Arriba, L.; de Andrés, A. Lip cancer in renal transplant patients. *Oral Oncol.* **2011**, *47*, 68–71. [CrossRef] [PubMed]
63. Motlokwa, P.K.; Tsima, B.M.; Martei, Y.M.; Ralefala, T.; Galebole, F.; Stephens-Shields, A.J.; Grover, S.; Gross, R. Disparities in Oral Cancer Stage at Presentation in a High HIV Prevalence Setting in Sub-Saharan Africa. *JCO Glob. Oncol.* **2022**, *8*, e2100439. [CrossRef] [PubMed]
64. Whiteside, T.L. Immunobiology and immunotherapy of head and neck cancer. *Curr Oncol Rep.* **2001**, *3*, 46–55. [CrossRef] [PubMed]
65. Wen, B.W.; Tsai, C.S.; Lin, C.L.; Chang, Y.J.; Lee, C.F.; Hsu, C.H.; Kao, C.H. Cancer risk among gingivitis and periodontitis patients: A nationwide cohort study. *QJM* **2014**, *107*, 283–290. [CrossRef] [PubMed]
66. Gupta, B.; Ariyawardana, A.; Johnson, N.W. Oral cancer in India continues in epidemic proportions: Evidence base and policy initiatives. *Int. Dent. J.* **2013**, *63*, 12–25. [CrossRef] [PubMed]
67. Dickenson, A.J.; Currie, W.J.; Avery, B.S. Screening for syphilis in patients with carcinoma of the tongue. *Br. J. Oral Maxillofac. Surg.* **1995**, *33*, 319–320. [CrossRef]
68. Mohd Bakri, M.; Mohd Hussaini, H.; Rachel Holmes, A.; David Cannon, R.; Mary Rich, A. Revisiting the association between candidal infection and carcinoma, particularly oral squamous cell carcinoma. *J. Oral Microbiol.* **2010**, *21*, 2. [CrossRef]
69. Garrote, L.F.; Herrero, R.; Reyes, R.M.; Vaccarella, S.; Anta, J.L.; Ferbeye, L.; Muñoz, N.; Franceschi, S. Risk factors for cancer of the oral cavity and oro-pharynx in Cuba. *Br. J. Cancer* **2001**, *85*, 46–54. [CrossRef]
70. Hassona, Y.; Scully, C.; Almangush, A.; Baqain, Z.; Sawair, F. Oral potentially malignant disorders among dental patients: A pilot study in Jordan. *Asian Pac. J. Cancer Prev.* **2014**, *15*, 10427–10431. [CrossRef]
71. Ben-David, Y.; Leiser, Y.; Kachta, O.; El-Naaj, I.A. Does long-term treatment with Doxil®predispose patients to oral cancer? *Int. J. Clin. Oncol.* **2013**, *18*, 554–555. [CrossRef]
72. Fahmy, M.S.; Sadeghi, A.; Behmard, S. Epidemiologic study of oral cancer in Fars Province, Iran. *Community Dent. Oral Epidemiol.* **1983**, *11*, 50–58. [CrossRef]
73. Sankaranarayanan, R.; Nair, M.K.; Mathew, B.; Balaram, P.; Sebastian, P.; Dutt, S.C. Recent results of oral cancer research in Kerala, India. *Head Neck.* **1992**, *14*, 107–112. [CrossRef]
74. Warnakulasuriya, S.; Kovacevic, T.; Madden, P.; Coupland, V.H.; Sperandio, M.; Odell, E.; Møller, H. Factors predicting malignant transformation in oral potentially malignant disorders among patients accrued over a 10-year period in South East England. *J. Oral Pathol. Med.* **2011**, *40*, 677–683. [CrossRef] [PubMed]
75. Túri, K.; Barabás, P.; Csurgay, K.; Léhner, G.Y.; Lőrincz, A.; Németh, Z.S. An analysis of the epidemiological and etiological factors of oral tumors of young adults in a Central-Eastern European population. *Pathol. Oncol. Res.* **2013**, *19*, 353–363. [CrossRef] [PubMed]
76. Gorsky, M.; Epstein, J.B.; Oakley, C.; Le, N.D.; Hay, J.; Stevenson-Moore, P. Carcinoma of the tongue: A case series analysis of clinical presentation, risk factors, staging, and outcome. *Oral Surg. Oral Med. Oral Pathol. Oral Radiol. Endod.* **2004**, *98*, 546–552. [CrossRef]
77. Hsue, S.S.; Wang, W.C.; Chen, C.H.; Lin, C.C.; Chen, Y.K.; Lin, L.M. Malignant transformation in 1458 patients with potentially malignant oral mucosal disorders: A follow-up study based in a Taiwanese hospital. *J. Oral Pathol. Med.* **2007**, *36*, 25–29. [CrossRef]
78. Saira; Ahmed, R.; Malik, S.; Khan, M.F.; Khattak, M.R. Epidemiological and clinical correlates of oral squamous cell carcinoma in patients from north-west Pakistan. *J. Pak. Med. Assoc.* **2019**, *69*, 1074–1078.
79. Yao, J.G.; Gao, L.B.; Liu, Y.G.; Li, J.; Pang, G.F. Genetic variation in interleukin-10 gene and risk of oral cancer. *Clin. Chim. Acta* **2008**, *388*, 84–88. [CrossRef]
80. De Benedittis, M.; Petruzzi, M.; Giardina, C.; Lo Muzio, L.; Favia, G.; Serpico, R. Oral squamous cell carcinoma during long-term treatment with hydroxyurea. *Clin. Exp. Dermatol.* **2004**, *29*, 605–607. [CrossRef] [PubMed]
81. Tsai, C.W.; Chang, W.S.; Lin, K.C.; Shih, L.C.; Tsai, M.H.; Hsiao, C.L.; Yang, M.D.; Lin, C.C.; Bau, D.T. Significant association of Interleukin-10 genotypes and oral cancer susceptibility in Taiwan. *Anticancer Res.* **2014**, *34*, 3731–3737.
82. Abhinav, R.P.; Williams, J.; Livingston, P.; Anjana, R.M.; Mohan, V. Burden of diabetes and oral cancer in India. *J. Diabetes Complicat.* **2020**, *34*, 107670. [CrossRef]
83. Satheeshkumar, P.S.; Mohan, M.P. Oral Helicobacter pylori infection and the risk of oral cancer. *Oral Oncol.* **2013**, *49*, e20–e21. [CrossRef] [PubMed]

84. Krüger, M.; Hansen, T.; Kasaj, A.; Moergel, M. The Correlation between Chronic Periodontitis and Oral Cancer. *Case Rep. Dent.* **2013**, *2013*, 262410. [CrossRef] [PubMed]
85. Hermsen, M.A.; Xie, Y.; Rooimans, M.A.; Meijer, G.A.; Baak, J.P.; Plukker, J.T.; Arwert, F.; Joenje, H. Cytogenetic characteristics of oral squamous cell carcinomas in Fanconi anemia. *Fam. Cancer* **2001**, *1*, 39–43. [CrossRef]
86. Moura, L.K.B.; Mobin, M.; Matos, F.T.C.; Monte, T.L.; Lago, E.C.; Falcão, C.A.M.; Ferraz, M.Â.A.L.; Santos, T.C.; Tapety, F.I.; Nunes, C.M.C.L.L.; et al. Bibliometric Analysis on the Risks of Oral Cancer for People Living with HIV/AIDS. *Iran J. Public Health* **2017**, *46*, 1583–1585. [PubMed]
87. Singh, P.K.; Ahmad, M.K.; Kumar, V.; Gupta, R.; Kohli, M.; Jain, A.; Mahdi, A.A.; Bogra, J.; Chandra, G. Genetic polymorphism of interleukin-10 (-A592C) among oral cancer with squamous cell carcinoma. *Arch. Oral Biol.* **2017**, *77*, 18–22. [CrossRef]
88. Tarvainen, L.; Suojanen, J.; Kyyronen, P.; Lindqvist, C.; Martinsen, J.I.; Kjaerheim, K.; Lynge, E.; Sparen, P.; Tryggvadottir, L.; Weiderpass, E.; et al. Occupational Risk for Oral Cancer in Nordic Countries. *Anticancer Res.* **2017**, *37*, 3221–3228. [PubMed]
89. Soulier, J. Fanconi anemia. *Hematol. Am. Soc. Hematol. Educ. Program.* **2011**, *2011*, 492–497. [CrossRef] [PubMed]
90. Sun, C.; Hu, Z.; Zhong, Z.; Jiang, Y.; Sun, R.; Fei, J.; Xi, Y.; Li, X.; Song, M.; Li, W.; et al. Clinical and prognostic analysis of second primary squamous cell carcinoma of the tongue after radiotherapy for nasopharyngeal carcinoma. *Br. J. Oral Maxillofac. Surg.* **2014**, *52*, 715–720. [CrossRef]
91. Hashibe, M.; Ritz, B.; Le, A.D.; Li, G.; Sankaranarayanan, R.; Zhang, Z.F. Radiotherapy for oral cancer as a risk factor for second primary cancers. *Cancer Lett.* **2005**, *220*, 185–195. [CrossRef]
92. Santos, A.M.; Marcu, L.G.; Wong, C.M.; Bezak, E. Risk estimation of second primary cancers after breast radiotherapy. *Acta Oncol.* **2016**, *55*, 1331–1337. [CrossRef]
93. Rafferty, M.A.; O'Dwyer, T.P. Secondary primary malignancies in head and neck squamous cell carcinoma. *J. Laryngol. Otol.* **2001**, *115*, 988–991. [CrossRef] [PubMed]
94. Lee, K.D.; Lu, C.H.; Chen, P.T.; Chan, C.H.; Lin, J.T.; Huang, C.E.; Chen, C.C.; Chen, M.C. The incidence and risk of developing a second primary esophageal cancer in patients with oral and pharyngeal carcinoma: A population-based study in Taiwan over a 25 year period. *BMC Cancer* **2009**, *9*, 373. [CrossRef] [PubMed]
95. Shanmugham, J.R.; Zavras, A.I.; Rosner, B.A.; Giovannucci, E.L. Alcohol-folate interactions in the risk of oral cancer in women: A prospective cohort study. *Cancer Epidemiol. Biomark. Prev.* **2010**, *19*, 2516–2524. [CrossRef] [PubMed]
96. De Araújo, R.L.; Lyko Kde, F.; Funke, V.A.; Torres-Pereira, C.C. Oral cancer after prolonged immunosuppression for multiorgan chronic graft-versus-host disease. *Rev. Bras. Hematol. Hemoter.* **2014**, *36*, 65–68. [CrossRef]
97. Rosenquist, K.; Wennerberg, J.; Schildt, E.B.; Bladström, A.; Göran Hansson, B.; Andersson, G. Oral status, oral infections and some lifestyle factors as risk factors for oral and oropharyngeal squamous cell carcinoma. A population-based case-control study in southern Sweden. *Acta Otolaryngol.* **2005**, *125*, 1327–1336. [CrossRef]
98. Douglas, C.M.; Jethwa, A.R.; Hasan, W.; Liu, A.; Gilbert, R.; Goldstein, D.; De Almedia, J.; Lipton, J.; Irish, J.C. Long-term survival of head and neck squamous cell carcinoma after bone marrow transplant. *Head Neck.* **2020**, *42*, 3389–3395. [CrossRef]
99. Farrar, M.; Sandison, A.; Peston, D.; Gailani, M. Immunocytochemical analysis of AE1/AE3, CK 14, Ki-67 and p53 expression in benign, premalignant and malignant oral tissue to establish putative markers for progression of oral carcinoma. *Br. J. Biomed. Sci.* **2004**, *61*, 117–124. [CrossRef]
100. Hsu, H.J.; Yang, Y.H.; Shieh, T.Y.; Chen, C.H.; Kao, Y.H.; Yang, C.F.; Ko, E.C. TGF-β1 and IL-10 single nucleotide polymorphisms as risk factors for oral cancer in Taiwanese. *Kaohsiung J. Med. Sci.* **2015**, *31*, 123–129. [CrossRef]
101. Danylesko, I.; Shimoni, A. Second Malignancies after Hematopoietic Stem Cell Transplantation. *Curr. Treat. Options Oncol.* **2018**, *19*, 9. [CrossRef]
102. Adhikari, J.; Sharma, P.; Bhatt, V.R. Risk of secondary solid malignancies after allogeneic hematopoietic stem cell transplantation and preventive strategies. *Future Oncol.* **2015**, *11*, 3175–3185. [CrossRef]
103. Demarosi, F.; Lodi, G.; Carrassi, A.; Soligo, D.; Sardella, A. Oral malignancies following HSCT: Graft versus host disease and other risk factors. *Oral Oncol.* **2005**, *41*, 865–877. [CrossRef] [PubMed]
104. Manavoğlu, O.; Orhan, B.; Evrensel, T.; Karabulut, Y.; Ozkocaman, V.; Ozyardimci, C. Second primary cancer due to radiotherapy and chemotherapy. *J. Environ. Pathol. Toxicol. Oncol.* **1996**, *15*, 275–278.
105. Takeuchi, Y.; Onizawa, K.; Wakatsuki, T.; Yamagata, K.; Hasegawa, Y.; Yoshida, H. Tongue cancer after bone marrow transplantation. *Oral Oncol.* **2006**, *42*, 251–254. [CrossRef]
106. Tomihara, K.; Dehari, H.; Yamaguchi, A.; Abe, M.; Miyazaki, A.; Nakamori, K.; Hareyama, M.; Hiratsuka, H. Squamous cell carcinoma of the buccal mucosa in a young adult with history of allogeneic bone marrow transplantation for childhood acute leukemia. *Head Neck* **2009**, *31*, 565–568. [CrossRef]
107. Kawano, K.; Goto, H.; Takahashi, Y.; Kaku, Y.; Oobu, K.; Yanagisawa, S. Secondary Squamous Cell Carcinoma of the Oral Cavity in Young Adults after Hematopoietic Stem Cell Transplantation for Leukemia: Report of Two Cases with Human Papillomavirus Infection. *Oral Sci. Int.* **2007**, *4*, 110–116. [CrossRef]
108. Inamoto, Y.; Shah, N.N.; Savani, B.N.; Shaw, B.E.; Abraham, A.A.; Ahmed, I.A.; Akpek, G.; Atsuta, Y.; Baker, K.S.; Basak, G.W.; et al. Secondary solid cancer screening following hematopoietic cell transplantation. *Bone Marrow Transplant.* **2015**, *50*, 1013–1023. [CrossRef] [PubMed]
109. Hernández, G.; Arriba, L.; Jiménez, C.; Bagán, J.V.; Rivera, B.; Lucas, M.; Moreno, E. Rapid progression from oral leukoplakia to carcinoma in an immunosuppressed liver transplant recipient. *Oral Oncol.* **2003**, *39*, 87–90. [CrossRef]

110. Torres-Pereira, C.C.; Stramandinoli-Zanicotti, R.T.; Amenábar, J.M.; Sassi, L.M.; Galbiatti Pedruzzi, P.A.; Piazzetta, C.M.; Bonfim, C. Oral squamous cell carcinoma in two siblings with Fanconi anemia after allogeneic bone marrow transplantation. *Spec. Care Dentist* **2014**, *34*, 212–215. [CrossRef] [PubMed]
111. Alotaiby, F.; Song, F.; Boyce, B.J.; Cao, D.; Zhao, Y.; Lai, J. Unusual Papillary Squamous Cell Carcinoma of the Tip of Tongue Presenting in a Patient Status Post Heart Transplant. *Anticancer Res.* **2018**, *38*, 4203–4206. [CrossRef]
112. Shiboski, C.H.; Schmidt, B.L.; Jordan, R.C. Tongue and tonsil carcinoma: Increasing trends in the U.S. population ages 20–44 years. *Cancer* **2005**, *103*, 1843–1849. [CrossRef] [PubMed]
113. Weng, X.; Xing, Y.; Cheng, B. Multiple and Recurrent Squamous Cell Carcinoma of the Oral Cavity After Graft-Versus-Host Disease. *J. Oral Maxillofac. Surg.* **2017**, *75*, 1899–1905. [CrossRef] [PubMed]
114. Sharma, R.N. Oral Carcinoma: A Clinical Study Of 122 Cases. *J. Indian Med. Assoc.* **1964**, *43*, 263–268. [PubMed]
115. Fu, X.; Chen, S.; Chen, W.; Yang, Z.; Song, M.; Li, H.; Zhang, H.; Yao, F.; Su, X.; Liu, T.; et al. Clinical analysis of second primary gingival squamous cell carcinoma after radiotherapy. *Oral Oncol.* **2018**, *84*, 20–24. [CrossRef]
116. García-Martín, J.M.; Varela-Centelles, P.; González, M.; Seoane-Romero, J.M.; Seoane, J.; García-Pola, M.J. Epidemiology of oral cancer. In *Oral Cancer Detection*; Panta, P., Ed.; Springer: Cham, Switzerland, 2019.
117. Tao, Y.; Sturgis, E.M.; Huang, Z.; Sun, Y.; Dahlstrom, K.R.; Wei, Q.; Li, G. A TGF-β1 genetic variant at the miRNA187 binding site significantly modifies risk of HPV16-associated oropharyngeal cancer. *Int. J. Cancer* **2018**, *143*, 1327–1334. [CrossRef] [PubMed]
118. Madrid, C.; Scully, C. Oral cancer: Comprehending the condition, causes, controversies, control and consequences. 17. Osteonecrosis. *Dent. Update* **2012**, *39*, 377–379. [CrossRef]
119. Dhanuthai, K.; Rojanawatsirivej, S.; Thosaporn, W.; Kintarak, S.; Subarnbhesaj, A.; Darling, M.; Kryshtalskyj, E.; Chiang, C.P.; Shin, H.I.; Choi, S.Y.; et al. Oral cancer: A multicenter study. *Med. Oral Patol. Oral Cir. Bucal.* **2018**, *23*, e23–e29. [CrossRef]
120. Geng, F.; Wang, Q.; Li, C.; Liu, J.; Zhang, D.; Zhang, S.; Pan, Y. Identification of Potential Candidate Genes of Oral Cancer in Response to Chronic Infection With Porphyromonas gingivalis Using Bioinformatical Analyses. *Front Oncol.* **2019**, *9*, 91. [CrossRef]
121. Pisani, L.P.; Estadella, D.; Ribeiro, D.A. The Role of Toll Like Receptors (TLRs) in Oral Carcinogenesis. *Anticancer Res.* **2017**, *37*, 5389–5394.
122. Okubo, M.; Kioi, M.; Nakashima, H.; Sugiura, K.; Mitsudo, K.; Aoki, I.; Taniguchi, H.; Tohnai, I. M2-polarized macrophages contribute to neovasculogenesis, leading to relapse of oral cancer following radiation. *Sci Rep.* **2016**, *6*, 27548. [CrossRef]
123. Dewan, K.; Kelly, R.D.; Bardsley, P. A national survey of consultants, specialists and specialist registrars in restorative dentistry for the assessment and treatment planning of oral cancer patients. *Br. Dent. J.* **2014**, *216*, E27. [CrossRef]
124. Mukhopadhyaya, R.; Rao, R.S.; Fakih, A.R.; Gangal, S.G. Detection of circulating immune complexes in patients with squamous cell carcinoma of the oral cavity. *J. Clin. Lab. Immunol.* **1986**, *21*, 189–193. [PubMed]
125. Adewole, R.A. Alcohol, smoking and oral cancer. A 10-year retrospective study at Base Hospital, Yaba. *West Afr. J. Med.* **2002**, *21*, 142–145.
126. Kashyap, T.; Pramanik, K.K.; Nath, N.; Mishra, P.; Singh, A.K.; Nagini, S.; Rana, A.; Mishra, R. Crosstalk between Raf-MEK-ERK and PI3K-Akt-GSK3β signaling networks promotes chemoresistance, invasion/migration and stemness via expression of CD44 variants (v4 and v6) in oral cancer. *Oral Oncol.* **2018**, *86*, 234–243. [CrossRef] [PubMed]
127. Moore, S.; Johnson, N.; Pierce, A.; Wilson, D. The epidemiology of lip cancer: A review of global incidence and aetiology. *Oral Dis.* **1999**, *5*, 185–195. [CrossRef]
128. Ueda, N.; Kamata, N.; Hayashi, E.; Yokoyama, K.; Hoteiya, T.; Nagayama, M. Effects of an anti-angiogenic agent, TNP-470, on the growth of oral squamous cell carcinomas. *Oral Oncol.* **1999**, *35*, 554–560. [CrossRef] [PubMed]
129. Chen, Y.; Wang, X.; Fang, J. Mesenchymal stem cells participate in oral mucosa carcinogenesis by regulating T cell proliferation. *Clin. Immunol.* **2019**, *198*, 46–53. [CrossRef]
130. Kikuchi, K.; Noguchi, Y.; de Rivera, M.W. Detection of Epstein-Barr virus genome and latent infection gene expression in normal epithelia, epithelial dysplasia, and squamous cell carcinoma of the oral cavity. *Tumour Biol.* **2016**, *37*, 3389–3404. [CrossRef]
131. Lenouvel, D.; González-Moles, M.Á.; Talbaoui, A. An update of knowledge on PD-L1 in head and neck cancers: Physiologic, prognostic and therapeutic perspectives. *Oral Dis.* **2020**, *26*, 511–526. [CrossRef]
132. Brown, A.M.; Lally, E.T.; Frankel, A.; Harwick, R.; Davis, L.W.; Rominger, C.J. The association of the IGA levels of serum and whole saliva with the progression of oral cancer. *Cancer* **1975**, *35*, 1154–1162. [CrossRef]
133. Johnson, N.W. Az oralis carcinomák etiológiája és rizikófaktorai, különös tekintettel a dohányzásra és az alkoholfogyasztásra [Aetiology and risk factors for oral cancer, with special reference to tobacco and alcohol use]. *Magy Onkol.* **2001**, *45*, 115–122.
134. Adams, S.; Lin, J.; Brown, D.; Shriver, C.D.; Zhu, K. Ultraviolet Radiation Exposure and the Incidence of Oral, Pharyngeal and Cervical Cancer and Melanoma: An Analysis of the SEER Data. *Anticancer Res.* **2016**, *36*, 233–237. [PubMed]
135. Kurokawa, H.; Tsuru, S.; Okada, M.; Nakamura, T.; Kajiyama, M. Evaluation of tumor markers in patients with squamous cell carcinoma in the oral cavity. *Int. J. Oral Maxillofac. Surg.* **1993**, *22*, 35–38. [CrossRef] [PubMed]
136. Talamini, R.; Vaccarella, S.; Barbone, F. Oral hygiene, dentition, sexual habits and risk of oral cancer. *Br. J. Cancer* **2000**, *83*, 1238–1242. [CrossRef]
137. La Rosa, G.R.M.; Gattuso, G.; Pedullà, E.; Rapisarda, E.; Nicolosi, D.; Salmeri, M. Association of oral dysbiosis with oral cancer development. *Oncol. Lett.* **2020**, *19*, 3045–3058. [CrossRef] [PubMed]

138. Das, D.; Ghosh, S.; Maitra, A. Epigenomic dysregulation-mediated alterations of key biological pathways and tumor immune evasion are hallmarks of gingivo-buccal oral cancer. *Clin. Epigenetics* **2019**, *11*, 178. [CrossRef]
139. Rajkumar, T.; Sridhar, H.; Balaram, P. Oral cancer in Southern India: The influence of body size, diet, infections and sexual practices. *Eur. J. Cancer Prev.* **2003**, *12*, 135–143. [CrossRef]
140. Khanna, S. Immunological and biochemical markers in oral carcinogenesis: The public health perspective. *Int. J. Environ. Res. Public Health* **2008**, *5*, 418–422. [CrossRef]
141. Engku Nasrullah Satiman, E.A.F.; Ahmad, H.; Ramzi, A.B.; Wahab, R.A.; Kaderi, M.A.; Harun, W.H.A.W.; Dashper, S. The role of Candida albicans candidalysin ECE1 gene in oral carcinogenesis. *J. Oral Pathol. Med.* **2020**, *49*, 835–841. [CrossRef]
142. Wu, T.S.; Tan, C.T.; Chang, C.C. B-cell lymphoma/leukemia 10 promotes oral cancer progression through STAT1/ATF4/S100P signaling pathway. *Oncogene.* **2015**, *34*, 1207–1219. [CrossRef]
143. Malinowska, K.; Morawiec-Sztandera, A.; Majsterek, I.; Kaczmarczyk, D. TC2 C776G polymorphism studies in patients with oral cancer in the Polish population. *Pol. J. Pathol.* **2016**, *67*, 277–282. [CrossRef]
144. Leuci, S.; Coppola, N.; Blasi, A. Oral Dysplastic Complications after HSCT: Single Case Series of Multidisciplinary Evaluation of 80 Patients. *Life* **2020**, *10*, 236. [CrossRef] [PubMed]
145. Anqi, C.; Takabatake, K.; Kawai, H.; Oo, M.W.; Yoshida, S.; Fujii, M.; Omori, H.; Sukegawa, S.; Nakano, K.; Tsuijigiwa, H.; et al. Differentiation and roles of bone marrow-derived cells on the tumor microenvironment of oral squamous cell carcinoma. *Oncol. Lett.* **2019**, *18*, 6628–6638. [CrossRef] [PubMed]
146. Furquim, C.P.; Pivovar, A.; Amenábar, J.M.; Bonfim, C.; Torres-Pereira, C.C. Oral cancer in Fanconi anemia: Review of 121 cases. *Crit. Rev.Oncol. Hematol.* **2018**, *125*, 35–40. [CrossRef]
147. Shah, A.T.; Wu, E.; Wein, R.O. Oral squamous cell carcinoma in post-transplant patients. *Am. J. Otolaryngol.* **2013**, *34*, 176–179. [CrossRef] [PubMed]
148. Elad, S.; Zadik, Y.; Zeevi, I.; Miyazaki, A.; de Figueiredo, M.A.; Or, R. Oral cancer in patients after hematopoietic stem-cell transplantation: Long-term follow-up suggests an increased risk for recurrence. *Transplantation* **2010**, *90*, 1243–1244. [CrossRef] [PubMed]
149. Abdelsayed, R.A.; Sumner, T.; Allen, C.M.; Treadway, A.; Ness, G.M.; Penza, S.L. Oral precancerous and malignant lesions associated with graft-versus-host disease: Report of 2 cases. *Oral Surg. Oral Med. Oral Pathol. Oral Radiol. Endod.* **2002**, *93*, 75–80. [CrossRef] [PubMed]
150. González-Moles, M.Á.; Ruiz-Ávila, I.; González-Ruiz, L.; Ayén, Á.; Gil-Montoya, J.A.; Ramos-García, P. Malignant transformation risk of oral lichen planus: A systematic review and comprehensive meta-analysis. *Oral Oncol.* **2019**, *96*, 121–130. [CrossRef]
151. Nagao, Y.; Sata, M.; Fukuizumi, K.; Harada, H.; Kameyama, T. Oral cancer and hepatitis C virus (HCV): Can HCV alone cause oral cancer?—A case report. *Kurume Med. J.* **1996**, *43*, 97–100. [CrossRef]
152. Nagao, Y.; Sata, M.; Noguchi, S. Detection of hepatitis C virus RNA in oral lichen planus and oral cancer tissues. *J. Oral Pathol. Med.* **2000**, *29*, 259–266. [CrossRef]
153. Nagao, Y.; Sata, M.; Tanikawa, K.; Itoh, K.; Kameyama, T. High prevalence of hepatitis C virus antibody and RNA in patients with oral cancer. *J. Oral Pathol. Med.* **1995**, *24*, 354–360. [CrossRef]
154. Nagao, Y.; Sata, M. Oral verrucous carcinoma arising from lichen planus and esophageal squamous cell carcinoma in a patient with hepatitis C virus-related liver cirrhosis-hyperinsulinemia and malignant transformation: A case report. *Biomed. Rep.* **2013**, *1*, 53–56. [CrossRef] [PubMed]
155. Gandolfo, S.; Richiardi, L.; Carrozzo, M. Risk of oral squamous cell carcinoma in 402 patients with oral lichen planus:A follow-up study in an Italian population. *Oral Oncol.* **2004**, *40*, 77–83. [CrossRef] [PubMed]
156. Wang, L.Y.; You, S.L.; Lu, S.N. Risk of hepatocellular carcinoma and habits of alcohol drinking, betel quid chewing and cigarette smoking: A cohort of 2416 HBsAg-seropositive and 9421 HBsAg-seronegative male residents in Taiwan. *Cancer Causes Control* **2003**, *14*, 241–250. [CrossRef]
157. Kao, C.H.; Sun, L.M.; Liang, J.A.; Chang, S.N.; Sung, F.C.; Muo, C.H. Relationship of zolpidem and cancer risk: A Taiwanese population-based cohort study. *Mayo Clin. Proc.* **2012**, *87*, 430–436. [CrossRef] [PubMed]
158. Tandle, A.T.; Sanghvi, V.; Saranath, D. Determination of p53 genotypes in oral cancer patients from India. *Br. J. Cancer* **2001**, *84*, 739–742. [CrossRef]
159. Shih, L.C.; Li, C.H.; Sun, K.T. Association of Matrix Metalloproteinase-7 Genotypes to the Risk of Oral Cancer in Taiwan. *Anticancer Res.* **2018**, *38*, 2087–2092.
160. Chiu, C.F.; Tsai, M.H.; Tseng, H.C.; Wang, C.L.; Tsai, F.J.; Lin, C.C.; Bau, D.T. A novel single nucleotide polymorphism in ERCC6 gene is associated with oral cancer susceptibility in Taiwanese patients. *Oral Oncol.* **2008**, *44*, 582–586. [CrossRef]
161. Park, J.Y.; Schantz, S.P.; Stern, J.C.; Kaur, T.; Lazarus, P. Association between glutathione S-transferase pi genetic polymorphisms and oral cancer risk. *Pharmacogenetics* **1999**, *9*, 497–504.
162. Hatagima, A.; Costa, E.C.; Marques, C.F.; Koifman, R.J.; Boffetta, P.; Koifman, S. Glutathione S-transferase polymorphisms and oral cancer: A case-control study in Rio de Janeiro, Brazil. *Oral Oncol.* **2008**, *44*, 200–207. [CrossRef]
163. Misra, C.; Majumder, M.; Bajaj, S.; Ghosh, S.; Roy, B.; Roychoudhury, S. Polymorphisms at p53, p73, and MDM2 loci modulate the risk of tobacco associated leukoplakia and oral cancer. *Mol Carcinog.* **2009**, *48*, 790–800. [CrossRef]
164. Sartor, M.; Steingrimsdottir, H.; Elamin, F. Role of p16/MTS1, cyclin D1 and RB in primary oral cancer and oral cancer cell lines. *Br. J. Cancer* **1999**, *80*, 79–86. [CrossRef] [PubMed]

165. Chiang, C.T.; Chang, T.K.; Hwang, Y.H. A critical exploration of blood and environmental chromium concentration among oral cancer patients in an oral cancer prevalent area of Taiwan. *Environ. Geochem. Health* **2011**, *33*, 469–476. [CrossRef] [PubMed]
166. Chen, W.C.; Chen, M.F.; Lin, P.Y. Significance of DNMT3b in oral cancer. *PLoS ONE* **2014**, *9*, e89956. [CrossRef] [PubMed]
167. Kang, D.; Gridley, G.; Huang, W.Y. Microsatellite polymorphisms in the epidermal growth factor receptor (EGFR) gene and the transforming growth factor-alpha (TGFA) gene and risk of oral cancer in Puerto Rico. *Pharmacogenet. Genom.* **2005**, *15*, 343–347. [CrossRef]
168. Rao, A.K.D.M.; Manikandan, M.; Arunkumar, G.; Revathidevi, S.; Vinothkumar, V.; Arun, K.; Tiwary, B.K.; Rajkumar, K.S. Prevalence of p53 codon 72, p73 G4C14-A4T14 and MDM2 T309G polymorphisms and its association with the risk of oral cancer in South Indians. *Gene Rep.* **2017**, *7*, 106–112. [CrossRef]
169. Yen, C.Y.; Liu, S.Y.; Chen, C.H.; Tseng, H.F.; Chuang, L.Y.; Yang, C.H.; Lin, Y.C.; Wen, C.H.; Chiang, W.F.; Ho, C.H. Combinational polymorphisms of four DNA repair genes XRCC1, XRCC2, XRCC3, and XRCC4 and their association with oral cancer in Taiwan. *J. Oral Pathol. Med.* **2008**, *37*, 271–277. [CrossRef]
170. Ramachandran, S.; Ramadas, K.; Hariharan, R.; Rejnish Kumar, R.; Radhakrishna Pillai, M. Single nucleotide polymorphisms of DNA repair genes XRCC1 and XPD and its molecular mapping in Indian oral cancer. *Oral Oncol.* **2006**, *42*, 350–362. [CrossRef]
171. Shukla, D.; Dinesh Kale, A.; Hallikerimath, S.; Vivekanandhan, S.; Venkatakanthaiah, Y. Genetic polymorphism of drug metabolizing enzymes (GSTM1 and CYP1A1) as risk factors for oral premalignant lesions and oral cancer. *Biomed. Pap. Med. Fac. Univ. Palacky Olomouc. Czech Repub.* **2012**, *156*, 253–259. [CrossRef]
172. Park, J.Y.; Muscat, J.E.; Ren, Q. CYP1A1 and GSTM1 polymorphisms and oral cancer risk. *Cancer Epidemiol. Biomark. Prev.* **1997**, *6*, 791–797.
173. Cha, I.H.; Park, J.Y.; Chung, W.Y.; Choi, M.A.; Kim, H.J.; Park, K.K. Polymorphisms of CYP1A1 and GSTM1 genes and susceptibility to oral cancer. *Yonsei Med. J.* **2007**, *48*, 233–239. [CrossRef]
174. Carneiro, N.K.; Oda, J.M.; Losi Guembarovski, R.; Ramos, G.; Oliveira, B.V.; Cavalli, I.J.; Ribeiro, E.M.d.S.F.; Goncalves, M.S.B.; Watanabe, M.A.E. Possible association between TGF-β1 polymorphism and oral cancer. *Int. J. Immunogenet.* **2013**, *40*, 292–298. [CrossRef] [PubMed]
175. Wang, L.-H.; Ting, S.-C.; Chen, C.-H.; Tsai, C.-C.; Lung, O.; Liu, T.-C.; Lee, C.-W.; Wang, Y.-Y.; Tsai, C.-L.; Lin, Y.-C. Polymorphisms in the apoptosis-associated genes FAS and FASL and risk of oral cancer and malignant potential of oral premalignant lesions in a Taiwanese population. *J. Oral Pathol. Med.* **2010**, *39*, 155–161. [CrossRef] [PubMed]
176. Chung, T.T.; Pan, M.S.; Kuo, C.L. Impact of RECK gene polymorphisms and environmental factors on oral cancer susceptibility and clinicopathologic characteristics in Taiwan. *Carcinogenesis* **2011**, *32*, 1063–1068. [CrossRef]
177. Shukla, D.; Dinesh Kale, A.; Hallikerimath, S.; Yerramalla, V.; Subbiah, V.; Mishra, S. Association between GSTM1 and CYP1A1 polymorphisms and survival in oral cancer patients. *Biomed. Pap. Med. Fac. Univ. Palacky Olomouc. Czech Repub.* **2013**, *157*, 304–310. [CrossRef]
178. Gunduz, E.; Gunduz, M.; Ouchida, M. Genetic and epigenetic alterations of BRG1 promote oral cancer development. *Int. J. Oncol.* **2005**, *26*, 201–210. [CrossRef] [PubMed]
179. Merrill, R.M.; Isakson, R.T.; Beck, R.E. The association between allergies and cancer: What is currently known? *Ann. Allergy Asthma Immunol.* **2007**, *99*, 102–150. [CrossRef] [PubMed]
180. Li, G.; Sturgis, E.M.; Wang, L.E. Association of a p73 exon 2 G4C14-to-A4T14 polymorphism with risk of squamous cell carcinoma of the head and neck. *Carcinogenesis* **2004**, *25*, 1911–1916. [CrossRef]
181. Twu, C.W.; Jiang, R.S.; Shu, C.H.; Lin, J.C. Association of p53 codon 72 polymorphism with risk of hypopharyngeal squamous cell carcinoma in Taiwan. *J. Formos. Med. Assoc.* **2006**, *105*, 99–104. [CrossRef]
182. Katoh, T. The frequency of glutathione-S-transferase M1 (GSTM1) gene deletion in patients with lung and oral cancer. *Sangyo Igaku.* **1994**, *36*, 435–439. [CrossRef]
183. Wang, Z. The role of COX-2 in oral cancer development, and chemoprevention/ treatment of oral cancer by selective COX-2 inhibitors. *Curr. Pharm. Des.* **2005**, *11*, 1771–1777. [CrossRef]
184. Liu, F.; Liu, L.; Li, B. p73 G4C14-A4T14 polymorphism and cancer risk: A meta-analysis based on 27 case-control studies. *Mutagenesis* **2011**, *26*, 573–581. [CrossRef] [PubMed]
185. Singh, A.P.; Shah, P.P.; Ruwali, M.; Mathur, N.; Pant, M.C.; Parmar, D. Polymorphism in cytochrome P4501A1 is significantly associated with head and neck cancer risk. *Cancer Investig.* **2009**, *27*, 869–876. [CrossRef] [PubMed]
186. Shillitoe, E.J. The role of viruses in squamous cell carcinoma of the oropharyngeal mucosa. *Oral Oncol.* **2009**, *45*, 351–355. [CrossRef] [PubMed]
187. Beppu, M.; Ikebe, T.; Shirasuna, K. The inhibitory effects of immunosuppressive factors, dexamethasone and interleukin-4, on NF-kappaB-mediated protease production by oral cancer. *Biochim. Biophys. Acta* **2002**, *1586*, 11–22. [CrossRef]
188. Van der Meij, E.H.; Epstein, J.B.; Hay, J.; Ho, V.; Lerner, K. Sweet's syndrome in a patient with oral cancer associated with radiotherapy. *Eur. J. Cancer B Oral Oncol.* **1996**, *32B*, 133–136. [CrossRef]
189. Uittamo, J.; Siikala, E.; Kaihovaara, P.; Salaspuro, M.; Rautemaa, R. Chronic candidosis and oral cancer in APECED-patients: Production of carcinogenic acetaldehyde from glucose and ethanol by Candida albicans. *Int. J. Cancer* **2009**, *124*, 754–756. [CrossRef]
190. Shillitoe, E.J. The role of immunology in the diagnosis, prognosis and treatment planning of oral cancer. *Proc. R. Soc. Med.* **1976**, *69*, 747–749.

191. Meurman, J.H. Infectious and dietary risk factors of oral cancer. *Oral Oncol.* **2010**, *46*, 411–413. [CrossRef]
192. Sanjaya, P.R.; Gokul, S.; Gururaj Patil, B.; Raju, R. Candida in oral pre-cancer and oral cancer. *Med. Hypotheses* **2011**, *77*, 1125–1128. [CrossRef]
193. Morris, L.G.; Patel, S.G.; Shah, J.P.; Ganly, I. Squamous cell carcinoma of the oral tongue in the pediatric age group: A matched-pair analysis of survival. *Arch. Otolaryngol. Head Neck Surg.* **2010**, *136*, 697–701. [CrossRef]
194. Hara, H.; Ozeki, S.; Nagata, T.; Okamoto, M.; Sasaguri, M.; Tashiro, H.; Jingu, K. Pulmonary tuberculosis in patients with oral cancer. *Gan No Rinsho.* **1988**, *34*, 1647–1653. [PubMed]
195. Laprise, C.; Shahul, H.P.; Madathil, S.A. Periodontal diseases and risk of oral cancer in Southern India: Results from the HeNCe Life study. *Int. J. Cancer.* **2016**, *139*, 1512–1519. [CrossRef] [PubMed]
196. Arantes, D.A.; Costa, N.L.; Mendonça, E.F.; Silva, T.A.; Batista, A.C. Overexpression of immunosuppressive cytokines is associated with poorer clinical stage of oral squamous cell carcinoma. *Arch. Oral Biol.* **2016**, *61*, 28–35. [CrossRef] [PubMed]
197. Hwang, P.H.; Lian, L.; Zavras, A.I. Alcohol intake and folate antagonism via CYP2E1 and ALDH1: Effects on oral carcinogenesis. *Med. Hypotheses* **2012**, *78*, 197–202. [CrossRef]
198. Mun, M.; Yap, T.; Alnuaimi, A.D.; Adams, G.G.; McCullough, M.J. Oral candidal carriage in asymptomatic patients. *Aust. Dent. J.* **2016**, *61*, 190–195. [CrossRef]
199. Krogh, P.; Hald, B.; Holmstrup, P. Possible mycological etiology of oral mucosal cancer: Catalytic potential of infecting Candida albicans and other yeasts in production of N-nitrosobenzylmethylamine. *Carcinogenesis* **1987**, *8*, 1543–1548. [CrossRef]
200. Yakin, M.; Gavidi, R.O.; Cox, B.; Rich, A. Oral cancer risk factors in New Zealand. *N. Z. Med. J.* **2017**, *130*, 30–38.
201. Sheu, J.J.; Keller, J.J.; Lin, H.C. Increased risk of cancer after Bell's palsy: A 5-year follow-up study. *J. Neurooncol.* **2012**, *110*, 215–220. [CrossRef]
202. Ma'aita, J.K. Oral cancer in Jordan: A retrospective study of 118 patients. *Croat. Med. J.* **2000**, *41*, 64–69.
203. Mäkinen, A.; Nawaz, A.; Mäkitie, A.; Meurman, J.H. Role of Non-Albicans Candida and Candida Albicans in Oral Squamous Cell Cancer Patients. *J. Oral Maxillofac. Surg.* **2018**, *76*, 2564–2571. [CrossRef]
204. Menicagli, R.; Bolla, G.; Menicagli, L.; Esseridou, A. The Possible Role of Diabetes in the Etiology of Laryngeal Cancer. *Gulf. J. Oncolog.* **2017**, *1*, 44–51.
205. Bhattathiri, N.V.; Bindu, L.; Remani, P.; Chandralekha, B.; Nair, K.M. Radiation-induced acute immediate nuclear abnormalities in oral cancer cells: Serial cytologic evaluation. *Acta Cytol.* **1998**, *42*, 1084–1090. [CrossRef] [PubMed]
206. D'Costa, J.; Saranath, D.; Sanghvi, V.; Mehta, A.R. Epstein-Barr virus in tobacco-induced oral cancers and oral lesions in patients from India. *J. Oral Pathol. Med.* **1998**, *27*, 78–82. [CrossRef] [PubMed]
207. Jin, X.; Lu, S.; Xing, X.; Wang, L.; Mu, D.; He, M.; Huang, H.; Zeng, X.; Chen, Q. Thalidomide: Features and potential significance in oral precancerous conditions and oral cancer. *J. Oral Pathol. Med.* **2013**, *42*, 355–362. [CrossRef] [PubMed]
208. Gall, F.; Colella, G.; Di Onofrio, V.; Rossiello, R.; Angelillo, I.F.; Liguori, G. Candida spp. in oral cancer and oral precancerous lesions. *New Microbiol.* **2013**, *36*, 283–288.
209. Vijayakumar, T.; Sasidharan, V.K.; Ankathil, R.; Remani, P.; Kumari, T.V.; Vasudevan, D.M. Incidence of hepatitis B surface antigen (HBsAg) in oral cancer and carcinoma of uterine cervix. *Indian J. Cancer* **1984**, *21*, 7–10.
210. Li, M.H.; Ito, D.; Sanada, M.; Odani, T.; Hatori, M.; Iwase, M.; Nagumo, M. Effect of 5-fluorouracil on G1 phase cell cycle regulation in oral cancer cell lines. *Oral Oncol.* **2004**, *40*, 63–70. [CrossRef]
211. Mawardi, H.; Elad, S.; Correa, M.E.; Stevenson, K.; Woo, S.B.; Almazrooa, S.; Haddad, R.; Antin, H.J.; Soiffer, R.; Treister, H. Oral epithelial dysplasia and squamous cell carcinoma following allogeneic hematopoietic stem cell transplantation: Clinical presentation and treatment outcomes. *Bone Marrow Transplant.* **2011**, *46*, 884–891. [CrossRef]
212. Gruter, M.O.; Brand, H.S. Oral health complications after a heart transplant: A review. *Br. Dent. J.* **2020**, *228*, 177–182. [CrossRef]
213. Sankaranarayanan, R.; Dinshaw, K.; Nene, B.M. Cervical and oral cancer screening in India. *J. Med. Screen.* **2006**, *13* (Suppl. 1), S35–S38.
214. Nagasaka, M.; Zaki, M.; Kim, H. PD1/PD-L1 inhibition as a potential radiosensitizer in head and neck squamous cell carcinoma: A case report. *J. Immunother. Cancer* **2016**, *4*, 83. [CrossRef] [PubMed]
215. Kapoor, V.; Aggarwal, S.; Das, S.N. 6-Gingerol Mediates its Anti-Tumor Activities in Human Oral and Cervical Cancer Cell Lines through Apoptosis and Cell Cycle Arrest. *Phytother. Res.* **2016**, *30*, 588–595. [CrossRef] [PubMed]
216. Ha, N.H.; Park, D.G.; Woo, B.H. Porphyromonas gingivalis increases the invasiveness of oral cancer cells by upregulating IL-8 and MMPs. *Cytokine* **2016**, *86*, 64–72. [CrossRef] [PubMed]
217. Ahmed, H.G. Aetiology of oral cancer in the Sudan. *J. Oral Maxillofac. Res.* **2013**, *4*, e3. [CrossRef] [PubMed]
218. Lucchese, A. Viruses and Oral Cancer: Crossreactivity as a Potential Link. *Anticancer Agents Med. Chem.* **2015**, *15*, 1224–1229. [CrossRef] [PubMed]

Disclaimer/Publisher's Note: The statements, opinions and data contained in all publications are solely those of the individual author(s) and contributor(s) and not of MDPI and/or the editor(s). MDPI and/or the editor(s) disclaim responsibility for any injury to people or property resulting from any ideas, methods, instructions or products referred to in the content.

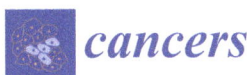

Systematic Review

Osteoradionecrosis of the Jaws Due to Teeth Extractions during and after Radiotherapy: A Systematic Review

Carlo Lajolo [1,2], Cosimo Rupe [1,2], Gioele Gioco [1,2,*], Giuseppe Troiano [3], Romeo Patini [1,2,*], Massimo Petruzzi [4], Francesco Micciche' [5,6] and Michele Giuliani [3]

1. Head and Neck Department, Fondazione Policlinico Universitario A. Gemelli IRCCS, 00168 Rome, Italy; carlo.lajolo@unicatt.it (C.L.); cosimorupe@gmail.com (C.R.)
2. School of Dentistry, Università Cattolica del Sacro Cuore, 00168 Rome, Italy
3. Department of Clinical and Experimental Medicine, University of Foggia, Via Rovelli 50, 71122 Foggia, Italy; giuseppe.troiano@unifg.it (G.T.); michele.giuliani@unifg.it (M.G.)
4. Interdisciplinary Department of Medicine, University of Bari, 70121 Bari, Italy; massimo.petruzzi@uniba.it
5. Dipartimento di Scienze Radiologiche, Radioterapiche ed Ematologiche, UOC di Radioterapia, Fondazione Policlinico Universitario A. Gemelli IRCCS, 00168 Rome, Italy; francesco.micciche@policlinicogemelli.it
6. Istituto di Radiologia, Università Cattolica del Sacro Cuore, 00168 Rome, Italy
* Correspondence: gioele.gioco01@icatt.it (G.G.); romeo.patini@unicatt.it (R.P.)

Simple Summary: Teeth extractions before or after radiotherapy (RT) could be procedures at high risk for osteoradionecrosis (ORN) onset. This systematic review was performed to investigate the ORN incidence following teeth extractions during and after RT for head and neck (H&N) cancer and to evaluate any other possible risk factor. The results highlight how post-RT teeth extractions are a major risk factor for ORN onset (ORN incidence of 5.8%), especially in the mandible, with a diminishing trend in the last years.

Abstract: Teeth extractions before or after radiotherapy (RT) could be procedures at high risk for osteoradionecrosis (ORN) onset. This systematic review was performed to investigate the ORN incidence following teeth extractions during and after RT for head and neck (H&N) cancer and to evaluate any other possible risk factor. Methods: This systematic review was conducted according to PRISMA protocol, and the PROSPERO registration number was CRD42018079986. An electronic search was performed on the following search engines: PubMed, Scopus, and Web of Science. A cumulative meta-analysis was performed. Results: Two thousand two hundred and eighty-one records were screened, and nine were finally included. This systematic review revealed an ORN incidence of 5.8% (41 patients out of 462, 95% CI = 2.3–9.4); 3 ORN developed in the maxilla. No other clinical risk factors were detected. Conclusion: Post-RT teeth extractions represent a major risk factor for ORN development, especially in the mandible, with a diminishing trend in the last years. Further research on other possible risk factors might improve this evidence.

Keywords: osteoradionecrosis; jaw; head and neck cancer; radiotherapy; tooth extraction

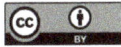

1. Introduction

Among the most common malignancies worldwide, head and neck (H&N) cancers represent the seventh one [1], and almost 75% of patients are treated with radiotherapy (RT), which is either curative or adjuvant or palliative [2]. Unfortunately, RT may cause several side effects, [3] among which osteoradionecrosis (ORN) of the jaws is the most serious.

Signs and symptoms of ORN can vary from pain, sequestration of necrotic bone, and fistulas, to more severe cases with the fracture of the mandible, which can result in sepsis, which is potentially life-threatening, or require major surgical procedures and provoke oral feeding difficulties [4].

ORN can be defined as exposed irradiated bone that fails to heal over a period of three months without evidence of persisting or recurrent tumor; nevertheless, the ORN definition remains a debated topic, due to the following issues: the possibility of ORN onset without bone exposure and the duration of bone exposure necessary to achieve a definite diagnosis, which varies from 1 to 6 months, according to the literature [5,6]. Furthermore, definitions retrieved in literature do not mention the possibility that patients could present jaw bones necrosis due to antiresorptive therapy (medication-related osteonecrosis of the jaws—MRONJ) [7], which may be administered for other tumors and must be excluded in the differential diagnosis or, at least, taken into debt consideration.

Hypovascularity and hypocellularity subsequent to bone irradiation [6] and the following fibro-atrophic process [8] seem to be crucial in the ORN pathogenesis, forming fragile tissues susceptible to necrosis, especially in cases of tissue damage, such as teeth extractions.

Teeth extractions after radiotherapy are recognized as the most important risk factor for the ORN onset [9–13], with a reported incidence ranging between 2% and 22% of patients [14,15], according to the different studied populations and the different diagnostic parameters.

Nabil et coll. (2011) [9] conducted a systematic review that revealed an overall ORN incidence of 7% in patients who underwent tooth extractions after RT; nevertheless, the high number of factors contributing to the ORN pathogenesis (i.e., tumour site, TNM, oncologic therapeutic protocol, oral general status, site of tooth extraction, flap elevation, antibiotics, and hyperbaric oxygen therapy) make the information necessary to prevent ORN onset after tooth extraction insufficient and inadequate, due to the complexity of the topic.

This systematic review was performed to assess (i) the ORN rate following post-radiotherapy tooth extractions; (ii) what is the time-lapse between RT and teeth extraction associated with a lower incidence of ORN; (iii) which other risk factors are associated with the ORN onset; (iv) whether any protocol could prevent or reduce the ORN rate; and (v) whether the ORN rate following the pre-RT tooth extraction is lower than the ORN rate following post-RT tooth extraction.

2. Methods

This systematic review was conducted following the Preferred Reporting Items for Systematic Reviews and Meta-Analyses (PRISMA) Statement criteria [16]. PROSPERO Registration was performed, and the following ID was assigned: CRD42018079986.

2.1. Inclusion and Exclusion Criteria

Inclusion and exclusion criteria are resumed in Table 1.

2.2. Search Strategy and Selection of Studies

An electronic search was performed on the following search engines: PubMed, Scopus, and Web of Science, without specifical filters, from January 1978 to November 2021.

The electronic search strategy was conducted by using a combination of the following MeSH terms and free text words: "Osteoradionecrosis" AND "Dentistry", "Osteoradionecrosis" AND "Prevention", "Osteoradionecrosis" AND "Tooth Extraction", and "Osteoradionecrosis" AND "Tooth Removal".

Two reviewers (G.T. and G.G.) assessed the studies' eligibility in a standardized independent manner. If there was any disagreement, it was evaluated by a third reviewer (C.L.) for the final decision. The screening process was conducted according to the PRISMA flow-diagram (Figure 1). A manual search was also conducted on the following journals: Oral Oncology, Clinical Oral Investigations, Oral Diseases, and European Journal of Oral Sciences. In addition, reference lists of the included articles were manually searched, in order to retrieve any possible full-length papers which could be included.

Table 1. Inclusion and exclusion criteria adopted for this systematic review.

Inclusion Criteria
Full papers, literature in English language, published after 1978 in peer-reviewed journals
Observational clinical studies, both prospective and retrospective (cohort and case-control), and RCTs
Minimum sample size of 10 patients who underwent tooth extractions after radiotherapy in an H&N district
No previous ORN at the extraction site
Mean 6 months follow-up after tooth extractions
Unhealed sockets followed up for at least 3 months
Exclusion criteria
Case reports, reviews, cross-sectional studies
Studies in which no clear definition of ORN was reported
Studies not specifying whether ORN developed at the extraction site.

Studies on therapies of patients with ORN were included only if the ORN was effectively due to dental extractions and if the total number of patients receiving tooth extractions was clearly stated. Because many definitions of ORN have been proposed, confusion exists regarding its diagnosis, mainly concerning the time of bone exposure. The assessment of the period of bone exposure is crucial to achieving an ORN diagnosis, because it is not possible to clinically distinguish between a delayed alveolar bone healing and a true ORN. In this revision, studies without a clear definition of ORN were excluded to avoid biases. Abbreviations: ORN, osteoradionecrosis; RCTs, randomized clinical trials; H&N, head and neck.

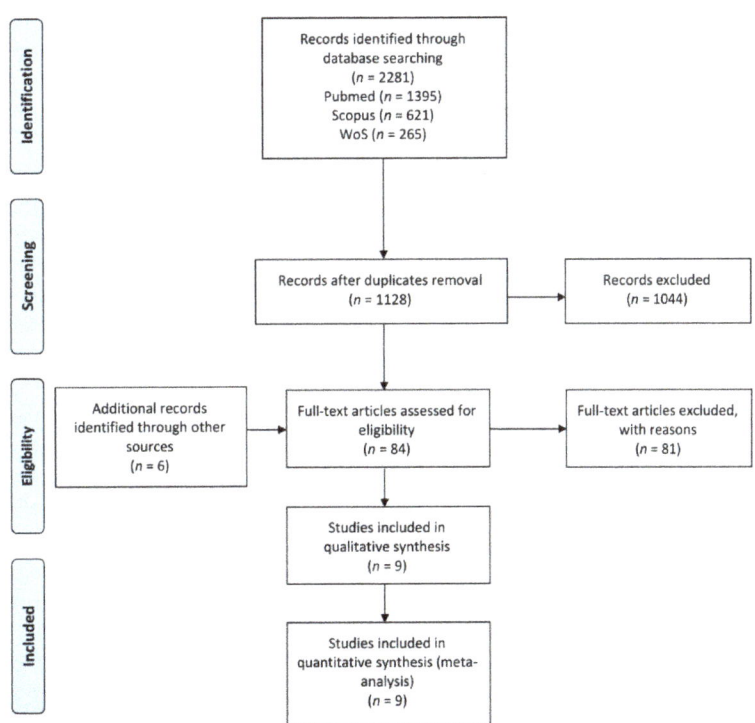

Figure 1. PRISMA flow-diagram of the selection process. Nine articles were finally included in the systematic review and meta-analysis. Adapted from Moher, D et al. (2010) [16]. For more information, visit www.prisma-statement.org (Accessed on 15 November 2021).

2.3. Data Collection

General information on the included papers (i.e., study design, year of publication, country, number of patients, ORN definition, and diagnostic process) and data related to patients (i.e., age and gender, tooth extraction protocol, extraction-related ORN, and other possible risk factors) were collected into a customized table.

2.4. Risk of Bias Assessment

The risk of bias assessment was performed throughout the modified Newcastle Ottawa scale [17] and the Jadad scale [18] (File S1, Supplementary Materials) by 2 reviewers (C.R. and C.L.). In case of disagreement, the final assessment was performed by a third reviewer (G.T.).

2.5. Statistical Analysis

A cumulative meta-analysis was performed with a random effects model in accordance to DerSimonian–Laird method. The pooled proportion (PP) of the rate of ORN occurrence was calculated. The results of the meta-analysis were presented throughout a forest plot graph. The software Open Meta-Analyst version 10 was used to perform the statistical analysis.

3. Results

3.1. Results of Search and Study Selection

The electronic search provided 2281 records (PubMed: 1395 papers, Scopus: 621 papers, Web of Science: 265 papers), and 84 papers were selected for full-paper evaluation. The manual search retrieved six additional articles which underwent a full-text evaluation; providing a total of 90 reviewed papers. Nine articles fulfilled the inclusion criteria and, thus, were included in qualitative and quantitative synthesis [11,12,14,15,19–23]. Table S1 (Supplementary Materials) reports the reasons for the exclusion of the other 81 full-length papers. The selection process is reported as a flow-diagram, following the PRISMA guidelines, in Figure 1.

3.2. Study Characteristics and Summary of Results

This systematic review includes seven retrospective cohort studies, one prospective study, and one clinical trial.

General information on the included papers (i.e., study design, year of publication, country, number of patients, ORN definition, and diagnostic process) is reported in Table 2.

Specific information regarding patients who underwent teeth extractions is presented in Table 3.

Teeth extractions were performed during and after RT on 462 patients out of a total of 800 subjects suffering from H&N cancer. Overall, among these patients, 41 received an ORN diagnosis at the extraction site in a mean follow-up of 40.6 months. The meta-analysis revealed a 5.8% ORN incidence (95% CI = 2.3–9.4, $p < 0.001$). The analysis showed the presence of a high rate of heterogeneity between the studies ($I^2 = 8466\%$). The pooled proportion (PP) and the box plot of the included articles are reported in Figure 2.

Three patients out of 41 developed ORN in the maxilla, while all of the others affected the mandible. Table S2 (Supplementary Materials) shows the details of reported ORN, although only few data could be retrieved.

Table 2. Population data of the selected articles: a total of 462 subjects underwent teeth extractions after RT.

Study	Study Design	Included Patients			Mean Age	Mean Follow-Up	RT Technique			Mean Dose §	Patients Receiving Tooth Extraction	Cases of ORN	ORN Due to Tooth Extraction
		Tot	M	F	Years	Months	EBR	IMRT	BT	Gy	n.	n.	n.
Morrish et al., 1981 [19]	R	100	60	40	65	23	100	0	0	66	18	22	9 [a]
Beumer et al., 1983 [15]	R	72	-	-	-	*	72	0	0	-	72	16	16 [a]
Marx et al., 1985 [20]	RCT	74	-	-	-	*	-	-	-	68	74	13	13 [b]
Epstein et al., 1987 [21]	R	146	103	43	54.7	60	140	0	6	-	54	8	3 [a]
Maxymiw et al., 1991 [12]	P	72	-	-	57.4	57.6	72	0	0	50	72	0	0 [b]
Lambert et al., 1997 [22]	R	47	-	-	-	35.3	-	-	-	60.6	46	0	0 [b]
David et al., 2001 [23]	R	24	13	11	61	10.3	-	-	-	-	24	0	0 [b]
Ben-David et al., 2007 [14]	R	176	128	48	55	35	0	176	0	54.6	13	0	0 [c]
Al-Bazie et al., 2016 [11]	R	89	55	34	41.8	63	-	-	-	65.4	89	0	0 [b]

* Although it was not possible to identify a mean value, the study was included because every patient received a follow-up of at least six months. § The prescribed dose to the tissues affected by the neoplasm. [a] Bone exposure longer than 3 months. [b] Bone exposure longer than 6 months. [c] Bone exposure is present in 2 consecutive follow-ups (6–8 weeks for the first two years, 3–4 months after the first 2 years). Abbreviations: Tot, Total; M, Male; F, Female; n., number; RCT, Randomized Clinical Trial; P, prospective; R, Retrospective; RT, radiotherapy; ORN, osteoradionecrosis; EBR, External Beam Radiotherapy; IMRT, Intensity Modulated Radiation Therapy; BT, Brachytherapy; Gy, Gray.

Table 3. Characteristics of patients who underwent teeth extraction: among 462 patients who received tooth extractions after RT, 41 ORN were diagnosed.

Study	Patients	Time from RT to Teeth Extraction	N. of Teeth Extraction	ORN Patients	ORN Sites		
		Months			Tot	Maxilla	Mandible
Morrish et al., 1981 [19]	18	-	-	9	9	-	-
Beumer et al., 1983 [15]	72	31	27	16	16	3	13
Marx et al., 1985 [20]	74	-	291	13	35	0	35
Epstein et al., 1987 [21]	54	32.4	173	3	3	0	3
Maxymiw et al., 1991 [12]	72	-	449	0	0	0	0
Lambert et al., 1997 [22]	46	-	704	0	0	0	0
David et al., 2001 [23]	24	-	54	0	0	0	0
Ben-David et al., 2007 [14]	13	-	-	0	0	0	0
Al-Bazie et al., 2016 [11]	89	15	232	0	0	0	0

Abbreviations: n., number; Tot, Total; ORN, osteoradionecrosis; RT, radiotherapy.

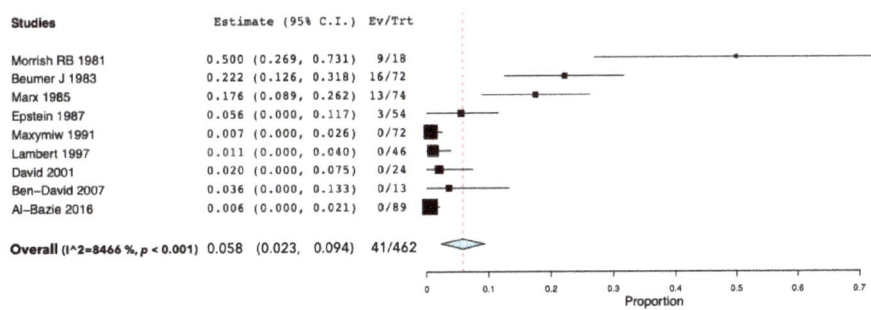

Figure 2. One-way forest plot of the selected articles shows the PP of the incidence of ORN in irradiated patients receiving teeth extractions during and after RT. Abbreviations: CI, Confidence Interval; Ev, Events; Trt, Total of Patients receiving teeth extractions; I^2, Higgins' Hindex.

3.3. Risk of Bias Assessment

The risk of bias assessment for the included papers is reported in Table 4. The methodological quality of the included studies was dis-homogeneous. Four articles out of nine reached a high score, such as Al-Bazie et al. (2016) [11,14], whereas others had an elevated risk of bias. Furthermore, the selection risk of bias was low, since all the inclusion criteria were strict, including only studies performed on a population of irradiated H&N cancer patients who received teeth extractions during and after RT. The shortcomings mostly concerned the comparability and the outcomes domains: in fact, no studies reported other confounders (i.e., antiresorptive drugs), and only a few studies reached one year of follow-up after teeth extractions and outlined the drop-out rate.

Table 4. Modified Newcastle-Ottawa Score and Jadad scale.

Cohort Studies	Selection				Comparability		Outcome			Modified Newcastle-Ottawa Score (Risk of Bias)
Author	Representativeness of cohort	Selection of non-exposed cohort	Ascertainment of exposure	Outcome of interest not present at onset	Control of confounding factors (extraction)	Control of confounding factors (field of radiation, timing, extraction protocol)	Assessment of outcome	Length of follow-up	Lost to follow-up	
Morrish et al., 1981 [19]	x	x	x	x	x			x	x	x	8
Beumer et al., 1983 [15]	x		x	x	x		x	x	x	x	7
Epstein et al., 1987 [21]	x	x	x	x	x		x	x			7
Maxymiw et al., 1991 [12]	x		x	x	x			x	x	x	7
Lambert et al., 1997 [22]	x		x	x	x			x	x		6
David et al., 2001 [23]	x		x	x	x			x	x	x	8
Ben-David et al., 2007 [14]	x	x	x	x	x			x	x	x	8
Al-Bazie et al., 2016 [11]	x		x	x	x		x	x	x	x	8

RCT Studies	Randomization			Blinding		Description of Withdrawal and Dropouts	Jadad Scale
Author	1 point if randomization is mentioned	1 point if the method of randomization is appropriate	Deduct 1 point if the method of randomization is inappropriate	1 point if blinding is mentioned	1 point if the method of blinding is appropriate	Deduct 1 point if the method of blinding is inappropriate	1 point if withdrawal and dropouts are described
Marx et al., 1985 [20]	x							

3.4. Results of Individual Studies

Results of individual studies among patients who underwent teeth extraction after radiotherapy are reported in Tables 2 and 3.

3.5. Excluded Studies

The reasons for the exclusion of the other 81 full-length papers are summarized in the Table S1 (Supplementary Materials), available electronically.

In particular, 22 studies did not reach an adequate sample size to be included; 17 studies provided an inadequate definition or diagnosis of ORN; 11 studies had a design not fulfilling the inclusion criteria (reviews, letters to editor); 15 studies analyzed a cohort not representative of the whole population of patients undergoing tooth extractions during or after RT; seven studies did not reach an adequate follow-up (six months after tooth extraction); nine studies diagnosed ORN cases, but it was not clear whether the ORN developed at post-extraction sites.

The study conducted by Schweiger et al. (1987) [24] was remarkable; nevertheless, it did not fulfill the inclusion criteria: the authors made an ORN diagnosis after one month of bone exposure. Notably, a medical examination conducted one month after tooth extraction may overestimate the ORN rate. In fact, the authors reported a higher risk of ORN incidence (8%) following post-RT dental extractions.

The study conducted by Saito et al. (2021) [25] was well conducted; nevertheless, as the authors declared in their discussion section, it was not possible to distinguish if ORN was present at the moment of the extraction or if it was a consequence of the post-RT dental extraction. This could have led to an overrating of ORN incidence (28.1%, as reported by the authors).

Another recent study, performed by Kubota et al., 2021 [26], showed good methodology. Nevertheless, the authors did not specify whether the ORN developed at the post-RT extraction site.

4. Discussion

The role of dentists in the H&N cancer supportive therapy is becoming fundamental. The main objectives of dental treatment in these patients, before radiotherapy, are the removal of oral foci and, after radiotherapy, the prevention and therapy of dental diseases and the side-effects of radio-chemotherapy involving the oral cavity. Development of more accurate radiotherapy techniques (e.g., IMRT) has decreased the number of side-effects in the oro-maxillofacial district [27]; nevertheless, ORN remains the most important event, and together with severe mucositis, which sometimes undermines a patient's life, it can occur in 2% to 22% of irradiated subjects [14,15]. Since teeth extractions performed after the RT represent the main risk factor for ORN onset, dentists should prevent dental diseases to minimize the number of extractions after the RT, and in the case where extraction is necessary, dentists should apply specific protocols to decrease the risk of the onset of ORN.

However, the possible progression of dental diseases, precipitated by the consequences of RT on oral and maxillofacial tissues (e.g., radio-induced caries), and the increase in life expectancy determine the possibility to perform dental extractions in patients who received radiotherapy for H&N cancer [1,28,29]. This systematic review showed an ORN rate of 5.8% in patients undergoing tooth extractions after RT, in accordance with the systematic review conducted by Nabil et coll. (2011) [9]. Comparing the final data obtained from this systematic review (5.8% of ORN in post-RT) with those of extractions performed before radiotherapy (2.2%), reported in a systematic review already conducted by our research group [30], it seems reasonable to consider post-RT extractions as a high-risk procedure and suggest performing them before starting RT. These results are in contrast with the findings emerging from another systematic review, which did not retrieve statistically significant differences in the ORN risk between patients undergoing tooth extractions before RT and patients undergoing tooth extractions after RT [31]. Although it is not easy to find an explanation for these differences in the results, it could be related to less restrictive inclusion and exclusion criteria adopted by Beaumont S et al. (2021). Nevertheless, both the reviews show how a thorough analysis of the risk factors needs to be performed, by means of new clinical trials, in order to reach a better understanding of the pathogenesis of ORN, as further discussed in the discussion section.

However, if we analyze the incidence of ORN in the papers included in this review, it is very uneven: notably, as presented in Figure 2, incidence varies from 50% to 5.6% in the articles prior to 1990 and is up to 0% in articles published from 1990 to today. Therefore, it seems that post-RT extractions no longer involve this risk, unlike pre-RT extractions, which despite a decreasing trend, still show a certain percentage of ORN, and this has been observed in recent studies too (e.g., 7.6% in Schuurhuis, 2011 and 13% in Batstone, 2012) [32,33]. Nevertheless, a recent study conducted by Kubota H et al. (2021) reported an ORN rate of 7.5% in patients who underwent radiotherapy during the last decade [26]. Further studies are needed in order to better clarify the real incidence of ORN. This different frequency of ORN for post-RT extractions, between studies conducted before and after 1990, appears notable but is difficult to fully understand.

Possible explanations are the introduction of the more advanced technique (IMRT) that could have contributed to the progressive reduction of this incidence. IMRT selectively irradiates the tumor, giving a significantly lower dose to healthy tissues. In the 1980s, the transition from traditional 2D to conformed 3D (3DCRT) treatment represented a critical advance in RT. In 3DCRT, simulation and treatment planning are based on computerized tomography (CT), reaching a precise definition of the area affected by neoplastic disease and a more accurate dose calculation. Afterwards, the introduction of IMRT, a highly specialized typology of conformative therapy, through the modulation of the beam flow, allowed the irradiation of the target site with a non-uniform intensity, increasing the dose only to cancer tissues. Furthermore, it allowed the use of multiple irradiation planes, including oblique and not coplanar planes, which together with the use of multilamellar collimators, ensure adequate irradiation of tumor tissues and the saving of healthy tissues, including alveolar bone. However, in many of the studies analyzed, the radiotherapy technique used was unknown.

Furthermore, the increased involvement of dentists in the management of H&N cancer patients could have improved oral conditions of patients post-RT: careful dental treatment before the beginning of RT (e.g., extraction of all teeth with uncertain prognosis), a thorough dental follow-up after the RT (e.g., interception of any possible dental diseases at early stages), and supportive therapies (i.e., oral hygiene recalls and professional fluoride therapy) may contribute to a better oral health after RT. The result of such careful management could mean (1) a lower number of extractions per patient, (2) less inflamed/infected foci, (3) a more accurate extraction planning, and (4) better general oral health conditions.

Our first consideration focuses on the critical issues of the definition and diagnosis of ORN. In accordance with the literature published in the last 15 years, we included only those studies that provided a clear definition of ORN and in which the ORN was diagnosed in the case of irradiated bone, exposed in the oral cavity, for a minimum of three months, with no local recurrences [5,6,34]. Most of the excluded studies, analyzed in full-text, provided no clear definition of the disease. We considered it essential that a clear definition of ORN was present in the study; in the literature, there are several definitions which differ from each other in the length of time of bone exposure and about the bone exposure as a main sign of ORN diagnosis. Although the bone exposure has to linger in post-extractive alveoli for a period of time such as to exclude delayed healing of the alveolus (i.e., dry socket), there is no agreement in defining the post-extraction time interval after which an ORN may be diagnosed. A short time interval could notably overestimate the real ORN rate; by contrast, a long time interval could underestimate the real rate of ORN because some ORN can heal spontaneously, going through bone sequestration, and therefore not be correctly diagnosed. Furthermore, some authors described the possibility that ORN occurs even without bone exposure [35]. Therefore, considering exposed bone as the only sign of ORN, the ORN rate could be underestimated due to a misdiagnosis or to a diagnostic delay. Further research should provide a clear definition of ORN so that it would be possible to compare the results and provide data with a stronger level of evidence.

Another relevant methodological bias that we found from the analysis of the literature concerns the outcome: most of the studies provided information on the number of patients with ORN without providing any information on the number of sites affected by ORN. Considering that ORN may occur in more than one site in the same patient, further research might provide a precise indication of the sites affected by ORN in relation to the post-extraction site. Moreover, to provide a specific risk of ORN onset at post-extractive alveoli, the studies should provide more precise information on the affected sites subjected to extraction (in the irradiated patient population). Contrariwise, most of the studies provided no information on either the sites undergoing post-RT extractions or on the number of post-extractive sites affected by ORN, except Marx et al. (1995) [20].

Some noteworthy clinical considerations concern the anatomical site of tooth extraction. Mandibular jaw appears to be a risk factor of ORN onset following teeth extractions. This systematic review reported only three cases of ORN in the maxilla, while all the other cases developed in the mandible. Unfortunately, it was not possible to clarify the ORN risk related to anatomical site, since the included articles did not report data regarding the anatomical site of extracted teeth in the overall population undergoing RT. Another clinical consideration concerns the surgical technique adopted for the extraction of teeth in patients that received irradiation. Non-surgical extractions are less invasive; however, the lifting of a flap allows the closure of the post-extraction site by first intention and the possibility to modify the bone morphology when necessary. Nowadays, little is known regarding whether any innovative surgical technique can decrease the ORN risk. Marx et coll. (1985) and Maxymiw et coll. (1991) performed all teeth extractions without lifting a flap [12,20]. The ORN rate found by these authors was somewhat discordant: Marx diagnosed 35 ORN out of 291 extracted teeth, and Maxymiw diagnosed no ORN out of 449 extracted teeth. However, the other included articles did not report sufficient data regarding teeth extraction techniques. Further studies are necessary to confirm whether the extraction technique influences the risk of ORN.

Another little-known aspect concerns the reasons to perform dental extractions in this specific cohort of patients: none of the included articles provided information on this matter. Notably, an assessment should be performed as to whether the motivation for a tooth to be extracted could favor the onset of ORN, bearing in mind that the non-extraction of teeth affected by inflammatory-infectious processes could represent a trigger for the onset of ORN, similar to what occurs for MRONJ [36]. By contrast, it seems reasonable that extractions of teeth affected by an inflammatory-infectious process may represent a higher ORN risk procedure. However, post-irradiated alveolar bone could be affected by spontaneous ORN, miming in the early stages an inflammatory-infectious process, overestimating the risk of ORN consequent to post-RT extraction. The articles included in this review do not provide information regarding this topic.

A necessary consideration is relative to the dose received by the post-extraction sites, which could be considered a risk factor for ORN onset. The patients affected by ORN received an average dose of 68 Gy. Unfortunately, it was not possible to define a threshold, since the included articles did not provide information for the specific post-extraction alveoli. Nevertheless, a reasonable opinion is that high-dose radiation therapy increases the risk of ORN.

A highly debated topic in the literature concerns the identification of a time interval after the end of the RT, beyond which the surgical procedures may be safer or associated with a lower risk. Although a reasonable judgement seems to be that postponing the extraction can reduce the risk of ORN, alterations of bone metabolism could persist or worsen several years after the end of radiation therapy. This systematic review showed that patients who developed ORN had a mean time interval from RT to dental extractions longer than the whole population (33 months vs. 24.7 months); these data, contrariwise to general opinion, seem to suggest that a longer time-lapse between RT and ORN could not prevent the ORN onset. However, this information was reported in only two of the four studies that diagnosed ORNs and refers to average values. Specifically, Beumer et al. (1983) [15] conducted dental extractions at different time intervals (7–60 months), and the time-interval from RT to dental extraction was not associated with a higher ORN risk. Although the most recent evidence seems to confirm this result [31] and some authors suggest performing tooth extractions in the immediate post-RT period [26], it is important to consider the possible existence of a "bimodal pattern" of RT damage, showing two different peaks of risk: 12 months after the end of RT and 24–60 months after RT [10]. At present, no controlled studies allow a conclusion regarding the existence of a time interval that reduces the risk of ORN; therefore, this topic warrants further investigation.

Among the risk factors to be evaluated in the estimate of the onset of ORN, the influence of any previous or ongoing medical therapy that may enhance the risk must also be considered. The increased number of patients undergoing medical treatments with antiresorptive, antiangiogenetic, and biological drugs (e.g., denosumab, bisphosphonates) for oncological or metabolic reasons makes it necessary to conduct an accurate interview of the medical history of each patient [37]. Studies included in this review provided no information on this regard. A critical clinical consideration pertains to the different perioperative medical support protocols reported in the literature to reduce the ORN risk. Among those protocols, antibiotics associated with antiseptic rinses are the most used. There is strong evidence that the deeper zones of necrotic bone are colonized by bacteria of the oral district, so much so that the pathogenetic idea of aseptic necrosis has been repeatedly challenged over time. In the study conducted by Al-Bazie et al. (2016) [11] and Maxymiw et al. (1991) [12], the antibiotic prophylaxis with amoxicillin and penicillin V was included in the protocol and was effective in the prevention of ORN, reporting an ORN rate of 0% (0 ORN out of 161 patients). Additionally, Marx et al. (1985) [20] and Epstein et al. (1987) [21] performed antibiotic prophylaxis; however, their studies showed a higher ORN rate of 35.4% and 5.56%, respectively (altogether, 16 ORN cases out of 91 patients, indicating an ORN rate of 17.58%). Further studies with a larger sample size are therefore needed to clarify the real usefulness of antibiotics in preventing ORN.

Hyperbaric oxygen therapy (HBO) is another peri-operative support provided. The rationale for using HBO is based on the impact of an increased amount of oxygen on hypoxic tissues. Locally, HBO increases the amount of growth factors, including those playing an active role in angiogenesis. Oxygen can also promote an antibacterial effect on the trauma site. Based on the available evidence, the effectiveness of HBO in preventing ORN is debated [38,39]. The articles included in this systematic review did not provide sufficient data regarding the effectiveness of HBO. Further trials are needed to resolve the controversy [37].

Another consideration should be done among new drugs proposed for ORN medical therapy (i.e., pentoxifylline, tocopherol) that could also represent a new approach to the prevention of ORNs [40]. Thus far, none of the studies has analyzed this aspect: future clinical studies might evaluate the preventive role of these drugs for ORN onset.

5. Conclusions

This systematic review highlights that dental extractions after RT are procedures at high risk of ORN, especially in the mandible. It was impossible to draw definitive conclusions about other clinical risk factors, including the time-lapse to respect between RT and tooth extractions. Data gathered from the analyzed literature presented a higher rate of ORN (5.8%) when compared with extractions performed before RT (2.2%) [30]; even if the general trend of ORN is decreasing for both pre- and post-RT extractions, studies performed on extraction after RT presented a peculiar bimodal trend: studies before 1990 show a much higher ORN rate compared with those performed after 1990, which are proximate to 0%. Reasons for this bimodal behaviour are not completely understood; possible explanations are that the introduction of the more advanced radiotherapy techniques and the greatest role of the dental clinician for H&N cancer supportive therapy could have improved oral conditions of patients after RT. Further research among other possible risk factors should be conducted to investigate their role in ORN development.

Supplementary Materials: The following are available online at https://www.mdpi.com/article/10.3390/cancers13225798/s1, File S1: Modified Newcastle-Ottawa quality assessment tool forms for observational studies, Table S1: Articles excluded from systematic review and reasons for their exclusions, Table S2: Details of reported ORN Patients. Gender, Age, and Tumor Site of ORN Patients are not reported because only a few data were retrieved.

Author Contributions: All authors contributed to the study conception and design. Material preparation, data collection, and analysis and the first draft of the manuscript were performed by C.L., G.G. and C.R. All authors commented on previous versions of the manuscript. All authors have read and agreed to the published version of the manuscript.

Funding: No funding to declare.

Institutional Review Board Statement: Not applicable.

Informed Consent Statement: Not applicable.

Data Availability Statement: Data are available upon request to the authors.

Conflicts of Interest: None of the authors have any conflicts of interest to declare.

References

1. Bray, F.; Ferlay, J.; Soerjomataram, I.; Siegel, R.; Torre, L.; Jemal, A. Global Cancer Statistics 2018: GLOBOCAN Estimates of Incidence and Mortality Worldwide for 36 Cancers in 185 Countries 2018. *CA Cancer J. Clin.* **2018**, *68*, 394–424. [CrossRef]
2. Ratko, T.; Douglas, G.; de Souza, J.; Belinson, S.; Aronson, N. *Radiotherapy Treatments for Head and Neck Cancer Update [Internet]*; (Comparative Effectiveness Review, No. 144.); Agency for Healthcare Research and Quality: Rockville, MD, USA, 2014. Available online: https://www.ncbi.nlm.nih.gov/books/NBK269018 (accessed on 14 November 2021).
3. Kielbassa, A.; Hinkelbein, W.; Hellwig, E.; Meyer-Lückel, H. Radiation-related damage to dentition. *Lancet Oncol.* **2006**, *7*, 326–335. [CrossRef]
4. Nadella, K.; Kodali, R.; Guttikonda, L.; Jonnalagadda, A. Osteoradionecrosis of the Jaws: Clinico-Therapeutic Management: A Literature Review and Update. *J. Maxillofac. Oral Surg.* **2015**, *14*, 891–901. [CrossRef]
5. Chronopoulos, A.; Zarra, T.; Ehrenfeld, M.; Otto, S. Osteoradionecrosis of the jaws: Definition, epidemiology, staging and clinical and radiological findings. A concise review. *Int. Dent. J.* **2018**, *68*, 22–30. [CrossRef]
6. Marx, R. Osteoradionecrosis: A new concept of its pathophysiology. *J. Oral Maxillofac. Surg.* **1983**, *41*, 283–288. [CrossRef]
7. Miniello, T.G.; Araújo, J.P.; Silva, M.L.G.; Paulo Kowalski, L.; Rocha, A.C.; Jaguar, G.C.; Abreu Alves, F. Influence of bisphosphonates on clinical features of osteoradionecrosis of the maxilla and mandible. *Oral Dis.* **2019**, *25*, 1344–1351. [CrossRef]
8. Delanian, S.; Lefaix, J. The radiation-induced fibroatrophic process: Therapeutic perspective via the antioxidant pathway. *Radiother. Oncol.* **2004**, *73*, 119–131. [CrossRef]
9. Nabil, S.; Samman, N. Incidence and prevention of osteoradionecrosis after dental extraction in irradiated patients: A systematic review. *Int. J. Oral Maxillofac. Surg.* **2011**, *40*, 229–243. [CrossRef]
10. Marx, R.; Johnson, R. Studies in the radiobiology of osteoradionecrosis and their clinical significance. *Oral Surg. Oral Med. Oral Pathol.* **1987**, *64*, 379–390. [CrossRef]
11. Al-Bazie, S.; Bahatheq, M.; Al-Ghazi, M.; Al-Rajhi, N.; Ramalingam, S. Antibiotic protocol for the prevention of osteoradionecrosis following dental extractions in irradiated head and neck cancer patients: A 10 years prospective study. *J. Cancer Res. Ther.* **2016**, *12*, 565–570. [CrossRef]
12. Maxymiw, W.; Wood, R.; Liu, F. Post-radiation dental extractions without hyperbaric oxygen. *Oral Surg. Oral Med. Oral Pathol.* **1991**, *72*, 270–274. [CrossRef]
13. Buglione, M.; Cavagnini, R.; Di Rosario, F.; Sottocornola, L.; Maddalo, M.; Vassalli, L.; Magrini, S.M. Oral toxicity management in head and neck cancer patients treated with chemotherapy and radiation: Dental pathologies and osteoradionecrosis (Part 1) literature review and consensus statement. *Crit. Rev. Oncol. Hematol.* **2016**, *97*, 131–142. [CrossRef] [PubMed]
14. Ben-David, A.; Diamante, M.; Radawski, J.; Vineberg, K.; Stroup, C.; Murdoch-Kinch, C.; Eisbruch, A. Lack of Osteoradionecrosis of the Mandible after IMRT for Head and Neck Cancer: Likely Contributions of both Dental Care and Improved Dose Distribution. *Int. J. Radiat. Oncol. Biol. Phys.* **2007**, *68*, 392–402. [CrossRef]
15. Beumer, J.; Harrison, R.; Sanders, B.; Kurrasch, M. Postradiation Dental Extractions: A Review of the Literature and A Report of 72 Episodes. *Head Neck Surg.* **1983**, *6*, 581–586. [CrossRef]
16. Moher, D.; Liberati, A.; Tetzlaff, J.; Altman, D.; Group, P. Preferred reporting items for systematic reviews and meta-analyses: The PRISMA statement. *Int. J. Surg.* **2010**, *8*, 336–341. [CrossRef] [PubMed]
17. Stang, A. Critical evaluation of the Newcastle-Ottawa scale for the assessment of the quality of nonrandomized studies in meta-analyses. *Eur. J. Epidemiol.* **2010**, *25*, 603–605. [CrossRef]
18. Jadad, A.; Moore, R.; Carroll, D.; Jenkinson, C.; Reynolds, D.; Gavaghan, D.; McQuay, H.J. Assessing the quality of reports of randomized clinical trials: Is blinding necessary? *Control. Clin. Trials* **1996**, *17*, 1–12. [CrossRef]
19. Morrish, R.J.; Chan, E.; Silverman, S.J.; Meyer, J.; Fu, K.; Greenspan, D. Osteonecrosis in patients irradiated for head and neck carcinoma. *Cancer* **1981**, *47*, 1980–1983. [CrossRef]
20. Marx, R.; Johnson, R.; Kline, S. Prevention of osteoradionecrosis: A randomized prospective clinical trial of hyperbaric oxygen versus penicillin. *J. Am. Dent. Assoc.* **1985**, *111*, 49–54. [CrossRef] [PubMed]
21. Epstein, J.; Rea, G.; Wong, F.; Spinelli, J.; Stevenson-Moore, P. Osteonecrosis: Study of the relationship of dental extractions in patients receiving radiotherapy. *Head Neck Surg.* **1987**, *10*, 48–54. [CrossRef]
22. Lambert, P.; Intriere, N.; Eichstaedt, R. Management of dental extractions in irradiated jaws: A protocol with hyperbaric oxygen therapy. *J. Oral Maxillofac. Surg.* **1997**, *55*, 268–274. [CrossRef]
23. David, L.; Sàndor, G.; Evans, A.; Brown, D. Hyperbaric oxygen therapy and mandibular osteoradionecrosis: A retrospective study and analysis of treatment outcomes. *J. Can. Dent. Assoc.* **2001**, *67*, 384.
24. Schweiger, J. Oral complications following radiation therapy: A five-year retrospective report. *J. Prosthet. Dent.* **1987**, *58*, 78–82. [CrossRef]
25. Saito, I.; Hasegawa, T.; Kawashita, Y.; Kato, S.; Yamada, S.I.; Kojima, Y.; Ueda, N.; Umeda, M.; Shibuya, Y.; Kurita, H.; et al. Association between dental extraction after radiotherapy and osteoradionecrosis: A multi-centre retrospective study. *Oral Dis.* **2021**, in press. [CrossRef]
26. Kubota, H.; Miyawaki, D.; Mukumoto, N.; Ishihara, T.; Matsumura, M.; Hasegawa, T.; Akashi, M.; Kiyota, N.; Shinomiya, H.; Teshima, M.; et al. Risk factors for osteoradionecrosis of the jaw in patients with head and neck squamous cell carcinoma. *Radiat. Oncol.* **2021**, *16*, 1. [CrossRef]

27. Gomez-Millan, J.; Fernández, J.; Medina Carmona, J. Current status of IMRT in head and neck cancer. *Rep. Pract. Oncol. Radiother.* **2013**, *20*, 361–365. [CrossRef]
28. Schuurhuis, J.; Stokman, M.; Witjes, M.; Dijkstra, P.; Vissink, A.; Spijkervet, F. Evidence supporting pre-radiation elimination of oral foci of infection in head and neck cancer patients to prevent oral sequelae. A systematic review. *Oral Oncol.* **2015**, *51*, 212–220. [CrossRef]
29. Brennan, M.; Woo, S.; Lockhart, P. Dental treatment planning and management in the patient who has cancer. *Dent. Clin. North Am.* **2008**, *52*, 19–37. [CrossRef] [PubMed]
30. Lajolo, C.; Gioco, G.; Rupe, C.; Troiano, G.; Cordaro, M.; Lucchese, A.; Giuliani, M. Tooth extraction before radiotherapy is a risk factor for developing osteoradionecrosis of the jaws: A systematic review. *Oral Dis.* **2020**, *27*, 1595–1605. [CrossRef]
31. Beaumont, S.; Bhatia, N.; McDowell, L.; Fua, T.; McCullough, M.; Celentano, A.; Yap, T. Timing of dental extractions in patients undergoing radiotherapy and the incidence of osteoradionecrosis: A systematic review and meta-analysis. *Br. J. Oral Maxillofac. Surg.* **2021**, *59*, 511–523. [CrossRef]
32. Schuurhuis, J.; Stokman, M.; Roodenburg, J.; Reintsema, H.; Langendijk, J.; Vissink, A.; Spijkervet, F.K. Efficacy of routine pre-radiation dental screening and dental follow-up in head and neck oncology patients on intermediate and late radiation effects. A retrospective evaluation. *Radiother. Oncol.* **2011**, *101*, 403–409. [CrossRef] [PubMed]
33. Batstone, M.; Cosson, J.; Marquart, L.; Acton, C. Platelet rich plasma for the prevention of osteoradionecrosis. A double blinded randomized cross over controlled trial. *Int. J. Oral Maxillofac. Surg.* **2012**, *41*, 2–4. [CrossRef]
34. Teng, M.; Futran, N. Osteoradionecrosis of the mandible. *Curr. Opin. Otolaryngol. Head Neck Surg.* **2005**, *13*, 217–221. [CrossRef]
35. Støre, G.; Boysen, M. Mandibular Osteoradionecrosis: Clinical behaviour and diagnostic aspects. *Clin. Otolaryngol. Allied Sci.* **2000**, *25*, 378–384. [CrossRef]
36. Saia, G.; Blandamura, S.; Bettini, G.; Tronchet, A.; Totola, A.; Bedogni, G.; Bedogni, A. Occurrence of bisphosphonate-related osteonecrosis of the jaw after surgical tooth extraction. *J. Oral Maxillofac. Surg.* **2010**, *68*, 797–804. [CrossRef]
37. Hinchy, N.; Jayaprakash, V.; Rossitto, R.; Anders, P.; Korff, K.; Canallatos, P.; Sullivan, M.A. Osteonecrosis of the jaw—Prevention and treatment strategies for oral health professionals. *Oral Oncol.* **2013**, *49*, 878–886. [CrossRef]
38. Shaw, R.; Butterworth, C. Hyperbaric oxygen in the management of late radiation injury to the head and neck. Part II: Prevention. *Br. J. Oral Maxillofac. Surg.* **2011**, *49*, 9–13. [CrossRef] [PubMed]
39. Chuang, S. Limited evidence to demonstrate that the use of hyperbaric oxygen (HBO) therapy reduces the incidence of osteoradionecrosis in irradiated patients requiring tooth extraction. *J. Evid. Based Dent. Pract.* **2012**, *12* (Suppl. S3), 248–250. [CrossRef] [PubMed]
40. Lyons, A.; Ghazali, N. Osteoradionecrosis of the jaws: Current understanding of its pathophysiology and treatment. *Br. J. Oral Maxillofac. Surg.* **2008**, *46*, 653–660. [CrossRef]

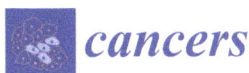

Systematic Review

Development and Validation of Prognostic Models for Oral Squamous Cell Carcinoma: A Systematic Review and Appraisal of the Literature

Diana Russo [1], Pierluigi Mariani [1], Vito Carlo Alberto Caponio [2], Lucio Lo Russo [2], Luca Fiorillo [3], Khrystyna Zhurakivska [2], Lorenzo Lo Muzio [2,4], Luigi Laino [1] and Giuseppe Troiano [2,*]

1. Multidisciplinary Department of Medical-Surgical and Dental Specialties, University of Campania "Luigi Vanvitelli", 80122 Napoli, Italy; dianarusso96@gmail.com (D.R.); marianipier@gmail.com (P.M.); luigi.laino@unicampania.it (L.L.)
2. Department of Clinical and Experimental Medicine, University of Foggia, 71122 Foggia, Italy; vitocarlo.caponio@unifg.it (V.C.A.C.); lucio.lorusso@unifg.it (L.L.R.); khrystyna.zhurakivska@unifg.it (K.Z.); lorenzo.lomuzio@unifg.it (L.L.M.)
3. Department of Biomedical and Dental Sciences and Morphological and Functional Imaging, Messina University, 98122 Messina, Italy; lfiorillo@unime.it
4. Consorzio Interuniversitario Nazionale per la Bio-Oncologia (C.I.N.B.O.), 66100 Chieti, Italy
* Correspondence: giuseppe.troiano@unifg.it; Tel.: +39-34889-86409; Fax: +39-0881-588081

Simple Summary: Prognostic models to choose the right treatment schedule are needed in order to translate into practice a personalized approach. None of these models have been still entered into the clinical practice for what concern oral squamous cell carcinoma (OSCC). In this manuscript we performed a systematic review and subsequent quality assessment of already development prognostic model for OSCC with the aim to take stock of the situation on their possible clinical use.

Abstract: (1) Background: An accurate prediction of cancer survival is very important for counseling, treatment planning, follow-up, and postoperative risk assessment in patients with Oral Squamous Cell Carcinoma (OSCC). There has been an increased interest in the development of clinical prognostic models and nomograms which are their graphic representation. The study aimed to revise the prognostic performance of clinical-pathological prognostic models with internal validation for OSCC. (2) Methods: This systematic review was performed according to the *Cochrane Handbook for Diagnostic Test Accuracy Reviews* chapter on searching, the PRISMA (Preferred Reporting Items for Systematic Reviews and Meta-Analysis) guidelines, and the Critical Appraisal and Data Extraction for Systematic Reviews of Prediction Modelling Studies (CHARMS). (3) Results: Six studies evaluating overall survival in patients with OSCC were identified. All studies performed internal validation, while only four models were externally validated. (4) Conclusions: Based on the results of this systematic review, it is possible to state that it is necessary to carry out internal validation and shrinkage to correct overfitting and provide an adequate performance for optimism. Moreover, calibration, discrimination and nonlinearity of continuous predictors should always be examined. To reduce the risk of bias the study design used should be prospective and imputation techniques should always be applied to handle missing data. In addition, the complete equation of the prognostic model must be reported to allow updating, external validation in a new context and the subsequent evaluation of the impact on health outcomes and on the cost-effectiveness of care.

Keywords: oral squamous cell carcinoma; nomograms; prognostic models; overall survival; prognosis; systematic review

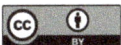

1. Background

Head and Neck Cancer (HNC) is the sixth most common type of cancer across the world with nearly 550,000 new cases per year. Most of HNCs are diagnosed as Oral

Squamous Cell Carcinomas (OSCC) and oral cancer ranks eighth among the most common causes of cancer-related deaths worldwide [1,2]. Both pharmacological and surgical protocols for OSCCs diagnosed in early stages are less aggressive and characterized by better outcomes, whilst in advanced stages, very high patients' morbidity and poor clinical outcomes are expected [3]. Despite the increased knowledge and the encouraging scientific findings of the past 20 years on such diseases, the overall 5-year survival rate for OSCC is still below 50% [4].

Nowadays, the Tumor-Node-Metastasis (TNM) staging system is employed worldwide to predict tumor prognosis and to guide physicians towards the correct treatment choice, however, survival outcomes in patients classified within the same TNM stage class could be dramatically different, with discrepancies in therapy response and tumor management [5].

One of the main limitations of OSCC-related TNM system is its main focus on the anatomical extension of the disease. However, within each staging group, the prognosis can be modified by tumor-related factors, such as genetics, patient age, sex, race or comorbidities. For this reason, the need for a more "personalized" approach to the oncologic patient was underlined in the recent eighth edition of the American Joint Committee On Cancer (AJCC) staging system [6]. It is, therefore, necessary to investigate further prognostic factors to construct prognostic models to carry out a personalized prognosis evaluation [7,8].

Recently, there has been an increased interest in the development of clinical prognostic models and, in particular, in nomograms which are their graphic representation [9]. These are a set of mathematical algorithms that can be used to predict patient outcomes by incorporating multiple variables. Clinic-pathological and genetic variables are mainly incorporated in OSCC prognostic models, showing interesting evidence of their role in patients' prognosis [10,11]. Purpose of these models is to estimate the probability or individual risk that a given condition, such as recurrence or death, will occur in a specific time by combining information from multiple prognostic factors of an individual [12].

Due to the recent interest in these new prognostic tools, and their potential important role in clinical practice, some guidelines have been defined for explanation and elaboration of clinically useful and correctly elaborated prognostic model. These Guidelines are reported in the Prognosis Research Strategy (PROGRESS) 3 and the Transparent Reporting of a multivariable prediction model for Individual Prognosis or Diagnosis (TRIPOD) [7,13]. In 2016 the AJCC developed the acceptance criteria for inclusion of risk models for individualized prognosis in the practice of precision medicine in the systematic reviews [14]. In the same year, Debray et al. developed a guide for systematic reviews and meta-analyzes of the performance of prognostic models [15]. Additionally, the Prediction Model Risk of Bias Assessment Tool (PROBAST) was also developed to assess the risk of bias and the applicability of diagnostic and prognostic prediction model studies [16].

In this scenario, this study presents a systematic review of clinical-pathological prognostic models with internal validation for OSCC, using the AJCC inclusion criteria and according to current published guidelines.

2. Materials and Methods

2.1. Protocol

This systematic review was performed according to the *Cochrane Handbook for Diagnostic Test Accuracy Reviews* chapter on searching [17], the PRISMA (Preferred Reporting Items for Systematic Reviews and Meta-Analysis) guidelines [18], and the Critical Appraisal and Data Extraction for Systematic Reviews of Prediction Modelling Studies (CHARMS) [19]. The reviews aim was to evaluate the prognostic performance of nomograms in patients with OSCC. This protocol was designed a priori and registered on the online database PROSPERO (CRD42020219937).

2.2. Search Strategy

Studies were identified by using different search engines: Medline/PubMed, ISI Web of Science and SCOPUS. In addition, partial research of the gray literature was carried out through Google Scholar. Furthermore, bibliographies of included studies were handed-revised to find further studies to include in this review. Search operations ended in October 2020. For the search strategy, MeSH terms and free text words were combined through Boolean operators as follow: (prognostic model OR prognostic index OR prediction model OR signature OR risk assessment OR prognostic assessment OR nomogram OR risk score OR model stratification) AND ((OSCC OR "oral cancer" OR tongue) NOT (gastric OR laryngeal OR pharynx OR endocrine OR colorectal OR breast OR prostate OR lung OR salivary OR review OR meta-analysis)).

2.3. Eligibility Criteria

To be included, studies had to fulfill the following criteria: (i) characteristics of the prognostic model had to be reported, together with their representative alternative presentation (e.g., scoring system, nomogram, etc.) for patient diagnosed with OSCC undergoing surgery with or without adjuvant therapy; (ii) at least one between with Overall Survival (OS) and Disease-Free Survival (DFS) had to be reported as outcome; (iii) studies had to follow TRIPOD and CHARMS checklist [13,19]; (iv) the prognostic model had to be internally validated; (v) and based on clinicopathological prognostic factors; (vi) that met all the thirteen inclusion criteria described by AJCC [9]; (vii) cohort studies, retrospective studies and studies that performed external validation of a pre-existing model were included; (viii) published in English; (ix) with available full text. We excluded: (i) case reports; case series; reviews and meta-analysis; (ii) studies that intend to modify existing prediction models and not to create new ones; (iii) studies including prognostic models that are not based on measurable markers in resected tumor tissue (saliva, blood, etc.); (iv) studies that met the three AJCC exclusion criteria [9].

2.4. Article Selection, Data Collection Process, and Data Items

Articles were independently selected by two of the authors (D.R., P.M.) in multiple steps. First, results of different databases were crossed, and duplicates were electronically removed by EndNote v.X9 software. Subsequently, a manual check was performed to furtherly remove previous undetected duplicates. The first screening for inclusion was performed by reading title and abstract. Full assessment for eligibility was furtherly carried out by full-text reading, judging each study as included, excluded or uncertain, according to the previously listed criteria. A third reviewer (G.T.) acted as an arbiter and calculated a value of k-statistic to ascertain the level of reviewers' agreement. In cases of disagreement, the same author (G.T.) took a final decision. From each of the selected articles, relevant information were extracted into a data extraction sheet using the TRIPOD and CHAMRS checklist, such as: author, year of publication, country where the study was carried out, the title of the paper, sample size, internal validation sample size, tumor localization sub-site, predictors (candidate and final) used to develop the models, outcome of the model (OS, DFS), method for the internal validation was carried out, modelling method, handling of missing data, model discrimination, model calibration, model presentation, handling of continuous predictors, presence of external validation, type of study.

2.5. Risk of Bias Assessment

Risk Of Bias (ROB) within individual studies was assessed by using Prediction model Risk Of Bias Assessment Tool (PROBAST) [16]. PROBAST can be used to assess any type of prognostic prediction model aimed at individualized predictions regardless of the predictors used. The tool comprises four domains—population, predictor, outcome, analysis, questions are answered as "yes", "probably yes", "probably no", "no", or "no information". Risk of bias is summarized as "low", "high", or "unclear". The degree of applicability is rated as "low", "high", or "unclear" concern. The "unclear" category should be used only when reported information is insufficient. In both cases, for both ROB and applicability, an overall judgment is provided. ROB was assessed separately for development (comprising internal validation) and external validation settings. For articles reporting both model development and external validation, the risk of bias was assessed independently.

3. Results

A total of 5972 records were identified in the initial search and were screened by title and abstract by two reviewers. Among these, 66 match our eligibility criteria and were furtherly assessed by full-text reading. At the end of selection process, 6 articles were considered suitable for inclusion in this systematic review [20–25]. Details on the selection process and reasons for exclusion are shown on Figure 1. The value of k-statistic resulted 0.87, indicating an excellent level of agreement between reviewers.

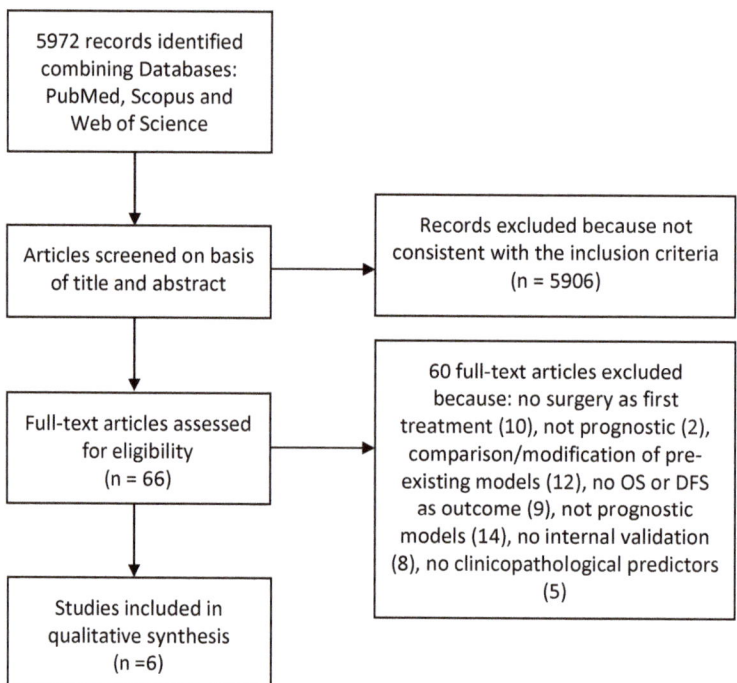

Figure 1. Flow-chart: 5972 records were identified in the initial search and, among them, 66 were further evaluated by reading the full text. At the end of the selection process, 6 articles were considered suitable for inclusion in this systematic review.

3.1. Study Characteristics and Model Development

All studies were published between 2014 and 2019. Prognostic models were mainly developed in China (50%, $n = 3$) [22,24,26], the remaining in India (33.3%; $n= 2$) [21,25] and in USA (16.6%; $n = 1$) [23] (Table 1). Patient data were collected retrospectively and hospital-based in four studies [21,23,25,26], while in two studies these were collected from the SEER database [22,24]. Data of patients' samples and tumor characteristics are summarized on Table 1.

Table 1. Features of the models included.

Authors	Year	Country	Title	Source of Data	Sample Size	Validation Saple Size	Tumor Site	Outcome	Study
Bobdey [20]	2016	India	Nomogram prediction for survival of patients with oral cavity squamous cell carcinoma	Hospital-based	609	None	Lip, tongue, gum; floor of the mouth; hard palate; cheek mucosa; vestibule of mouth; retromolar trigone	5 years Overall Survival	Retrospective study
Li [21]	2017	China	Nomograms to estimate long-term overall survival and tongue cancer-specific survival of patients with tongue squamous cell carcinoma	Population-based	7587	191	Tongue	5 and 8 years Overall Survival	Retrospective study
Montero [22]	2014	USA	Nomograms for preoperative prediction of prognosis in patients with oral cavity squamous cell carcinoma	Hospital-based	1617	None	Buccal mucosa; tongue; floor of mouth; hard palate; upper gum; lower gum; retromolar trigone	5 years Overall Survival	Retrospective study
Sun [23]	2019	China	Nomograms to predict survival of stage IV tongue squamous cell carcinoma after surgery	Population-based	1085	465	Tongue	3 and 5 years Overall Survival	Retrospective study
Bobdey [24]	2018	India	A Nomogram based prognostic score that is superior to conventional TNM staging in predicting outcome of surgically treated T4 buccal mucosa cancer: Time to think beyond TNM	Hospital-based	205	198	Buccal mucosa	3 years Overall Survival	Retrospective study
Chang [25]	2018	China	"A Prognostic Nomogram Incorporating Depth of Tumor Invasion to Predict Long-term Overall Survival for Tongue Squamous Cell Carcinoma with R0 Resection"	Hospital-based	235	223	Tongue	5 years Overall Survival	Retrospective study

The main investigated prognostic factor was age (100%; $n = 6$) [21–26], in four articles T stage [22,23,25,26], N status [22,24–26] and sex [21–23,26] are inspected, while three studies looked into histological grade [22,24,26] and subsite of the tumor onset [23,24,26]. Main final factors that were found to be independently associated with OS were age and race. Candidates and final prognostic factors included in prognostic models are reported on Table 2. None of the studies evaluated DFS, while OS resulted to be the main outcome (Table 1). Multivariable Cox proportional hazards was used as developer model in 50% of studies [22,24,26], alternatively to a combined modelling method using multivariable Cox proportional hazard regression models and stepdown reduction methods [21,23,25]. Only Montero et al. reported how missing data were handled, by implementation of an imputation technique [22].

Table 2. Predictors included in the prognostic models.

Author Year	Candidate Predictors	Final Predictors
Bobdey 2016 [20]	Age	Age
	Bone infiltration	Clinical lymph node status
	Clinical lymph node status	Comorbidities
	Comorbidities	Differentiation
	Differentiation	Perineural invasion
	Perineural invasion	Stage
	Sex	Tumor thicknesss
	Stage	
	Tumor thicknesss	
Li 2017 [21]	Age	Age
	Grade	Grade
	M stage	M stage
	Martial status	Martial status
	N stage	N stage
	Race	Race
	Radiotherapy	T stage
	Sex	
	T stage	
Montero 2014 [22]	Age	Age
	Alcohol use	Clinical lymph node status
	Clinical lymph node status	Comorbidities
	Comorbidities	Race
	Invasion of other structures	Tobacco use
	Race	Tumor size
	Sex	
	Tobacco use	
	Tumor site	
	Tumor size	
Sun 2019 [23]	Age	Age
	Chemotherapy	M stage
	Grade	Martial status
	M stage	N stage
	Martial status	Race
	N stage	Radiotherapy
	Race	T stage
	Radiotherapy	Tumor site
	T stage	
	Tumor site	

Table 2. *Cont.*

Author Year	Candidate Predictors	Final Predictors
Bobdey 2017 [24]	Age Bone infiltration Differentiation Extracapsular spread N stage Perineural invasion Status of surgical margin T stage	Bone infiltration N stage Perineural invasion
Chang 2018 [25]	Age Alcohol use Body mass index Clinical tumor stage Crossing the midline of the tongue Diabetes Depth of invasion Grade Hypertension M stage Metabolic syndrome N stage Neck dissection Race Sex T stage Tobacco use Treatment Tumor site	Age Depth of invasion N stage Neck dissection

In most of the prognostic models (66%, $n = 4$) [22,23,25,26], continuous predictors were dichotomized or categorized, hence the nonlinearity of continuous predictors was assessed. For two prognostic models, cubic splines were used to test for the presence of, a non-linear association between continuous predictors and the predicted outcome [23,26].

All the studies used a nomogram as final presentation [21–26]. Methodological characteristics of prognostic models developed are summarized on Table 3.

3.2. Validation of the Models

Internal validation was performed in all studies by 1000-time bootstrapping [21–23,25,26], except Sun et al. who employed a combined 500-time bootstrapping and 5-fold cross-validation methodology [23].

As a method of discrimination, C-statistics has been used in five studies [21–25]; only one study performed AUC [26].

Four studies reported assessed calibration of the model by means of calibration plots [22–24,26], while two did not describe their calibration method [21,25].

In all studies, predictive accuracy was quantified by calculation of the Concordance index (C-index) for each outcome, all the included studies had a C-index higher than 0.6 [21–26]. External validation was performed in four studies and C-index was found to be higher than 0.6 in all the articles included [22,24–26]. Methodological features of the development and validation of prognostic models are listed on Table 3.

Table 3. Methodological characteristics of prognostic models developed.

Authors and Year	Internal Validation	Modelling Method	Handling of Missing Data	Model Discrimination	Model Calibration	Model Presentation	Handling of Continuous Predictors	Non-Linearity	Internal Validation C-Index	External Validation C-Index
Bobdey 2016 [20]	1000-time bootstrapping	Multivariable Cox proportional hazards regression models and stepdown reduction method	n/a	C-statistic	n/a	Nomogram	Mixed: Continuous; Categorical/dichotomous	none	0.7263	none
Li 2017 [21]	1000-time bootstrapping	Multivariable Cox proportional hazards regression models	n/a	C-statistic	Calibration plot	Nomogram	Categorical/dichotomous	n/a	0.709	0.691
Montero 2014 [22]	1000-time bootstrapping	Multivariable Cox proportional hazards regression models and stepdown reduction method	Imputation	C-statistic	Calibration plot	Nomogram	Categorical/dichotomous	Cubic splines	0.67	none
Sun 2019 [23]	Combination of methods: 500-time bootstrapping; 5-fold cross-validation	Multivariable Cox proportional hazards regression models	n/a	C-statistic	Calibration plot	Nomogram	Mixed: Continuous; Categorical/dichotomous	none	0.705	0.664
Bobdey 2017 [24]	1000-time bootstrapping	Multivariable Cox proportional hazards regression models and stepdown reduction method	n/a	C-statistic	n/a	Nomogram	Categorical/dichotomous	n/a	0.7266	0.740
Chang 2018 [25]	1000-time bootstrapping	Multivariable Cox proportional hazards regression models	n/a	AUC	Calibration plot	Nomogram	Categorical/dichotomous	Cubic splines	0.78	0.71

3.3. Risk of Bias

PROBAST was used to assess the risk of bias of included studies. Four models presented a low overall bias level [21,22,24,26], while two reported a high overall bias level [23,25]. The overall applicability level resulted to be low in all studies [21–24,26], except one [25]. Four out of six studies performed external validation of the models [22,24–26]. The overall risk of bias was low in three out of four models [22,24,26]. In the external validations, applicability was found to be low in all studies [22,24–26]. The risk of bias for each domain of the developed models and the external validations is shown, respectively, on Figures 2 and 3. The applicability for each domain, both for the developed models and for the external validations, is reported in Tables 4 and 5.

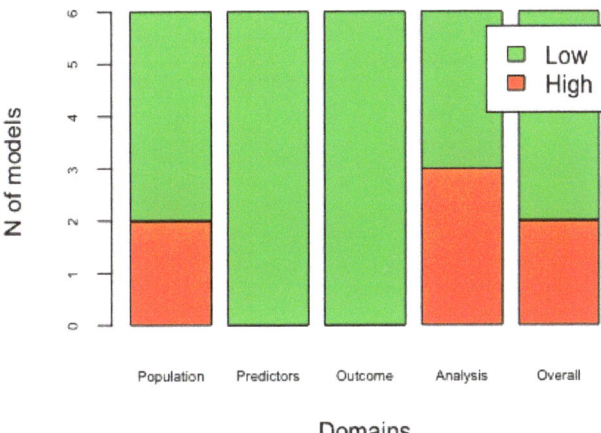

Figure 2. Risk of bias of the developed prognostic models: For each of the six prognostic models included in this systematic review, four domains of bias (population, predictors, outcomes, analysis) were evaluated as "high" or "low". In this way, the overall risk of bias of each article was assessed.

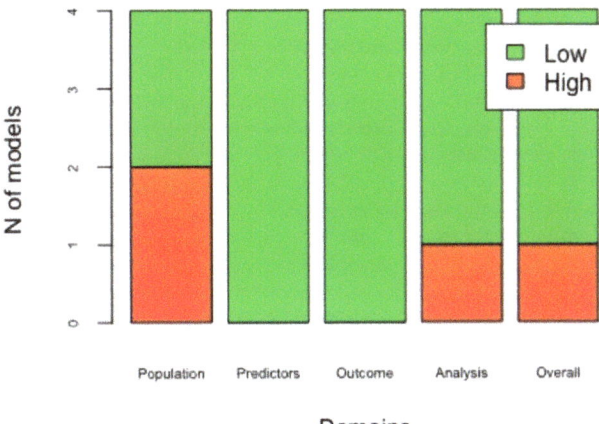

Figure 3. Risk of bias of models' external validations: For each of the four externally validated prognostic models included in this systematic review, four domains of bias (population, predictors, outcomes, analysis) were assessed as "high" or "low". In this way, the overall risk of bias of each article was assessed.

Table 4. Applicability of the developed prognostic models.

Author Year	Domain 1	Domain 2	Domain 3	Overall
Bodbey 2016 [20]	Low	Low	Low	Low
Li 2017 [21]	Low	Low	Low	Low
Montero 2014 [22]	Low	Low	Low	Low
Sun 2019 [23]	Low	Low	Low	Low
Bobdey 2017 [24]	Low	Low	High	High
Chang 2018 [25]	Low	Low	Low	Low

For each of the six prognostic models included in this systematic review, four domains (population, predictors, outcomes, analysis) were evaluated as "high" or "low". In this way, the overall applicability of each article was assessed.

Table 5. Applicability of models' external validations.

	PROBAST_External Validation_Applicability			
Author Year	Domain 1	Domain 2	Domain 3	Overall
Li 2017 [21]	Low	Low	Low	Low
Sun 2019 [23]	Low	Low	Low	Low
Bobday 2017 [24]	Low	Low	High	Low
Chang 2018 [25]	Low	Low	Low	Low

For each of the four externally validated prognostic models included in this systematic review, four domains (population, predictors, outcomes, analysis) were assessed as "high" or "low". In this way, the overall applicability of each article was assessed.

4. Discussions

An accurate prediction of cancer survival is very important for counseling, treatment planning, follow-up and postoperative risk assessment in patients with OSCC [27]. Although the use of prognosis models is still relatively new for OSCC, these models are already widely used for other human diseases [28–31]. It is now well known that cancer-related outcomes are influenced by several factors that are not included in the TNM system. The vast majority of these factors has not been incorporated into the staging system because they may not predict outcome "independently" in multivariate prognosis models, however many of them may work in tandem and have varying degrees of influence on each other [32,33].

This systematic review has yielded a detailed picture of prognostic models for predicting OS in patients with OSCC. Six studies included in this review correctly developed models according to the TRIPOD, all the included studies carried out internal validation of the model and four models were also externally validated [21–26]. The majority of models assessed OS in patients with squamous cell carcinoma of the tongue [22,24,26], two assessed all possible sites of tumor onset [21,23], and one model only assessed the buccal mucosa cancer [25]. All models rated OS at five years, except for Bobdey et al [25]. who only rated it at three years; furthermore, Li et al. and Sun et al., also evaluated OS at eight and three years respectively [21,23]. Among the clinical factors, those most included in the models are age, race, martial state, comorbidities and smoking; while among the histopathological ones the most investigated were T stage, N stage and M stage.

This systematic review showed methodological differences in model development. It is well known that the performance of a prognostic model is overestimated when it is just assessed in the patient sample that was used to build the model [34]. Internal validation provides a better estimate of model performance in new patients when done by adjusting overfitting, that is the difference between the accuracy of the apparent prediction and the accuracy of the prediction measured on an independent test set. Resampling techniques are a set of methods to provide an assessment of accuracy for the developed prognostic prediction models [35]. As an exception, Sun et al. [23] used a combined bootstrapping and cross-validation method, although all other studies used 1000-time bootstrapping as a resampling technique. Nevertheless, an evaluation of a model's performance by using bootstrapping or cross-validation is not enough to overcome overfitting, such type of studies should also apply shrinkage, which is a method used adjust the regression coefficients [36,37]. However, none of the studies used this technique, probably because its usefulness for models with a low number of predictors is unclear [13].

Another important finding from our review is that one-third of the studies did not report on model calibration [38]. Calibration reflects the agreement between the model's predictions and the observed outcomes. It is preferably reported graphically, usually with a calibration plot [39]. Another key aspect of the characterization of a prognostic model is discrimination, that is, the ability of a forecasting model to differentiate between those who experience the outcome event or not [13]. The most used measure for discrimination is the Concordance Index (C-index), which reflects the probability that for any pair of individuals randomly, one with and one without the outcome, the model assigns a higher probability to the individual with the outcome [40]. For survival models, many c-indices have been proposed, so it is important to underline that, from our results, the most commonly used is the discrimination model proposed by Harrell [41]. In any case, discrimination can vary in a range from 0 to 1 and is considered good when higher than 0.5, considering that all the studies included in this systematic review presented a C-index at least higher than 0.6, all of them showed a good prognostic accuracy [42]. In addition, improvements in study design and analysis are crucial to allow evidence of more reliable prognostic factors that can be incorporated into new prognostic models, or to update existing models, to improve discrimination [43]. Another important finding was the almost total lack of handling of the missing data, except for Montero et al. [22] who carried out the multivariate imputations by chained equations (MICE) [44] before conducting multivariable regression statistical analysis [23]. The absence of a mention of the missing data leads to a so-called "full case analysis". Including only participants with complete data, as well as being inefficient as it reduces the sample, can also lead to biased results due to a subsample [12]. Additionally, in only two prognostic models, continuous predictors were dichotomized or categorized, and the non-linearity of continuous predictors was examined using restricted cubic splines [23,26].

In the end, only four prognostic models performed external validation, in none of these the population in which the validation was performed was specifically reported and this data also negatively influenced the risk of bias. External validation is preferable to internal validation for testing the transportability of a model since it is impossible for the population, or distribution of predictors, in an independent population to be the same as in the model development population [45]. Secondly, to improve the generalizability of a model, it should ideally be validated in different contexts with different population [46]. Furthermore, in the literature, there are currently no external validation by independent researchers of prognostic models for OS in patients with OSCC. A reliable model should be tested by independent researchers in different contexts to ensure the generalizability of prognostic models [15].

Most of the prognostic models in the literature describe the development of the model, a small number report external validation studies and currently, there are no studies considering clinical impact or utility [7]. Identifying accurate prognostic models and performing impact studies to investigate their influence on decision making, patient outcomes and costs is a fundamental component of stratified medicine because it contributes evidence at multiple stages in translation [47].

Multivariable Cox proportional hazards regression models were used to developing the models, as indicated for survival data [48]. All included prognostic models used nomogram as model presentation, yet none of the prognostic models reported the original mathematical regression formula. This turns out to be highly limiting, firstly because this presentation format is not a simplification of a developed model, but rather a graphical presentation of the original mathematical regression formula, and secondly, because re-calibration, and updating of the original formula is necessary to perform validation [49]. Furthermore, it would be advisable to provide readers with the appropriate tools for the interpretation and application of the nomogram [30].

All the studies included in this systematic review had a retrospective design, and therefore showed issues related to missing data and a lack of consistency in predictor and outcome measurement [16]. In addition, both the single-institutional studies and the SEER database lacks critical information. The former, being the cohort of similar patients, may not be relevant in predicting the risk of other patient populations. The second lacks information that could be relevant to prognosis such as comorbidities, chemotherapy and tobacco smoking [50]. Prospective cohort studies should be performed for predictive modeling since they enable not only clear and consistent definitions but also prospective measurement of predictors and outcomes [13,50].

The recognition of the methodological limitations found in the developed models and their external validation were evaluated as a high risk of bias, as indicated in the PROBAST. Domain four (analysis domain) is the one that most influenced the overall risk of bias [16,51].

5. Limitations

The main limitations related to this systematic review are due to the very strict inclusion criteria to ensure the high accuracy of the contents. Certainly, having selected only internally validated models and articles written in English has strongly restricted the number of studies included. However, as this is the first systematic review of the literature on prognostic models for OSCC patients, this was done to provide clinicians and researchers with a clear picture of the correct model development method. Future systematic reviews should include a greater number of outcomes (cancer-specific survival, recurrence-free survival, etc.) and include biomolecular prognostic factors in addition to clinicopathological one.

6. Conclusions

Based on the findings of this systematic review, the following recommendations could be reported: (i) model development studies should weight for overfitting by carrying out internal validation (by resampling techniques such as bootstrapping) and using shrinkage techniques, (ii) model calibration and discrimination should always be examined, (iii) imputation techniques for missing data handling should always be applied, (iv) non-linearity of continuous predictors should be examined, (v) the complete equation of the prognostic model should always be reported to allow external validation and updating by independent research groups; (vi) prospective studies should be performed to reduce the risk of bias (vii) external validation in a new context and impact assessment on health outcomes and cost effectiveness of care should be carried out.

Author Contributions: D.R. and P.M. contributed to data acquisition and drafted the manuscript; V.C.A.C., K.Z., L.L.R., L.F. and L.L.M. contributed to data analysis and interpretation; K.Z., L.L. and G.T. contributed to conception, design and critically revised the manuscript. All authors read and approved the final manuscript. All authors have read and agreed to the published version of the manuscript.

Funding: This research did not receive any specific grant from funding agencies in the public, commercial, or not-for-profit sectors.

Institutional Review Board Statement: Not applicable.

Informed Consent Statement: Not applicable.

Data Availability Statement: The data presented in this study are freely available in the article.

Conflicts of Interest: The authors declare no conflict of interest.

References

1. Jiang, X.; Wu, J.; Wang, J.; Huang, R. Tobacco and oral squamous cell carcinoma: A review of carcinogenic pathways. *Tob. Induc. Dis.* **2019**, *17*, 1–9. [CrossRef]
2. Fitzmaurice, C.; Abate, D.; Abbasi, N.; Abbastabar, H.; Abd-Allah, F.; Abdel-Rahman, O.; Abdelalim, A.; Abdoli, A.; Abdollahpour, I.; Abdulle, A.S.M.; et al. Global, Regional, and National Cancer Incidence, Mortality, Years of Life Lost, Years Lived With Disability, and Disability-Adjusted Life-Years for 29 Cancer Groups, 1990 to 2017. *JAMA Oncol.* **2019**, *5*, 1749. [CrossRef]
3. Vassiliou, L.V.; Acero, J.; Gulati, A.; Hölzle, F.; Hutchison, I.L.; Prabhu, S.; Testelin, S.; Wolff, K.D.; Kalavrezos, N. Management of the clinically N0 neck in early-stage oral squamous cell carcinoma (OSCC). An EACMFS position paper. *J. Cranio-Maxillofac. Surg.* **2020**, *48*, 711–718. [CrossRef] [PubMed]
4. Almangush, A.; Mäkitie, A.A.; Triantafyllou, A.; de Bree, R.; Strojan, P.; Rinaldo, A.; Hernandez-Prera, J.C.; Suárez, C.; Kowalski, L.P.; Ferlito, A.; et al. Staging and grading of oral squamous cell carcinoma: An update. *Oral Oncol.* **2020**, *107*, 104799. [CrossRef]
5. Rahman, N.; MacNeill, M.; Wallace, W.; Conn, B. Reframing Histological Risk Assessment of Oral Squamous Cell Carcinoma in the Era of UICC 8th Edition TNM Staging. *Head Neck Pathol.* **2021**, *15*, 202–211. [CrossRef]
6. Moeckelmann, N.; Ebrahimi, A.; Tou, Y.K.; Gupta, R.; Low, T.H.; Ashford, B.; Ch'ng, S.; Palme, C.E.; Clark, J.R. Prognostic implications of the 8th edition American Joint Committee on Cancer (AJCC) staging system in oral cavity squamous cell carcinoma. *Oral Oncol.* **2018**, *85*, 82–86. [CrossRef]
7. Steyerberg, E.W.; Moons, K.G.M.; van der Windt, D.A.; Hayden, J.A.; Perel, P.; Schroter, S.; Riley, R.D.; Hemingway, H.; Altman, D.G. Prognosis Research Strategy (PROGRESS) 3: Prognostic Model Research. *PLoS Med.* **2013**, *10*, e1001381. [CrossRef] [PubMed]
8. Riley, R.D.; Moons, K.G.M.; Snell, K.I.E.; Ensor, J.; Hooft, L.; Altman, D.G.; Hayden, J.; Collins, G.S.; Debray, T.P.A. A guide to systematic review and meta-analysis of prognostic factor studies. *BMJ* **2019**, *364*, k4597. [CrossRef]
9. Tham, T.; Machado, R.; Herman, S.W.; Kraus, D.; Costantino, P.; Roche, A. Personalized prognostication in head and neck cancer: A systematic review of nomograms according to the AJCC precision medicine core (PMC) criteria. *Head Neck* **2019**, *41*, 2811–2822. [CrossRef] [PubMed]
10. Mattavelli, D.; Lombardi, D.; Missale, F.; Calza, S.; Battocchio, S.; Paderno, A.; Bozzola, A.; Bossi, P.; Vermi, W.; Piazza, C.; et al. Prognostic nomograms in oral squamous cell carcinoma: The negative impact of low neutrophil to lymphocyte ratio. *Front. Oncol.* **2019**, *9*, 339. [CrossRef]
11. Troiano, G.; Caponio, V.C.A.; Botti, G.; Aquino, G.; Losito, N.S.; Pedicillo, M.C.; Zhurakivska, K.; Arena, C.; Ciavarella, D.; Mastrangelo, F.; et al. Immunohistochemical Analysis Revealed a Correlation between Musashi-2 and Cyclin-D1 Expression in Patients with Oral Squamous Cells Carcinoma. *Int. J. Mol. Sci.* **2019**, *21*, 121. [CrossRef]
12. Heus, P.; Damen, J.A.A.G.; Pajouheshnia, R.; Scholten, R.J.P.M.; Reitsma, J.B.; Collins, G.S.; Altman, D.G.; Moons, K.G.M.; Hooft, L. Uniformity in measuring adherence to reporting guidelines: The example of TRIPOD for assessing completeness of reporting of prediction model studies. *BMJ Open* **2019**, *9*, e025611. [CrossRef] [PubMed]
13. Moons, K.G.M.; Altman, D.G.; Reitsma, J.B.; Ioannidis, J.P.A.; Macaskill, P.; Steyerberg, E.W.; Vickers, A.J.; Ransohoff, D.F.; Collins, G.S. Transparent Reporting of a multivariable prediction model for Individual Prognosis Or Diagnosis (TRIPOD): Explanation and Elaboration. *Ann. Intern. Med.* **2015**, *162*, W1–W73. [CrossRef]
14. Kattan, M.W.; Hess, K.R.; Amin, M.B.; Lu, Y.; Moons, K.G.; Gershenwald, J.E.; Gimotty, P.A.; Guinney, J.H.; Halabi, S.; Lazar, A.J.; et al. American Joint Committee on Cancer acceptance criteria for inclusion of risk models for individualized prognosis in the practice of precision medicine. *CA Cancer J. Clin.* **2016**, *66*, 370–374. [CrossRef]
15. Debray, T.P.A.; Damen, J.A.A.G.; Snell, K.I.E.; Ensor, J.; Hooft, L.; Reitsma, J.B.; Riley, R.D.; Moons, K.G.M. A guide to systematic review and meta-analysis of prediction model performance. *BMJ* **2017**, *356*, i6460. [CrossRef] [PubMed]
16. Wolff, R.F.; Moons, K.G.M.; Riley, R.D.; Whiting, P.F.; Westwood, M.; Collins, G.S.; Reitsma, J.B.; Kleijnen, J.; Mallett, S. PROBAST: A Tool to Assess the Risk of Bias and Applicability of Prediction Model Studies. *Ann. Intern. Med.* **2019**, *170*, 51–58. [CrossRef]
17. Bossuyt, P.; Davenport, C.; Deeks, J.; Hyde, C.; Leeflang, M.; Scholten, R. Cochrane Handbook for Systematic Reviews of Diagnostic Test Accuracy Chapter 11 Interpreting Results and Drawing Conclusions. 2013, pp. 1–31. Available online: http://srdta.cochrane.org/ (accessed on 5 September 2021).
18. Moher, D.; Liberati, A.; Tetzlaff, J.; Altman, D.G.; Altman, D.; Antes, G.; Atkins, D.; Barbour, V.; Barrowman, N.; Berlin, J.A.; et al. Preferred reporting items for systematic reviews and meta-analyses: The PRISMA statement. *PLoS Med.* **2009**, *6*, e1000097. [CrossRef]
19. Moons, K.G.M.; de Groot, J.A.H.; Bouwmeester, W.; Vergouwe, Y.; Mallett, S.; Altman, D.G.; Reitsma, J.B.; Collins, G.S. Critical Appraisal and Data Extraction for Systematic Reviews of Prediction Modelling Studies: The CHARMS Checklist. *PLoS Med.* **2014**, *11*, e1001744. [CrossRef] [PubMed]
20. Bobdey, S.; Balasubramaniam, G.; Mishra, P. Nomogram prediction for survival of patients with oral cavity squamous cell carcinoma. *Head Neck* **2016**, *38*, 1826–1831. [CrossRef] [PubMed]
21. Li, Y.; Zhao, Z.; Liu, X.; Ju, J.; Chai, J.; Ni, Q.; Ma, C.; Gao, T.; Sun, M. Nomograms to estimate long-term overall survival and tongue cancer-specific survival of patients with tongue squamous cell carcinoma. *Cancer Med.* **2017**, *6*, 1002–1013. [CrossRef]
22. Montero, P.H.; Yu, C.; Palmer, F.L.; Patel, P.D.; Ganly, I.; Shah, J.P.; Shaha, A.R.; Boyle, J.O.; Kraus, D.H.; Singh, B.; et al. Nomograms for preoperative prediction of prognosis in patients with oral cavity squamous cell carcinoma. *Cancer* **2014**, *120*, 214–221. [CrossRef]

23. Sun, W.; Cheng, M.; Zhuang, S.; Chen, H.; Yang, S.; Qiu, Z. Nomograms to predict survival of stage IV tongue squamous cell carcinoma after surgery. *Medicine* **2019**, *98*, e16206. [CrossRef]
24. Bobdey, S.; Mair, M.; Nair, S.; Nair, D.; Balasubramaniam, G.; Chaturvedi, P. A Nomogram based prognostic score that is superior to conventional TNM staging in predicting outcome of surgically treated T4 buccal mucosa cancer: Time to think beyond TNM. *Oral Oncol.* **2018**, *81*, 10–15. [CrossRef]
25. Chang, B.; He, W.; Ouyang, H.; Peng, J.; Shen, L.; Wang, A.; Wu, P. A prognostic nomogram incorporating depth of tumor invasion to predict long-term overall survival for tongue squamous cell carcinoma with R0 resection. *J. Cancer* **2018**, *9*, 2107–2115. [CrossRef]
26. Chang, W.C.; Chang, C.F.; Li, Y.H.; Yang, C.Y.; Su, R.Y.; Lin, C.K.; Chen, Y.W. A histopathological evaluation and potential prognostic implications of oral squamous cell carcinoma with adverse features. *Oral Oncol.* **2019**, *95*, 65–73. [CrossRef] [PubMed]
27. Feng, Q.; May, M.T.; Ingle, S.; Lu, M.; Yang, Z.; Tang, J. Prognostic Models for Predicting Overall Survival in Patients with Primary Gastric Cancer: A Systematic Review. *Biomed Res. Int.* **2019**, *2019*, 5634598. [CrossRef] [PubMed]
28. Wesdorp, N.J.; van Goor, V.J.; Kemna, R.; Jansma, E.P.; van Waesberghe, J.H.T.M.; Swijnenburg, R.J.; Punt, C.J.A.; Huiskens, J.; Kazemier, G. Advanced image analytics predicting clinical outcomes in patients with colorectal liver metastases: A systematic review of the literature. *Surg. Oncol.* **2021**, *38*, 101578. [CrossRef]
29. Bradley, A.; Van Der Meer, R.; McKay, C.J. A systematic review of methodological quality of model development studies predicting prognostic outcome for resectable pancreatic cancer. *BMJ Open* **2019**, *9*, e027192. [CrossRef] [PubMed]
30. Kreuzberger, N.; Damen, J.A.; Trivella, M.; Estcourt, L.J.; Aldin, A.; Umlauff, L.; Vazquez-Montes, M.D.; Wolff, R.; Moons, K.G.; Monsef, I.; et al. Prognostic models for newly-diagnosed chronic lymphocytic leukaemia in adults: A systematic review and meta-analysis. *Cochrane Database Syst. Rev.* **2020**. [CrossRef]
31. Wang, S.; Guan, X.; Ma, M.; Zhuang, M.; Ma, T.; Liu, Z.; Chen, H.; Jiang, Z.; Chen, Y.; Wang, G.; et al. Reconsidering the prognostic significance of tumour deposit count in the TNM staging system for colorectal cancer. *Sci. Rep.* **2020**, *10*, 89. [CrossRef]
32. Brierley, J.; O'Sullivan, B.; Asamura, H.; Byrd, D.; Huang, S.H.; Lee, A.; Piñeros, M.; Mason, M.; Moraes, F.Y.; Rösler, W.; et al. Global Consultation on Cancer Staging: Promoting consistent understanding and use. *Nat. Rev. Clin. Oncol.* **2019**, *16*, 763–771. [CrossRef]
33. Dijkland, S.A.; Retel Helmrich, I.R.A.; Steyerberg, E.W. Validation of prognostic models: Challenges and opportunities. *J. Emerg. Crit. Care Med.* **2018**, *2*, 91. [CrossRef]
34. Bellou, V.; Belbasis, L.; Konstantinidis, A.K.; Tzoulaki, I.; Evangelou, E. Prognostic models for outcome prediction in patients with chronic obstructive pulmonary disease: Systematic review and critical appraisal. *BMJ* **2019**, *367*, l5358. [CrossRef]
35. Iba, K.; Shinozaki, T.; Maruo, K.; Noma, H. Re-evaluation of the comparative effectiveness of bootstrap-based optimism correction methods in the development of multivariable clinical prediction models. *BMC Med. Res. Methodol.* **2021**, *21*, 9. [CrossRef]
36. Zhang, Z.; Cortese, G.; Combescure, C.; Marshall, R.; Lee, M.; Lim, H.; Haller, B. Overview of model validation for survival regression model with competing risks using melanoma study data. *Ann. Transl. Med.* **2018**, *6*, 325. [CrossRef]
37. Steyerberg, E.W.; Vickers, A.J.; Cook, N.R.; Gerds, T.; Gonen, M.; Obuchowski, N.; Pencina, M.J.; Kattan, M.W. Assessing the performance of prediction models: A framework for traditional and novel measures. *Epidemiology* **2010**, *21*, 128–138. [CrossRef]
38. Austin, P.C.; Harrell, F.E.; van Klaveren, D. Graphical calibration curves and the integrated calibration index (ICI) for survival models. *Stat. Med.* **2020**, *39*, 2714–2742. [CrossRef]
39. Pencina, M.J.; D'Agostino, R.B. Evaluating discrimination of risk prediction models: The C statistic. *J. Am. Med. Assoc.* **2015**, *314*, 1063–1064. [CrossRef]
40. Harrell, F.E.; Lee, K.L.; Mark, D.B. Prognostic/Clinical Prediction Models: Multivariable Prognostic Models: Issues in Developing Models, Evaluating Assumptions and Adequacy, and Measuring and Reducing Errors. In *Tutorials in Biostatistics*; John Wiley & Sons, Ltd.: Chichester, UK, 2005; Volume 1, pp. 223–249. [CrossRef]
41. Brentnall, A.R.; Cuzick, J. Use of the concordance index for predictors of censored survival data. *Stat. Methods Med. Res.* **2018**, *27*, 2359–2373. [CrossRef]
42. Riley, R.D.; Hayden, J.A.; Steyerberg, E.W.; Moons, K.G.M.; Abrams, K.; Kyzas, P.A.; Malats, N.; Briggs, A.; Schroter, S.; Altman, D.G.; et al. Prognosis Research Strategy (PROGRESS) 2: Prognostic Factor Research. *PLoS Med.* **2013**, *10*, e1001380. [CrossRef]
43. van Buuren, S.; Groothuis-Oudshoorn, K. mice: Multivariate Imputation by Chained Equations in R. *J. Stat. Softw.* **2011**, *45*, 1–67. [CrossRef]
44. Ramspek, C.L.; Jager, K.J.; Dekker, F.W.; Zoccali, C.; van Diepen, M. External validation of prognostic models: What, why, how, when and where? *Clin. Kidney J.* **2021**, *14*, 49–58. [CrossRef] [PubMed]
45. Kundu, S.; Mazumdar, M.; Ferket, B. Impact of correlation of predictors on discrimination of risk models in development and external populations. *BMC Med. Res. Methodol.* **2017**, *17*, 63. [CrossRef]
46. Hingorani, A.D.; Van Der Windt, D.A.; Riley, R.D.; Abrams, K.; Moons, K.G.M.; Steyerberg, E.W.; Schroter, S.; Sauerbrei, W.; Altman, D.G.; Hemingway, H.; et al. Prognosis research strategy (PROGRESS) 4: Stratified medicine research. *BMJ* **2013**, *346*, e5793. [CrossRef]
47. Bradburn, M.J.; Clark, T.G.; Love, S.B.; Altman, D.G. Survival Analysis Part II: Multivariate data analysis—An introduction to concepts and methods. *Br. J. Cancer* **2003**, *89*, 431–436. [CrossRef]
48. Steyerberg, E.W.; Vergouwe, Y. Towards better clinical prediction models: Seven steps for development and an ABCD for validation. *Eur. Heart J.* **2014**, *35*, 1925–1931. [CrossRef]

49. Duggan, M.A.; Anderson, W.F.; Altekruse, S.; Penberthy, L.; Sherman, M.E. The Surveillance, Epidemiology, and End Results (SEER) Program and Pathology. *Am. J. Surg. Pathol.* **2016**, *40*, e94–e102. [CrossRef]
50. Zamanipoor Najafabadi, A.H.; Ramspek, C.L.; Dekker, F.W.; Heus, P.; Hooft, L.; Moons, K.G.M.; Peul, W.C.; Collins, G.S.; Steyerberg, E.W.; van Diepen, M. TRIPOD statement: A preliminary pre-post analysis of reporting and methods of prediction models. *BMJ Open* **2020**, *10*, e041537. [CrossRef]
51. Zhao, R.; Jia, T.; Qiao, B.; Liang, J.; Qu, S.; Zhu, L.; Feng, H.; Xing, L.; Ren, Y.; Wang, F.; et al. Nomogram predicting long-term overall survival and cancer-specific survival of lip carcinoma patients based on the SEER database: A retrospective case-control study. *Medicine* **2019**, *98*, e16727. [CrossRef]

MDPI
St. Alban-Anlage 66
4052 Basel
Switzerland
www.mdpi.com

Cancers Editorial Office
E-mail: cancers@mdpi.com
www.mdpi.com/journal/cancers

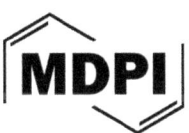

Disclaimer/Publisher's Note: The statements, opinions and data contained in all publications are solely those of the individual author(s) and contributor(s) and not of MDPI and/or the editor(s). MDPI and/or the editor(s) disclaim responsibility for any injury to people or property resulting from any ideas, methods, instructions or products referred to in the content.

www.ingramcontent.com/pod-product-compliance
Lightning Source LLC
LaVergne TN
LVHW070410100526
838202LV00014B/1431